ADVAI   S

Pa
PI   e

This book is dedicated to Professor Oded Bar-Or, who died on 8 December 2005.

For Elsevier:
Commissioning Editor: Dinah Thom
Project Manager: Emma Riley
Designer: Stewart Larking
Illustration Manager: Bruce Hogarth
Illustrator: Ethan Danielson

ADVANCES IN **SPORT** AND **EXERCISE** SCIENCE SERIES

Paediatric Exercise Physiology

Edited by

Neil Armstrong PhD DSc

Deputy Vice-Chancellor, Professor of Paediatric Physiology and Director of the Children's Health and Exercise Research Centre, University of Exeter, Exeter, UK

SERIES EDITORS

Neil Spurway PhD

Emeritus Professor of Exercise Physiology, University of Glasgow, Glasgow, UK

Don MacLaren PhD

Professor of Sports Nutrition, School of Sport and Exercise Sciences, Liverpool John Moores University, Liverpool, UK

Foreword by

N. C. Craig Sharp BVMS DSc

Emeritus Professor of Sports Science, Brunel University, Isleworth, Middlesex, UK

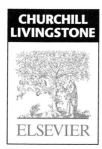

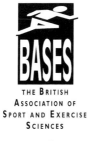

CHURCHILL LIVINGSTONE

ELSEVIER

THE BRITISH ASSOCIATION OF SPORT AND EXERCISE SCIENCES

EDINBURGH LONDON NEW YORK OXFORD PHILADELPHIA ST LOUIS SYDNEY TORONTO 2007

Contributors

Neil Armstrong PhD DSc
Professor of Paediatric Physiology, Director of the Children's Health and Exercise Research Centre, University of Exeter, Exeter, UK

Adam D. G. Baxter-Jones PhD
Professor, College of Kinesiology, University of Saskatchewan, Saskatoon, Saskatchewan, Canada

Michael Chia PhD
Associate Professor, Head of Physical Education and Sports Science, National Institute of Education, Nanyang Technological University, Singapore

Mark B. A. De Ste Croix PhD
Principal Lecturer, Faculty of Sport, Health and Social Care, University of Gloucestershire, Gloucester, UK

Roger G. Eston DPE
Professor of Human Physiology, Children's Health and Exercise Research Centre, University of Exeter, Exeter, UK

Samantha G. Fawkner PhD
Lecturer, School of Life Sciences, Heriot-Watt University, Edinburgh, UK

Clark A. Mundt MSc
Research Scholar, College of Kinesiology, University of Saskatchewan, Saskatoon, Saskatchewan, Canada

Gaynor Parfitt PhD
Senior Lecturer, Children's Health and Exercise Research Centre, University of Exeter, Exeter, UK

Lauren B. Sherar MSc
Research Scholar, College of Kinesiology, University of Saskatchewan, Saskatoon, Saskatchewan, Canada

Keith Tolfrey PhD
Reader in Paediatric Exercise Physiology, Department of Exercise and Sport Science, Manchester Metropolitan University, Alsager, UK

Jos W. R. Twisk PhD
*Senior Researcher, Department of Clinical Epidemiology and Biostatistics,
University Medical Centre and Institute of Health Sciences, Vrije University,
Amsterdam, The Netherlands*

Joanne R. Welsman PhD
*Senior Research Fellow, Deputy Director of the Children's Health and Exercise
Research Centre, University of Exeter, Exeter, UK*

Craig A. Williams PhD
*Senior Lecturer, Associate Director of the Children's Health and Exercise Research
Centre, University of Exeter, UK*

Richard J. Winsley PhD
*Lecturer, Associate Director of the Children's Health and Exercise Research Centre,
University of Exeter, Exeter, UK*

Foreword

It is now well accepted that, physiologically, children are not simply small adults. Nevertheless, the ways in which they seem to differ from adults do not always meet agreement. Take, for example, the question 'Do children perceive a given level of exertion as harder or easier than adults?' – as evidenced, for example, by the Borg RPE scale. This has been susceptible to a variety of differing interpretations. I would suggest from my own (relatively limited) experience that young children perceive treadmill running as correspondingly easier than adults – but others would indeed disagree.

On the anaerobic fatigue side, often, working with England U-8, U-10 and U-12 boys squash squads, I would notice that if one set them the task of presumed anaerobic 'shadow-training' on the court – i.e. periods of 30 s of high intensity corner-to-corner running, alternating with 30 s periods of active rest – these age groups would (if one let them) complete sets of 15 or even 20 repetitions. Whereas the older squads – U-14, U-16 and U-19 – would simply slow from fatigue at around 10 repetitions. Is this due to a different maturational lactate response?

Knowing that the surface area of an 8-year-old may be some 40% greater, relatively, than that of an adult can help explain why such children may be at higher risk of appropriate thermoregulatory upset in cold water or hot sunshine; and may also help in understanding how children can survive total ice-cold water immersion for periods of over half an hour, their rate of cooling being so rapid that the cryogenic effect is actually life-saving.

Nevertheless, knowing something is not always the same as acting on it. From an early age I coached my son Duncan at squash. Once when he was about 8 years old, I was feeding a long succession of balls for him to learn the overhead backhand volley. Gradually he learned the skill, and was striking the ball well, when he lowered his racket and said: 'Do you mind if we stop, I'm getting too hot!' Then I looked at my red-faced wee son and realized that, although I of all people should have known of the much poorer sweat and general thermoregulatory response of his age group, I had completely overlooked it in my pleasure at his grasping the technique.

Oded Bar-Or's 1983 text *Pediatric Sports Medicine for the Practitioner* was an absolutely seminal publication for those of us even peripherally in the field of children and exercise, containing as it did such a wealth of paediatric physiology. A few years ago, Professor Bar-Or was spending a sabbatical period with Professor Armstrong in Exeter, and I was visiting. Somehow the question of which was the leading paediatric exercise laboratory came up. 'Well, yours is', I said to Bar-Or. 'No', he said, turning to Neil, 'Yours is now.' No higher compliment could have been paid, and it is noteworthy that in the current volume, 11 of the 14 chapters are by staff or graduates of the Exeter

Children's Health and Exercise Research Centre, displaying a comprehensive range of materials from both their own research and the literature, relating to the physical performance of children and adolescents.

The list of 14 topics is exactly what one would want, ranging from growth, scaling and metabolism, through strength and high intensity exercise to pulmonary and cardiac function, oxygen kinetics and aerobic fitness. The environment, perceived exertion, responses to training, and the young athlete lead on to the final, vital chapter on physical activity and health. A knowledge of children's physiology is relevant to many aspects of work with young people, including medicine, sports science, sport, teaching, physical education – and general parenting; and the range and quality of the exercise science contained in the text form a database from which genuine advice of all types and at all levels can be sought and provided.

Given that children are the veritable stem cells of society, the thrust of a book leaning through their physiology into sport, activity and health cannot be over-estimated in importance, especially at a time when there are worryingly adverse trends in children's fitness, fatness and disease. Abundant paediatric medical and physiological data are scattered through the scientific literature, but naturally with a marked lack of integration. Here the data are not only well presented and reviewed, but synthesized into a coherent overall story in the book as a whole.

The publication of *Paediatric Exercise Physiology* will provide a great deal of critically evaluated information and approachable interest to a broad spectrum of readers. Editor Neil Armstrong and his 13 contributors are to be very warmly congratulated on a worthy successor to Oded Bar-Or's superb text.

N. C. Craig Sharp

Preface

This book will be of interest to scientists, physicians, paramedics, lecturers, teachers, and coaches working with children and adolescents, but it is primarily addressed to final year undergraduate and postgraduate sport and exercise science students. An understanding of the basic principles of exercise physiology is assumed and the primary objective of the book is to provide a state-of-the-art overview of the rapidly emerging field of paediatric exercise physiology.

Chapter topics have been chosen to provide comprehensive coverage of the content of taught modules in paediatric exercise physiology within a sport and exercise science programme. Each chapter begins with a list of learning objectives and concludes with a summary and a review of key points. Chapters are self-contained with selected references for readers interested in particular topics but also cross-referenced to other chapters where specific issues are examined in detail. A list of further reading is provided at the end of each chapter for those who wish to pursue the topic in more depth. The writers are all experienced lecturers and researchers in paediatric exercise physiology and 11 of the 14 chapters are authored by staff or graduates of the Children's Health and Exercise Research Centre at the University of Exeter.

The dramatic increase in published research over the last decade has enhanced understanding of the physiology of the exercising child, but in relation to research with adults data are sparse. Children and adolescents are not mini-adults and research techniques and equipment developed for use with adults are often not appropriate for young people. The involvement of children in non-therapeutic research raises ethical issues which have been debated at length elsewhere (e.g. Nicholson R H 1986 *Medical Research with Children*, Oxford University Press), and, although reference to ethical research is made where relevant throughout the text, detailed discussion is beyond the scope of this book. However, researchers must consider carefully whether the procedures they employ are ethical for use with young participants. Several techniques used almost routinely with adults (e.g. muscle biopsies) are not normally acceptable for research with healthy children, and paediatric physiologists must seek innovative experimental solutions to research questions.

Research with children presents many challenges and much remains to be learnt about physiological responses to exercise in relation to age, growth, maturation and sex. If this book stimulates interest in the physiology of the exercising child and encourages sport and exercise scientists to engage in research programmes devoted to enhancing understanding of paediatric exercise physiology, it will have served its purpose.

Exeter 2006   **Neil Armstrong**

Chapter 1

Growth and maturation

Adam D. G. Baxter-Jones and Lauren B. Sherar

CHAPTER CONTENTS

LEARNING OBJECTIVES

After studying this chapter you should be able to:
1. define childhood growth, maturation and development
2. understand the difference between cross-sectional, longitudinal and mixed longitudinal research design
3. interpret distance and velocity curves for height and body mass
4. describe growth changes in height, body mass and body proportions
5. understand why controlling for biological maturation is important in paediatric studies
6. determine age at peak height velocity from a longitudinal data set
7. describe the advantages and disadvantages of different maturity indicators in controlling for biological maturation
8. list some of the key regulators of growth and maturation
9. describe some differences in growth and performance among maturity groups (i.e. early, average and late maturers)
10. describe gender differences in growth and maturation.

INTRODUCTION

Paediatric exercise science examines the acute and chronic responses of the child and adolescent to exercise and/or physical activity. Morphological parameters and physiological functions such as heart volume, lung function, aerobic power and muscular strength develop with increasing age and body size. Furthermore, physical fitness (e.g. muscular, motor and cardiorespiratory fitness) also changes with growth and maturation. Therefore, variations in growth and maturation of a child can have profound effects upon aspects of physical activity, physical fitness and physical performance. To fully understand paediatric exercise physiology a student needs a sound understanding of the general principles of childhood growth and maturation, otherwise termed auxology. This chapter outlines the basic concepts of growth and maturation, and reviews some of the possible biological maturity indicators that can be used to control for the confounding effects of growth and maturation.

The terms growth, biological maturation and development are often used synonymously in the paediatric literature. Although interrelated, the concepts have fundamental and semantic differences. Growth refers to changes in size of an individual, as a whole or in parts. As children grow, they become taller and heavier, they increase their lean and fat tissues, and their organs increase in size. Changes in size are a result of three cellular processes: (1) an increase in cell number, or hyperplasia, (2) an increase in cell size, or hypertrophy, and (3) an increase in intercellular substances, or accretion. All three occur during growth but the predominance of one process over another varies with chronological age and the tissue involved (Malina et al 2004).

Maturation has been described as the process of being mature, or progress toward the mature state (Malina et al 2004). The process of maturing has two components, timing and tempo. The former refers to when specific maturational events occur (e.g. age when menarche is attained, age at the beginning of breast development, age at the appearance of pubic hair, or age at maximum growth in height during the adolescent growth spurt (peak height velocity; PHV)). Tempo refers to the rate at which maturation progresses (i.e. how quickly or slowly an individual passes from the initial stages of sexual maturation to the mature state). Maturation occurs in all biological systems in the body but at different rates. Furthermore, the timing and tempo of maturity vary considerably among individuals, with children of the same chronological age differing dramatically in their degree of biological maturity.

Development refers to the acquisition of behavioural competence (the learning of appropriate behaviours expected by society) and is culture specific. As children experience life at home, school, church, sports, recreation, and other community activities, they develop cognitively, socially, emotionally, morally, and so on. Children and adolescents learn to behave in culturally appropriate manners. Development can also be thought of within the biological context. Here development refers to the processes of differentiation and specialization occurring during the prenatal life. Apart from during prenatal life, the term development is seen most frequently in the behavioural literature and although an essential component it will not be covered in any detail in this book.

It is important to recognize that growth, maturation, and development occur simultaneously and interact; however, they may not follow the same time line. A young person could be advanced in terms of social and emotional development but delayed in biological maturation, or vice versa. In the growth and development literature, life leading up to maturity is split into three stages: the prenatal period, childhood and adolescence. The period of prenatal life is vitally important to the child's well-being; however, it will not be covered in this chapter, as discussion will focus on the first two decades of postnatal life. The terms adolescence and puberty are used frequently in the paediatric literature to explain the later period of growth and maturity, often with no clear distinction in their definitions. Some authors refer to adolescence when talking about psychosocial changes and puberty when talking about the physical changes. However, as most of the literature uses these terms interchangeably, this book will use adolescence synonymously with puberty.

Study design

The majority of studies of paediatric growth are cross-sectional. Cross-sectional studies take single measurements from individuals who differ in chronological age. Cross-sectional studies are attractive as they can be carried out quickly and include larger numbers of children. Unfortunately, cross-sectional studies only give a static picture of the population variation in growth variables and provide little information about individual growth patterns over time. Most of the seminal growth research has been longitudinal in design. Longitudinal studies measure the same subjects over time, allowing one to ascertain part of or the entire growth pattern of an individual. A pure longitudinal design is where a cohort of children born within the same year is followed continuously and assessed on at least three separate occasions. A compromise between cross-sectional and longitudinal design is the mixed-longitudinal design. In this design either a number of relatively short longitudinal studies are interlocked covering a whole age range (e.g. 8–10 years, 9–11 years, 10–13 years, etc.), or some individuals are measured repeatedly and others are measured only once. In both of these cases information is provided on status and rate of growth. However, sophisticated statistical techniques are required to accurately interpret the data (see Ch. 2). The advantage of longitudinal over cross-sectional designs is that within-individual variance can be obtained and thus the timing and tempo of an individual's pattern of growth identified. When conducting longitudinal research it is important to remember that two measures separated by a time period do not constitute longitudinal data; true longitudinal data have at least three measures and thus two velocities. Unfortunately, longitudinal research is often impractical for paediatric exercise research as the process is laborious, expensive and time-consuming for both the participants and investigators. This means that most knowledge in paediatric exercise science is based on cross-sectional research.

GROWTH

Body dimensions and proportions

Different parts of the body grow at different rates and different times. It has been proposed (Scammon 1930) that all tissues and systems follow four patterns of growth: (1) neurological (e.g. brain and head), (2) genital (e.g. reproductive organs), (3) general (e.g. stature, heart size), and (4) lymphoid (e.g. lymph glands, tonsils, appendix). These patterns of growth are shown in Figure 1.1. The data shown are relative, as size attained by each type of tissue at each age is expressed as a percentage of the total increment between birth and 20 years of age (100%). Brain and head growth are the most rapid from birth, with steady growth from about 7 years of age and a slight spurt during adolescence. By 2 years of age, brain and head reach nearly 50% of their adult size, with full adult size being reached by 8 to 10 years of age. The genital curve includes primary sex characteristics (e.g. uterus, vagina, fallopian tubes in females;

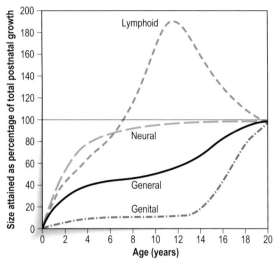

Figure 1.1 Scammon growth curves of different parts and tissues of the body. All curves are of size attained plotted as percentage of total gain from birth to 20 years. Size at 20 years is 100% on the vertical scale. (From Scammon 1930, with the permission of University of Minnesota Press.)

prostate and seminal vesicles in males) and secondary sex characteristics (e.g. breasts in females, facial hair in males, and axillary and pubic hair in both sexes). The genital curve shows some growth during infancy followed by reduced growth during child-hood; by 10 to 12 years of age reproductive organs are only 10% of their adult size. During adolescence (puberty) there is a rapid growth in genital tissues. The general curve of growth includes many tissues and systems in the body, such as skeletal tissue, the respiratory system and the digestive system to name a few. The general curve follows an 'S', or sigmoidal curve of growth. The 'S' shape reflects a rapid growth dur-ing infancy and early childhood, steady growth during mid-childhood, rapid growth during early adolescence and a levelling off in late adolescence. At 10–12 years of age children are roughly 84% of their adult height. The lymphoid tissues are involved with the immunological capacities of the child and show a different growth curve from the rest of the body. There is a remarkable increase in size of the lymphoid tissue until the early adolescent years (approximately 11 to 13 years). The relative size of the tissue then steeply declines during puberty, probably as a result of the upregulation of sex hormones during this period.

Growth during childhood and adolescence occurs distal to proximal. For example, the hands and feet experience accelerated growth first, followed by the calf and the forearm, the hips and the chest, and lastly the shoulders. Thus, during childhood there may be a period where youths appear to have large hands and feet in relation to the rest of their body. However, once the adolescent spurt has ended, hands and feet are a little smaller in proportion to arms, legs and stature. Most body dimensions, with the exception of subcutaneous adipose tissue and the dimensions of the head and face, follow a growth pattern similar to that of stature; however, there are wide variations in the timing of growth spurts. From childhood to adolescence, the lower extremities (legs) grow faster than the upper body (trunk). This results in sitting height contributing less to stature as age progresses. During the adolescent growth spurt the legs experience a growth spurt earlier than the trunk. Thus, for a period during early adolescence, a youth will have relatively long legs, but the appearance of long-leggedness disappears with the later increase in trunk length. Sex differences in leg length and sitting height are small during childhood. For a short time during the early part of adolescence girls, on average, have a slightly longer leg length than boys. Boys' leg length exceeds girls' by about 12 years of age, but boys do not catch up in sitting height until about 14 years of age. The longer period of pre-adolescent growth in boys is largely responsible for the fact that men's legs are longer than women's in relation to trunk length.

Stature

Standing height or stature is a linear measurement of the distance from the floor, or standing surface, to the top of the skull and is the most widely used indicator of somatic growth because of its relative ease in measurement. The terms stature and height are used synonymously in the paediatric literature and in this book. Stature is made up of sitting height (distance from the sitting surface to the top of the head) and leg length, or subischial length (distance between the hip joint and the floor). The exact landmark of the hip joint is sometimes hard to locate so leg length is most often calculated by subtracting sitting height from standing height. Stature varies during the course of the day, with readings being higher in the morning and decreasing throughout the day. Shrinkage during the day occurs because the intervertebral discs become compressed as result of weight-bearing. The diurnal variation may be as much as 1 cm or more (Malina et al 2004).

By linking together an individual's height data at successive ages a distance graph is produced that describes the height achieved at any age. An example is shown in Figure 1.2A. This type of graph has been named a height distance curve, or a height-for-age curve. When interpreting these graphs it is important to remember that although the curve in Figure 1.2A appears to be somewhat smooth, growth is not a continuous process. If the measurements were taken on a more frequent basis than every 6 months (i.e. bi-weekly) one would see that growth actually occurs in short bursts of activity (saltation), with intervening periods of no growth (statis). Also, growth is not a linear process; individuals do not grow the same amount in each calendar year. For example, there is relatively rapid growth during infancy, steady growth during childhood, rapid growth in adolescence and slow growth as an individual reaches maturity (sigmoidal curve). These patterns of rates of growth are better reflected when the velocity (or rate) of growth is plotted and a curve fitted.

An example of a height velocity curve is shown in Figure 1.2B. A velocity curve better reflects the child's state of growth at any particular time than does the distance curve (Fig. 1.2A). During the first year of life, infants grow at a fast rate, approximately 25 cm per year. During the first half of the year the velocity may be even faster, around 30 cm per year. During the second year of life there is growth of another 12–13 cm in stature so that by the age of 2 years the child has attained about 50% of adult stature. From then on there is a steady deceleration in growth, dropping to a rate of about 5–6 cm per year before the initiation of peak height velocity (PHV). Peak height velocity refers to the maximum rate of growth in stature during the adolescent growth period. Girls, on average, attain PHV approximately 2 years earlier than boys, with their onset of PHV occurring between 8.2 and 10.3 years. On average PHV is reached between 11.3 and 12.2 years. Corresponding ages for boys are 10.0–12.1 years and 13.3–14.4 years (Malina et al 2004). There is also another distinct but smaller increase

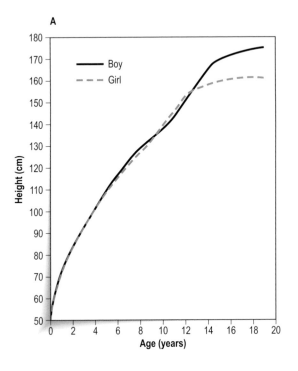

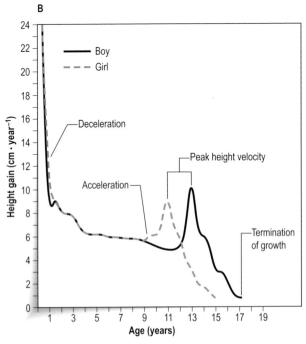

Figure 1.2 Growth in height of a typical boy and girl between 3 and 18 years of age. Figure 1.2A shows a plot of the height for age data (distance curve). Figure 1.2B shows the yearly increments in height (velocity curve). (Data from Malina et al 2004.)

in growth rate, usually between the ages of 6.5 and 8.5 years (Fig. 1.2B). This is called the juvenile or mid-growth spurt.

On average, males are usually 13 cm taller than females upon reaching their final adult height. Up until the initiation of PHV the sex differences in height are small. Therefore, boys achieve their height advantage during the adolescent period. Specifically, boys, on average, experience about 2 years more pre-adolescent growth, approximately 5 cm per year, than girls. This is roughly 10 cm of growth that girls do not experience. Boys also achieve a slightly greater (on average 2 cm) magnitude of height at PHV. Both of these growth differences cause males, on average, to have a greater adult stature. Girls stop growing in stature by about 16 years of age and boys by about 18 or 19 years of age. However, these ages may be spuriously young as many growth studies stop measuring youth at 17 or 18 years of age and it is known that many people continue to grow into their early to mid twenties.

These curves of growth in height (Fig. 1.2) reflect the growth patterns found in all healthy children who live in a normal environment. As mentioned, individuals will differ in absolute height of growth velocity (i.e. adult heights) and in the timing of the adolescent growth spurt; however, to reach their destined final height each individual will go through a similar pattern of human growth.

Body mass

Body mass is made up of a composite of tissues, including both fat and fat-free tissue, that accrue at different rates and times. Changes in body mass can thus be a result of changes in fat or fat-free mass, but also changes in body water (dehydration or over hydration). The relative proportions and distributions of fat and fat-free components depend on age, sex, and other environmental and genetic factors. Body mass is a very sensitive and thus fluctuating measurement, in the sense that it can change from one day to another due to minor alterations in body composition. Furthermore, body mass, like stature, also shows diurnal variation. An individual is lightest in the morning, after voiding the bladder. Throughout the day body mass increases and is affected by diet and physical activity. In menstruating adolescent girls the phase of the menstrual cycle can also affect body mass.

The average distance and velocity curve for the development of body mass in males and females is shown in Figure 1.3. As seen with the development of height (Fig. 1.2), body mass follows a four-phase growth pattern: rapid growth in infancy and early childhood, rather steady gain during mid-childhood, rapid gain during adolescence, and usually a slower increase into adulthood. During the first year of life body mass doubles and by the end of the second year it has quadrupled. Most children show the lowest annual increment in body mass around 2–3 years of age; from this point to the onset of adolescence body mass increases, but at a slower rate. At the onset of adolescence there is a rapid gain in the velocity of body mass development. The precise timing of the adolescent growth spurt in body mass is generally less clear than it is for height. It has been estimated that peak velocity in body mass normally occurs 0.2–0.4 years after PHV in boys and 0.3–0.9 years after PHV in girls (Armstrong & Welsman 1997).

Boys and girls follow the same pattern in body mass development. Before the adolescent growth spurt boys are slightly heavier than girls. Girls then experience an earlier growth spurt and thus for a short time are heavier. As soon as boys go through their adolescent growth spurt they catch up and thus become and remain heavier than girls. It is important to remember that there is a normal range of individual

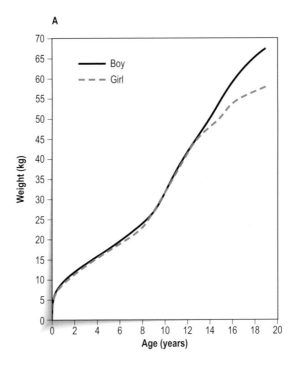

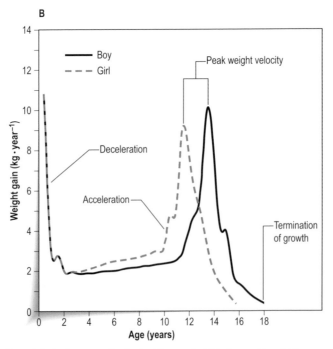

Figure 1.3   Growth in body mass of a typical boy and girl between 3 and 18 years of age. Figure 1.3A shows a plot of the body mass for age data (distance curve). Figure 1.3B shows the yearly increments in body mass (velocity curve). (Data from Malina et al 2004.)

variation in body mass resulting in some girls being heavier than most boys at virtually all ages. In boys, the growth spurt in body mass is primarily due to gains in muscle mass and skeletal tissue, with fat mass remaining fairly stable. Girls, however, experience a less dramatic rise in muscle mass and skeletal tissue but experience a continuous rise in fat mass during adolescence. The increase in body fat during adolescence contributes to the changing shape and thus centre of gravity of the female adolescent. These adaptations may adversely affect performance in some activities such as gymnastics.

Body proportions

During adolescence girls and boys experience very different changes in body shape. Boys experience a broadening of the shoulders relative to the hips and girls experience a broadening of the hips relative to the shoulders. These sex differences are evident during childhood but become accentuated during adolescence. During the adolescent growth spurt boys gain more in shoulder (biacromial) breadth (about 2.3 cm), whereas girls gain slightly more in hip (bicristal) breadth (about 1.2 cm). Boys catch up to girls in their bicristal breadth in late adolescence (Malina et al 2004).

The timing and speed of these changes in body dimensions may have a dramatic effect on several aspects of physical performance. An increase in shoulder width can result in increased muscle mass in the upper body in boys. This is one reason why sex differences in strength are much greater in the upper compared to the lower body. Furthermore, this greater upper body muscle, combined with longer arms, could explain why older boys are better at throwing, racquet sports and rowing than girls. Girls tend to have a lower centre of gravity, due to the relative broadening of the hips, which may contribute to their better sense of balance (Armstrong & Welsman 1997).

CONTROLLING FOR BIOLOGICAL MATURITY

Often within exercise physiology there is an interest in examining the trainability of the child, or the association between physical activity and health outcomes. However, interpretation of these outcomes must consider the process of normal growth and maturation before any definitive conclusion can be reached. Unless body size and biological maturity indicators are considered, one cannot definitively identify the independent effects of physical activity or training on the outcome. Biological maturity can be controlled by aligning individuals by maturity status (or biological age), which requires an assessment of maturity. When considering how to assess biological maturation it is first important to understand that 1 year of chronological time does not equal 1 year of maturational time. Whilst every individual passes through the same stages of maturity they do so at differing rates, resulting in children of the same chronological age differing in their degree of maturity. This is reflected in Figure 1.4. Both boys are 14 years of age but differ considerably in their degree of maturity, with the boy on the left being an early maturer and the boy on the right being a late maturer. A second point to understand is that the size of an individual is not an accurate indicator of maturity. Certainly, in very general terms, size is associated with maturity, in that a bigger individual is likely to be chronologically older and thus more mature than a smaller individual. However, it is well recognized that size does not play a part in the assessment of maturity. This is covered later when the use of height as an indicator of maturity is discussed.

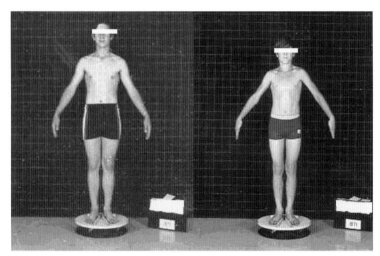

Figure 1.4   Two boys photographed at the same chronological age (14 years). The boy on the left is an early maturer and the boy on the right is a late maturer. Data taken from two individuals who participated in the Saskatchewan Growth and Development Study, 1964–1973 (Mirwald 1978).

To adequately control for maturity an indicator of maturity needs to be incorporated into the research methodology. The maturity indicator chosen can be any definable and sequential change in any part of the body that is characteristic of the progression of the body from immaturity to maturity (Cameron 2002). The most commonly used methods involve an assessment of skeletal age, secondary sex characteristics, menarcheal status and/or somatic characteristics. The technique of choice varies with the study design. Each method, with its associated limitations, will be briefly reviewed.

Skeletal age

A skeletal age assessment requires an X-ray, usually of the hand and wrist or knee, and is the only method that spans the entire growth period, from birth to maturity. During prenatal life all children start off with a skeleton of cartilage which develops through childhood and adolescence into a fully developed skeleton of bone. Therefore, the assessment of skeletal maturity is based on the observation that an individual more advanced in maturity will have greater bone development and a smaller amount of cartilage than a less mature child. Skeletal age assessment involves estimating the level of skeletal maturity that a child has attained at a given point in time relative to reference data for healthy children. Thus, an early maturing individual would have an older skeletal age compared to their chronological age. Although a number of techniques exist to assess skeletal maturity, two protocols, the atlas technique of Greulich & Pyle (1959) and the Tanner–Whitehouse 'bone specific scoring' technique (Tanner et al 1983), have dominated the literature. Both techniques use the left hand and wrist to estimate the skeletal age of a child; however, it is important to note that scores derived from these two methods are not equivalent. The methods differ in their scoring system and the populations on which they are based. A full description of these methods can be found in Malina and colleagues' (2004) comprehensive textbook. Skeletal ages ranging from 9 to 16 years have been demonstrated in groups of 13- and 14-year-olds, thus illustrating the wide variation in skeletal age evident in children of a similar chronological age (Kemper & Verschuur 1981). This variation emphasizes why using a common chronological age as a pubertal cut-off point, for example all children less than 12 years of age classified as prepubertal, is not tenable. Although the assessment of skeletal age is considered the best maturational index, it is costly, requires specialized equipment and interpretation, and the ethics of exposing children to repeated radiation must be considered carefully. Furthermore, discrepancies of one or more years between skeletal ages of the knee and of the hand–wrist have been documented in individual youths. This questions whether the skeletal maturity of the hand and wrist represents the maturity of the whole skeleton and highlights the discrepancies between skeletal age and chronological age.

Age at peak height velocity

Landmarks on an individual's height growth curve can be used as an indicator of maturity. The most commonly used somatic milestone in longitudinal studies of child-hood growth is the age at peak height velocity (APHV), although take-off (or initiation of PHV) and cessation of growth have also been used. To obtain APHV whole year height velocity (cm per year) increments are plotted and mathematical curve fitting procedures are used to identify the age when the maximum velocity in statural growth occurs. Girls usually reach PHV around 12 years and boys around 14 years of age. However, the timing of this event in relation to chronological age shows great variance. A British study found that girls reached PHV anywhere between 9.3 and 15.0 years and boys anywhere between 12.0 and 15.8 years (Malina et al 2004). Once APHV has been determined, individuals can be aligned by biological maturity age (years from APHV) rather than chronological age. For example, at APHV an individual has a biological maturity age equal to 0.0 years. At 11.8 years an individual who reaches PHV at 13.8 years will have a biological maturity age of –2.0 years. Alternatively, individuals can be characterized as early, average or late maturers depending on the age at which PHV is attained. Early maturers are those whose APHV occurs greater than 1 year prior to the mean age, whilst late maturers are those whose APHV occurs more than 1 year after the mean age; the remainder are classified as average maturers.

To facilitate a better understanding of the utility of APHV as an indicator of maturity, the following is a worked example (Table 1.1). To calculate an individual's APHV it is necessary to have serial measures of height and the age of the individual when the measurement was taken. This is shown in column A and B of Table 1.1. Next one has to calculate the years that have elapsed between present and previous meas-urement of height (the age increment). This is calculated by subtracting the age at the previous testing occasion from the age at the present testing time (A6 – A4). Next one has to calculate the midpoint age (in years) between the previous and present testing occasion (the age centre). This is calculated by adding together the age at the previous testing occasion and the age at present testing occasion and dividing by 2 ((A6 + A4)/2). Next the gain in height (cm) between the two testing occasions is calculated (a simple height increment). This is calculated by subtracting the height at the previous testing occasion from the height at the present testing occasion (B6 – B4). Lastly, the gain in height (cm) previously calculated is adjusted for the time elapsed between testing occasions (a whole year height increment). To find out when PHV occurs you find the whole year velocity column (column F) and read off the highest

Table 1.1   A worked example of calculating age at peak height velocity

	A	B	C	D	E	F
1	Distance			Velocity		
2						
3	Age at test (years)	Height (cm)	Age increment (years)	Age centre (years)	Simple height increment (cm)	Whole year height increment (cm)
4	7.450	124.0				
5			A6 – A4	(A6 + A4)/2	B6 – B4	(B6 – B4) /A6 – A4)
6	8.406	128.5				
7			A8 – A6	(A8 + A6)/2	B8 – B6	(B8 – B6) /(A8 – A6)
8	9.389	133.0				
9			0.94	9.86	6.0	6.4
10	10.332	139.0				
11			1.09	10.88	5.2	4.8
12	11.422	144.2				
13			0.94	11.89	6.4	6.8
14	12.362	150.6				
15			0.93	12.83	7.3	7.9
16	13.291	157.9				
17			1.1	13.84	10.6	9.7
18	14.389	168.5				
19			0.932	14.855	3.3	3.5

(a) Proportional allotment determination of age at peak height velocity (APHV):

$$APHV = \frac{A + VA - (VA - 1)}{[VA - (VA - 1)] + [VA - (VA + 1)]} - 0.5$$

Where:
A = age centre at peak velocity
VA = whole year height increment value at peak
(VA – 1) = whole year height increment value 1 year before peak
(VA + 1) = whole year height increment value 1 year after peak.

(b) Sample calculation of determination of APHV:

$$13.84 + \frac{9.7 - 7.9}{(9.7 - 7.9) + (9.7 - 3.5)} - 0.5$$

$$=$$

$$13.84 + \frac{1.8}{(1.8 + 6.2)} - 0.5 = 13.57 \text{ years}$$

value and the age-centred value. In the worked example the largest magnitude of height gain, or PHV, was 9.7 cm when age centre was 13.29 years. It should be noted that the highest value for height has to be followed by a smaller value to ensure that a peak in height has been reached. To get a truer assessment of APHV it is necessary to adjust for the fact that the individual reached APHV somewhere between the two testing occasions, which in the example is roughly 1 year apart. This is done through proportional allotment, and is demonstrated in the worked example. Proportional allotment uses the age centre and the whole year height increment value 1 year before peak, at peak, and 1 year after peak to estimate the age (between the two testing occasions) that PHV was reached. In the example, when APHV is adjusted using proportional allotment the individual is estimated to reach PHV at 13.57 years.

Predicting age at peak height velocity

To obtain APHV, serial data are required and therefore this indicator of maturity has previously been limited to longitudinal studies. Mirwald and colleagues (2002) developed sex-specific multiple regression equations, based on the growth patterns of the upper body and legs, which predict years from PHV. When years from PHV are considered in relation to current age, APHV can be estimated. The prediction equations require measures of stature, trunk length and leg length, as well as body mass and chronological age. Using these growth indicators APHV can be predicted within ±1 year, in 95% of cases. To facilitate a better understanding of the practical utility of the method, an example of how to predict the APHV of a boy aged 12.1 years is shown in Table 1.2. Sitting height, leg length (subtract sitting height from standing height), weight and chronological age are entered into the sex-specific regression equation (Mirwald et al 2002) to predict years from PHV. The equation predicts that the boy is −1.64 years from APHV. Subtracting years from PHV from age (12.1 years) gives a predicted APHV of 13.74 years. This APHV falls within a year of the average APHV for a boy (14 years), thus this boy could be considered an average maturer. A website (http://www.usask.ca/kinesiology/research_index.php) is available in which a child's APHV can be estimated by using the methodology described above. This method of assessing maturity is quick, non-invasive, and inexpensive to administer and can be used in cross-sectional studies. The added advantage to this technique is

Table 1.2   A worked example of predicting years from peak height velocity for a boy

Maturity offset = −9.236 + (0.0002708 × leg length and sitting height interaction) + (−0.001663 × age and leg length interaction) + (0.007216 × age and sitting height interaction) + (0.02292 × weight by height ratio)
Age: 12.1 years
Height: 150.0 cm
Weight: 39.0 kg
Leg length: 70.2 cm
Sitting height: 79.1 cm
Leg length and sitting height interaction: 70.2 × 79.1 = 5559.84
Age and leg length interaction: 12.1 × 70.2 = 849.42
Age and sitting height interaction: 12.1 × 79.1 = 957.11
Weight by height ratio: (39.0/150.0) × 100 = 26.0

Maturity offset = −9.236 + (0.0002708 × 5559.84) + (−0.001663 × 849.42) + (0.007216 × 957.11) + (0.02292 × 26.0)
        = −1.64 years from PHV
Age at PHV = 12.1 years + 1.64 = 13.74 years = average maturer

that it predicts a maturity benchmark that exists in both boys and girls; therefore, it allows for comparisons of maturity between boys and girls.

Predictions based on morphological age

The height attained at any given chronological age can be compared to reference norms to assess maturity. Individuals are assigned a morphological age based on their height for age. For example, statural growth of three males measured at 7, 14 and 40 years of age is presented in Figure 1.5 and will be used to indicate how height for age can be used to assess maturity. At 7 years of age boy 'A' and boy 'C' are about the same height whilst boy 'B' is 10 cm shorter. By 14 years of age boys 'A' and 'C' are still about the same height but boy 'B' is nearly 18 cm shorter. Using a morphological age scale boy 'B' at 14 years of age would be identified as a late maturer. The major disadvantage of this method is that it does not take into account the variability of height. For example, boy 'B' could be classified as a late maturer because he is shorter (i.e. he will also be shorter than average as an adult). Thus, it is now well recognized that using height for age in this way does not accurately assess biological maturity.

Expressing measured height in terms of percentage of final adult height accounts for the natural variability in height among individuals. In Figure 1.5, although in absolute terms boy 'B' appears to be small for his age, when presented as a percentage of final adult height there is no difference between boys 'B' and 'C' at 7 and 14 years of age. This is because at 40 years of age boy 'A' and 'B' are the same height and boy 'C' is 15 cm taller. Since roughly 92% of adult stature is reached at PHV (Tanner 1962) individuals could be classified into two maturity groups, pre- or post-PHV. Since the average age of PHV in boys is 14 years, boy 'A' at 14 years of age would be classified

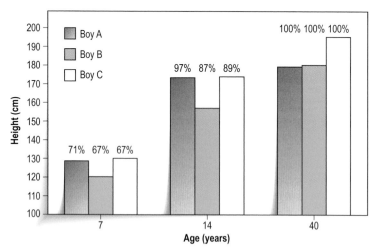

Figure 1.5   Height and percentage adult height for three males at 7, 14 and 40 years of age. (From A D G Baxter-Jones, J C Eisenmann, and L B Sherar, 2005, Controlling for maturation in pediatric exercise science, *Pediatric Exercise Science*, 17(1): page 24, figure 3. © 2005 by Human Kinetics. Reprinted with permission from Human Kinetics (Champaign, IL). Data were taken from three individuals who participated in the Saskatchewan Growth and Development Study. Data reference: Mirwald R L. Saskatchewan Growth and Development Study. In: *Kinanthropometry II*. M Ostyn, G Beunen, and J Simon (eds). Baltimore: University Park Press, 1980, pp. 289–305.)

as an early maturer (percentage adult stature >92%) and boys 'B' and 'C' as average maturers (percentage adult stature <92%). The disadvantage of this technique is that an adult height value is required during childhood and thus maturity status can only be assessed retrospectively.

Expressing current height as a percentage of adult height can be used in cross-sectional studies if adult height is predicted. A hurdle in the prediction of adult height is, however, accounting for individual variation in the timing and tempo of the adolescent growth spurt and sexual maturation in youths of the same chronological age. Growth in stature is known to have a distinct and measurable end point; however, as mentioned previously, children differ greatly in the rate at which they pass through the various phases of growth. Some children have a rapid tempo of growth and attain adult stature at a relatively early age, while others have a slow tempo and finish growing relatively late. Therefore, an accurate method of estimating adult height needs to incorporate an indicator of biological maturity for errors of prediction to be reduced. Many equations have been developed to predict adult height. The most commonly used methods are those of Bayley & Pinneau (1952), Roche et al (1975a, 1975b) and Tanner et al (1983, 2001). These methods all include an assessment of skeletal age to account for maturity differences. Unfortunately, the assessment of skeletal age is costly and requires exposure to radiation, which may hinder widespread use of these predictive equations outside of the clinical setting. In an effort to develop a non-intrusive and inexpensive method of predicting adult height, the modified Roche–Wainer–Thissen (RWT) method (Roche et al 1983) and the Khamis–Roche method (Khamis & Roche 1994) were developed. These two methods estimate adult stature from current age, stature, body mass, and mid-parent stature (adjusted mean height of the parents). However, these non-intrusive methods do not include a measure of biological maturity. Although the inclusion of mid-parent height has been shown to reduce error in the prediction, the heights of both parents are not always available.

A method of predicting adult height has been developed which is valid, non-intrusive, inexpensive and simple to administer (Sherar et al 2005). The method requires measures of height and a prediction of years from PHV (Mirwald et al 2002). Based on APHV individuals are classified as early, average or late maturers. Using maturity reference values obtained from sex-specific cumulative height velocity curves, the distance left to grow, depending on how far an individual is from PHV, can be obtained. Adding the distance left to grow to present height gives a prediction of adult height. As in other methods, there is error associated with this method. Although the error varies depending on prediction technique the error usually falls between 3 and 5 cm (Malina et al 2004).

Menarcheal status

Age at menarche (the first menstrual period) is the most commonly reported developmental milestone of female adolescence in both cross-sectional and longitudinal studies. Three methods (prospective, status quo, and recall) are commonly used to establish age at menarche. The best and most reliable is to follow individuals and note the date menarche occurs. However, this method is limited in that longitudinal data are required. Alternatively, normative values can be established by the status quo method. This involves asking a large number of girls (usually aged between 8 and 18 years) when they were born and whether they have started their menstrual flow. From their ages and their answers (yes or no) it is possible to calculate mean and standard deviation values for age of menarche. The third method is the recall method. A simple questionnaire is used to establish if an individual has experienced menarche;

if the answer is yes, they are asked to indicate the date or month. The retrospective method is useful for individuals after 17 years of age, when almost all girls have attained menarche.

Although age at menarche is a widely used maturity indicator in female studies, its use is limited to later adolescence as menarche usually occurs after PHV. Most studies, especially in athletes, use the recall method which has the limitation of recall error. Estimated mean ages are biased, since not all subjects have yet reached menarche. Furthermore, age of menarche has little use in gender comparison studies as no corresponding maturity indicator exists in males.

Secondary sex characteristics

Sexual maturation is a continuous process that extends from sexual differentiation in the embryo through puberty to full sexual maturity. The assessment of maturity in growth studies is based on the development of secondary sex characteristics during the pubertal period. Secondary sex characteristics most frequently assessed are breast development in girls, penis and testes development in boys, and pubic hair development in both sexes. Facial hair, axillary hair, voice change, body odour and body shape are other aspects of pubertal change that have been indexed. Secondary sex characteristics are used because they are a visible manifestation of sexual maturity at a given period of time.

Secondary sex staging divides the process of breast development in girls, genitalia development in boys, and pubic hair development in both sexes, into five stages. These secondary sex stages are commonly referred to as 'Tanner stages', although the technique was first documented by Reynolds & Wines (1948, 1951) and later described in more detail by Tanner (1962). The scale is usually used in conjunction with a series of photographs or drawings which are available in several texts (Malina et al 2004, Tanner 1962). Stage 1 indicates the prepubertal state – the absence of the development of each characteristic. Stage 2 indicates the initial overt development of each characteristic. Stages 3 and 4 indicate continued maturation of each characteristic and are somewhat difficult to evaluate. Stage 5 indicates the adult or mature state.

Traditionally, determination of sexual maturity has been obtained through direct visual observation. This approach is appropriate for clinical settings, but poses problems for the assessment of children in a non-clinical setting as the method invades the privacy of the child or adolescent involved. To address these concerns youngsters have been asked to rate their own stage of sexual maturity by comparing themselves to standardized photographs or drawings. Correlations between self-ratings and physician ratings are moderate to high. Nonetheless, there are still concerns that youngsters overestimate early stages and underestimate later stages of sexual development.

The first overt sign of pubertal development in boys is usually the enlargement of the testes accompanied by changes in texture and colour of the scrotal skin. The penis then begins to enlarge and pubic hair appears. In females the first sign of sexual maturity is breast development, followed by pubic hair development. However, in about one third of girls pubic hair appears before the breast bud. A textbook by Malina and colleagues (2004) includes an extensive review of the usual age ranges of boys entering the genital stages and girls entering the breast stages and both sexes entering the pubic hair stages. The review includes samples of girls and boys from different European and North American countries. The average age of entering genital stage 2 (G2) in boys ranges anywhere between 9.2 and 12.4 years, depending on the sample. The onset of pubic hair development (PH2) on average occurs anywhere between 11.2

years and 13.4 years. In comparison, PHV normally occurs when most boys are in G4 and PH4 (between 13.8 and 14.1 years). Elongation of the larynx (voice breaking) usually occurs late in puberty, about 1 year after the attainment of PHV. The first spontaneous ejaculation of seminal fluid during wakefulness has been reported to occur between 12.5 years and 16.5 years. Axillary hair appears usually after PH4; however, occasionally axillary hair may appear before the onset of pubic hair. Facial hair usually appears after the complete development of both pubic hair and genitalia. These wide age ranges illustrate the individual variation in entering, progressing through, and completing puberty.

Similar variability observed in males is seen in the onset, progression and completion of female sexual maturity. The advent of breast stage 2 (B2) is usually followed closely by the appearance of pubic hair (PH2). The progression of breast development and pubic hair development show considerable independence so, of girls in B3, 25% may be in PH1 and 10% in PH5 (Tanner 1962). The range of average ages reported by Malina and colleagues (2004) for the onset of breast stage 2 (B2) varied from 8.9 years to 11.6 years and for pubic hair stage 2 (PH2) from 8.8 years to 12.1 years. In comparison menarche occurs late in the sequence of events, an average of 1 year after PHV (between 12.8 and 13.5 years). Again there is considerable independence of menarche from pubertal characteristics; although most girls are in B4 some are in B3 and a small percentage may be in B2. Likewise most girls are in PH3 or PH4, while some may be in PH1. The majority of girls experience menarche at the time of maximum deceleration of growth in stature. Thus, menarche is closely associated with the timing of PHV, although the hormonal significance of this is unknown.

The various timings of these pubertal events is illustrated in Figure 1.6 using data from the Saskatchewan Pediatric Bone Mineral Accrual Study (PBMAS) (Bailey 1997). The figure shows that a number of pubertal events are occurring at the same time, all under the control of various endocrine systems and ultimately controlled by genetic expression. However, the timing of pubertal events varies between individuals of the same sex.

As well as individual variation there is also a marked sex difference in the timing of somatic and sexual maturation. Girls enter and end puberty approximately 2 years before boys. Pubertal events do not occur in the same sequence between the sexes. For example, when comparing pubic hair growth to statural growth PHV is a relatively early event in girls and a relatively late event in boys (Sherar et al 2004). Boys' PHV occurs, on average, during pubic hair stage 4 and 5, whereas girls' PHV usually occurs during pubic hair stage 3 and 4. This suggests that the timing of sexual and somatic maturation is not the same between girls and boys.

Aligning individuals by secondary sex characteristics is used frequently in paediatric exercise science literature because it does not require longitudinal observations, is easy to administer, cost-effective, and non-invasive (with the replacement of physician assessment with self-assessment). However, a common misuse of secondary sex characteristics when controlling for maturity is to analyse categories as if they were continuous variables. For example, an individual in the early phase of stage 3 of pubic hair development is rated the same as an individual in the late phase of this stage. It is rare that the point in time at which one stage changes to another stage is actually measured; what is actually being reported is the interval between two stages. This provides even less information when you consider that the length of time it takes to move through a stage varies considerably among individuals. In addition, there is no relationship between the age at which a secondary sex characteristic begins and the length of time that it takes to pass through the stage. Another concern with the use of secondary sex staging relates to possible misuse in alignment of individuals. Many

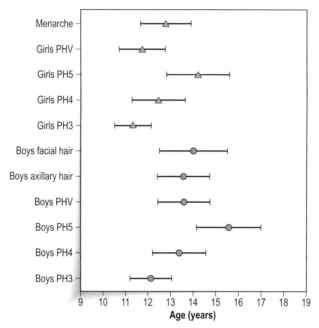

Figure 1.6   Average age of attainment of pubic hair (PH) stages 3–5 and peak height velocity (PHV). In boys only, axillary hair and facial hair growth. In girls only, menarche. Values are means (circles) and two standard deviations (bars). (From A D G Baxter-Jones, J C Eisenmann, and L B Sherar, 2005, Controlling for maturation in pediatric exercise science, *Pediatric Exercise Science*, 17(1): page 26, figure 4. © 2005 by Human Kinetics. Reprinted with permission from Human Kinetics (Champaign, IL). Data were taken from the Saskatchewan Pediatric Bone Mineral Accrual Study. Data reference: Bailey D A. The Saskatchewan Pediatric Bone Mineral Accrual Study: bone mineral acquisition during the growing years. *International Journal of Sports Medicine* 18:191–194, 1997.)

paediatric studies align boys and girls on: (a) the same secondary sex characteristics, (b) different secondary sex characteristic, or (c) more than one secondary sex characteristic to develop a composite score of sexual development. The assumption behind these strategies is that the order and timing of the appearance of the same secondary sex characteristic and/or different sex characteristics are identical in both sexes. It further presumes that the sequence of the appearance of secondary sex characteristics between sexes with other maturity indicators is also identical. However, as previously described, there is considerable difference in timing and tempo of somatic and sexual development between sexes during adolescence. This means that all three of these alignment strategies are inappropriate when making comparisons between boys and girls. Furthermore different maturity events occur at different times during adolescence. For example, genitalia development and breast development occur early in adolescence; whereas menarche in girls, and axillary and facial hair in boys, occur late in adolescence. The current standards for secondary sex staging ignore this difference in timing of secondary sex characteristics. An individual who is at stage 3 for breast development will not necessarily be at stage 3 for pubic hair development. Likewise, a boy at stage 3 for genital development is not necessarily of the same biological age as a girl who is at stage 3 for breast development. Hence, it is unfounded to make comparisons between individuals using different secondary sex characteristics. It is thus important for researchers to detail which secondary sex characteristic is being used as the maturity indicator.

When controlling for the confounding effects of biological maturity between genders, boys and girls are most often aligned on pubic hair stages, as this is the only sex characteristic that is present in both boys and girls (apart from axillary hair growth, which proves to be problematic if girls remove underarm hair). In addition to the other cautions previously outlined, one should be aware that pubic hair development represents the onset of adrenarche (an increased secretion of sex hormones by the adrenal cortex) and not necessarily the onset of true pubertal development. As stated previously, onset of breast development in girls and testicular volume in boys is the first true sign of centrally mediated puberty. Thus if individuals are aligned on pubic hair development only, caution should be taken when interpreting individuals classified into the early stages.

Hormonal indicators of maturity

Secondary sexual development and somatic development reflects to a large extent the external manifestations of hormonal changes; hence, circulating concentrations of hormones may serve as an indicator of maturity status. Confirmation studies have shown that salivary and serum levels of adrenal and gonadal hormones are closely related to the development of secondary sex characteristics. However, serum estimates are limited to the clinical setting as they require blood samples that are drawn at regular intervals under carefully controlled conditions and relatively sophisticated biochemical assays. Second, large diurnal fluctuations and inter-individual variation may limit the precision in estimating biological maturity. Third, the simple presence of a hormone does not necessarily imply that it is physiologically active. Finally, different tissues respond differently to circulating hormones and thus a hormonal marker may not be a reflection of whole body maturity.

Relationship between indicators

Correlations between the timing of maturity indicators are generally moderate to high, suggesting that there is a general maturity factor underlying the tempo of growth and maturation during adolescence in both boys and girls. However, there is sufficient variation to suggest that no single system (i.e. sexual, skeletal or somatic) provides a complete description of the tempo of maturation during adolescence. Furthermore, although sexual maturation and skeletal development are associated, an individual in one stage of secondary sexual development cannot be assumed to be in a set stage of skeletal development. The apparent discord among the aforementioned indicators reflects individual variation in the timing and tempo of sexual and somatic maturity, and the methodological concerns in the assessment of maturity that have been previously outlined.

REGULATION OF GROWTH AND MATURATION

As covered previously, the pubertal years are characterized by the maturation of secondary sex characteristics, the attainment of reproductive function, and a physical growth spurt. The hormonal initiation and regulation of these events have been well documented (Tanner 1962, 1989). In summary, late in childhood, the hypothalamus stimulates the anterior pituitary gland to release gonadatrophic hormones; the follicle-stimulating hormones (FSH) and the luteinizing hormone (LH) from the pituitary. Therefore, one of the first detectable signs of biological maturity, which precedes the morphological changes, is an increase in circulating concentrations of LH secretion during sleep, with concentrations beginning to rise first in girls, reflecting their earlier onset of puberty, and then in boys. In boys, LH stimulates the production and secretion of testosterone by the testes and FSH stimulates sperm production. In girls, FSH and LH are responsible for ovulation and stimulation of oestrogen by the ovaries. As puberty progresses, the release of LH gradually progresses into the waking periods of the day. With sexual maturity, LH secretion remains constant during the day and night in males and develops a cyclical pattern, just before menarche, in females.

During puberty there is large increase in the secretion of testosterone in males. Testosterone and dihydrotestosterone, an androgen that is derived from testosterone, are responsible for growth of the testes, penis, scrotum, prostate and seminal vesicles, the pubic, axillary and facial hair, the growth of muscles and voice change. The ovaries secrete female sex hormones, collectively known as oestrogens, with the main one being oestradiol. A large increase in oestradiol during puberty causes growth and maturation of females' primary and secondary sexual characteristics. These characteristics include ovaries, uterus, vagina, fallopian tubes, external features of female genitalia, breasts, pubic and axillary hair. During puberty oestrogens and androgens also have effects on muscle growth, fat accumulation, skeletal maturation and changes in shape (i.e. growth of parts of the pelvis in females).

The regulation of growth and maturation involves the complex and continuous interaction of genes, hormones, nutrients, and the physical environment. A genotype is the group of genes making up an individual. An individual's genotype can be thought of as a potential for growth and maturation. Whether a child achieves that potential, however, depends on the conditions into which the child is born and subsequently raised. A child's phenotype is the observed physical or physiological characteristics/ traits that are produced by the genotype in conjunction with the environment. Hormones are essential for a child to reach their full genetic potential. Physical activity is an environmental factor known to influence growth and maturation. The relationship between physical activity and growth and maturation has received much interest for two main reasons. The first is that physical activity is viewed as exerting a favourable influence on growth and maturation because of its influence on the balance between energy intake from the diet and energy expenditure. Daily imbalances between intake over expenditure accumulate over time and contribute to the development of excess mass and obesity, as well as to mass loss. Thus, physical activity can be seen as essential in maintaining the development of healthy body weight. A second point of interest is whether physical activity has a stimulatory or inhibitory influence on growth and maturation. In the past this has been a hot topic in elite gymnasts, with concerns that high levels of intensive training stunt the natural somatic growth and sexual maturity of the child and adolescent athlete. The relationship between physical activity and growth and maturation is discussed in Chapter 13. Additional environmental factors that are known to influence growth and maturation include illness, socioeconomic status of the family, family size, nutritional status, climate and others. For a comprehensive overview of the factors affecting growth and maturation read the textbooks by Malina et al (2004) and Cameron (2002).

MATURITY–ASSOCIATED VARIATION IN BODY SIZE AND FUNCTION

As highlighted throughout the chapter, children of the same age can vary considerably in their degree of biological maturity, or maturity status. A child's maturity status will influence measures of growth and performance. Early maturing individuals of both sexes are taller and heavier than average maturing and late maturing individuals of the same chronological age. If a youth's height was expressed as a percentage of his adult height, early maturing individuals would be closest to their adult height at all ages during adolescence. Early maturing individuals also have a greater mass for height at each age. The height advantage of the early maturing individual is primarily due to an earlier attainment of PHV and also a greater magnitude of peak height gain. Studies have repeatedly shown little or no correlation between the timing of the adolescent growth spurt (i.e. maturity status) and adult stature, suggesting that early, average and late maturing children reach, on average, the same adult height. This is not the same for mass. Early maturing individuals have, on average, greater body mass as young adults. Early maturing individuals and late maturing individuals also vary in body shape. Late maturers tend to have relatively longer legs (i.e. legs account for a greater percentage of adult stature) than early maturers. Furthermore, early maturing girls and boys tend to have relatively wider hips and relatively narrower shoulders. In contrast, late maturing individuals tend to have relatively narrower hips and relatively wider shoulders.

The average age at which the peak velocity in growth of lean mass and fat mass occurs is earliest in early maturers, later in average maturers, and latest in late maturers (Iuliano-Burns et al 2001). In both sexes early maturing youngsters have, on average, larger measurements of muscle and fat. The differences between children of contrasting maturity groups are primarily due to size differences, because early maturers are taller and heavier than late maturers of the same chronological age. When muscle widths are expressed relative to height the differences between maturity groups are often eliminated. However, there is some evidence that during the later adolescent years early maturing boys have larger muscle widths even after taking into account height differences. On the other hand, early maturing individuals of both sexes appear to have greater fat widths at all ages through adolescence, even when height differences are controlled (Malina et al 2004). In summary, at any given chronological age during adolescence, early maturing boys and girls are on average taller, heavier, have greater fat-free mass (especially in boys), total body fat, and per cent body fat (especially in girls) than their less mature peers. The maturity-associated differences in body size and body composition are especially marked during adolescence and influence strength and aerobic power.

Strength increases during adolescence are associated with the natural development in lean mass, and generally reach a peak at the same time as PHV in girls and a year after PHV in boys. Studies have shown that early maturing boys are stronger than late maturing boys during adolescence. Early maturing girls tend to be slightly stronger than late maturing girls early in adolescence (11 through 13 years of age), but as adolescence continues the difference between maturity groups disappears. When strength is expressed relative to height, the difference among maturity groups persists in boys, probably due to the early maturers' rapid growth in muscle mass. On the other hand, when strength is expressed relative to height in girls the differences between maturity groups disappear. This is discussed in more detail in Chapter 3.

It has been shown that early maturing individuals, when compared to late maturing individuals of the same chronological age, have a higher absolute peak $\dot{V}O_2$. Although the size advantage of the early maturing individual is reflected in a greater peak $\dot{V}O_2$, a maturity effect, independent of body size, has been demonstrated. This difference in peak $\dot{V}O_2$ between contrasting maturity groups is more pronounced in males than in females which may be due to males developing greater muscle mass, red blood cells, haemoglobin, lung capacity, pulmonary ventilation, and oxygen uptake than females during adolescence (Kemper & Verschuur 1981). When both early and late maturers are fully grown, and have achieved the same stature, the differences in peak $\dot{V}O_2$ disappear. This is developed further in Chapter 8.

THE IMPORTANCE OF CONTROLLING FOR BIOLOGICAL MATURITY

Paediatric exercise science examines the acute and chronic responses of the child and adolescent to exercise and/or physical activity. Of primary interest are the physiological changes, physical activity and health-related outcomes during childhood and adolescence, and the aforementioned differences between sexes, and between children and adults. The previous section highlights the changes in body size and function (i.e. aerobic power and strength) with biological age. Because children of the same age do not all follow the same tempo and timing of biological maturity (i.e. there are early, average and late maturers) it is essential to consider biological maturity when studying paediatric exercise physiology. The following uses a behavioural example of physical activity participation to illustrate the importance of controlling for biological age. Many studies have found that participation in physical activity decreases during adolescence and that the decline in physical activity is more pronounced in girls than in boys. However, most studies investigate the development of physical activity over chronological age without taking into account biological age. Figure 1.7A shows the physical activity development of boys and girls by chronological age. In both sexes physical activity decreases with increasing chronological age, and girls' physical activity is lower than boys. Figure 1.7B shows the same data, but this time aligned on biological age (years from PHV). When aligned on biological age there is still a decline in physical activity in both sexes; however, the sex differences are no longer apparent (apart from 3 years before PHV). Although only one study, these data suggest maturity differences between sexes (i.e. on average, girls mature earlier than boys) as one reason why girls are consistently documented to participate in less physical activity than boys during adolescence. This example highlights the importance of controlling for variation in biological maturity in paediatric studies.

SUMMARY

Within the paediatric literature the term maturity ordinarily refers to the extent to which the individual has progressed to the mature state. The process of maturation is continuous throughout childhood and adolescence. Girls, on average, experience the onset of puberty about 2 years in advance of boys, and for a shorter period are often taller and heavier than boys. Although all young people follow the same pattern of growth from infancy to full maturity, there is considerable variation, both between and within sexes, in the timing and magnitude of these changes. For example, in young people of the same chronological age some may be fully mature while others are still waiting for the onset of puberty.

During adolescence, sex differences in physique increase greatly, which is due chiefly to the differential action of sex hormones. Adolescent boys become considerably larger and acquire broader shoulders, whereas girls enlarge their pelvic diameter

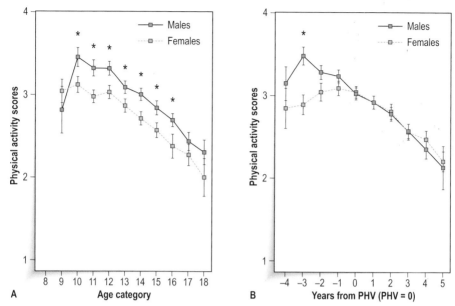

Figure 1.7 Physical activity (PA) (1: low; 5: high) development of boys and girls by chronological age and biological age (years from age at PHV). (A) Mean PA (± SEM) by chronological age bands. (B) Mean PA (± SEM) by biological age bands; *$P < 0.05$. (Thompson A M, Baxter-Jones A D, Mirwald R L, Bailey D A 2003 Comparison of physical activity in male and female children: does maturation matter? *Medicine and Science in Sports and Exercise* 35:1684–1690, with the permission of Lippincott, Williams & Wilkins.)

and have increased deposits of fat in various places such as the breast. Boys also lay down a considerably greater amount of lean tissue than do girls. The increase in skeletal size and muscle mass leads to increased strength in males. Within an age group, early maturers are on average, taller and heavier and have a larger fat-free mass (especially boys) and fat mass (especially girls) than late maturers.

The effects of a child's maturation, in a biological context, may mask or be greater than the effects associated with exposure to physical activity or exercise. The paediatric exercise scientist must therefore include an assessment of biological age in the study design so that its confounding effects can be controlled. The three most universally used indicators of biological maturity are maturation of the skeleton (skeletal age based on assessment of the bones of the hand and wrist), appearance of secondary sex characteristics (genitals in boys; breasts in girls, and pubic hair in both sexes), and the timing of maximum growth in height during the adolescent growth spurt (age at peak height velocity). Indicators of skeletal, sexual and somatic maturation are moderately to highly correlated during adolescence. However, no one indicator gives a complete description of the tempo of growth and maturation. It is recommended that for gender-specific comparisons any of the discussed methods are appropriate. However, for studies that make gender comparisons, either skeletal age or one of the somatic indices should be used.

KEY POINTS

1. Growth, biological maturation and development are terms used interchangeably in the paediatric literature. Growth refers to changes in the size of an individual, as a whole or in parts. Biological maturation is the progress towards the mature state. Development is either the acquisition of behavioural competence or the process of differentiation during prenatal life.

2. There are three types of study design utilized in paediatric growth studies: cross-sectional, longitudinal and mixed-longitudinal. Cross-sectional studies take single measurements from individuals who differ in chronological age. Longitudinal studies measure the same individual over a period of time, and require at least three serial measures on each individual. In a mixed-longitudinal study, either a number of relatively short longitudinal studies are interlocked to cover a wide age range, or some individuals are repeatedly measured and others are measured only once. Cross-sectional studies cannot provide information on an individual's timing and tempo of growth.

3. Tissues and systems of the body follow four patterns of growth: neurological, genital, general and lymphoid.

4. Males are on average 13 cm taller than females upon reaching their final height. This is primarily due to boys experiencing, on average, 2 years more pre-adolescent growth and a greater magnitude of height gain at peak height velocity.

5. During adolescence boys experience a broadening of the shoulders relative to the hips and girls experience a broadening of the hips relative to the shoulders. This can contribute to better upper body strength in boys and a better sense of balance (due to a lower centre of gravity) in girls during adolescence.

6. Every healthy individual follows the same pattern of growth from infancy to maturity; however, there is considerable variation both between and within sexes in the timing and the magnitude of these changes. This results in children of the same age differing in their degree of maturity. The most commonly used methods of assessing biological maturity involve assessment of skeletal age, secondary sex characteristics, menarcheal status and/or somatic characteristics.

7. Although correlations between the timing of maturity indicators are generally moderate to high, there is sufficient variation to suggest that no single system provides a complete description of the tempo of biological maturation during adolescence. The discord among indicators reflects individual variation in the timing and tempo of sexual and somatic maturation and methodological concerns in assessment.

8. Within an age group, early maturers are, on average, taller and heavier and have a larger fat-free mass (especially boys) and fat mass (especially girls) than late maturers. However, early, average and late maturers reach, on average, the same adult height.

9. The effects of a child's biological maturation may mask or be greater than the effects associated with exposure to physical activity or exercise. Therefore, biological maturation should be considered in studies of paediatric exercise physiology.

10. Individual growth and maturation depends on both a child's genotype and phenotype. A genotype is the genetic make-up of the child. A child's phenotype is the physical or physiological characteristics that are produced by the genotype in conjunction with the environment.

11. Pubertal events are initiated and regulated by the stimulation of the ovaries and the testes by gonadatrophins (namely follicle-stimulating hormone and luteinizing hormone) secreted by the anterior pituitary and the elevated production of the sex steroids by the gonads. The sex steroids have effects on muscle growth, fat accumu-

lation and changes in shape during adolescence. Hence many of the sex differences in physique during adolescence are due chiefly to the action of hormones.

References

Armstrong N, Welsman J 1997 Young people and physical activity. Oxford University Press, Oxford

Bailey D A 1997 The Saskatchewan Pediatric Bone Mineral Accrual Study: bone mineral acquisition during the growing years. International Journal of Sports Medicine 18:191–194

Baxter-Jones A D G, Eisenmann J C, Sherar L B 2005 Controlling for maturation in pediatric exercise science. Pediatric Exercise Science 17:18–30

Bayley N, Pinneau S R 1952 Tables for predicting adult height from skeletal age: revised for use with the Greulich–Pyle hand standards. Journal of Pediatrics 40:423–441

Cameron N 2002 Human growth and development. Academic Press, San Diego

Greulich W W, Pyle S I 1959 Radiographic atlas of the skeletal development of the hand and wrist. Stanford University Press, Palo Alto, CA

Iuliano-Burns S, Mirwald R L, Bailey D A 2001 Timing and magnitude of peak height velocity and peak tissue velocities for early, average, and late maturing boys and girls. American Journal of Human Biology 13:1–8

Kemper H C, Verschuur R 1981 Maximal aerobic power in 13- and 14-year-old teenagers in relation to biologic age. International Journal of Sports Medicine 2:97–100

Khamis H J, Roche A F 1994 Predicting adult stature without using skeletal age: The Khamis–Roche method. Pediatrics 94:504–507

Malina R M, Bouchard C, Bar-Or O 2004 Growth, maturation and physical activity, 2nd edn. Human Kinetics, Champaign, IL

Mirwald R L 1978 Saskatchewan growth and development study. In: Ostyn M, Beunen G, Simons J (eds) Kinanthropometry II. University Park Press, Baltimore, p 289–305

Mirwald R L, Baxter-Jones A D, Bailey D A, Beunen G P 2002 An assessment of maturity from anthropometric measurements. Medicine and Science in Sports and Exercise 34:689–694

Reynolds E L, Wines J V 1948 Individual differences in physical changes associated with adolescence in girls. American Journal of Diseases of Children 75:329–350

Reynolds E L, Wines J V 1951 Physical changes associated with adolescence in boys. American Journal of Diseases of Children 82:529–547

Roche A F, Wainer H, Thissen D 1975a Monographs in paediatrics, 3rd edn. Karger, Basel

Roche A F, Wainer H, Thissen D 1975b The RWT method for prediction of adult stature. Pediatrics 56:1026–1033

Roche A F, Tyleshevski F, Rogers E 1983 Non-invasive measurements of physical maturity in children. Research Quarterly for Exercise and Sport 54:364–371

Scammon R E 1930 The measurement of the body in childhood. In: Harris J A, Jackson C M, Paterson D G, Scammon R E (eds) The measurement of man. University of Minnesota Press, Minneapolis, p 173–215

Sherar L B, Baxter-Jones A D, Mirwald R L 2004 Limitations to the use of secondary sex characteristics for gender comparisons. Annals of Human Biology 31:586–593

Sherar L B, Mirwald R L, Baxter-Jones A D G, Thomis M 2005 Prediction of adult height using maturity based cumulative height velocity curves. Journal of Pediatrics 14:508–514

Tanner J M 1962 Growth at adolescence, 2nd edn. Blackwell Scientific Publications, Oxford

Tanner J M 1989 Foetus into man. Physical growth from conception to maturity, 2nd edn. Castlemead Publications, London

Tanner J M, Whitehouse R H, Cameron N et al 1983 Assessment of skeletal maturity and prediction of adult height, 2nd edn. Academic Press, New York

Tanner J M, Healy M J R, Goldstein H, Cameron N 2001 Assessment of skeletal maturity and prediction of adult height (TW2 Method), 3rd edn. Saunders, London

Thompson A M, Baxter-Jones A D, Mirwald R L, Bailey D A 2003 Comparison of physical activity in male and female children: does maturation matter? Medicine and Science in Sports and Exercise 35:1684–1690

Further reading

Kemper H C G Amsterdam growth and health longitudinal study: A 23-year follow-up from teenager to adult about lifestyle and health. In: Borms J, Hebbelinck M, Hills A P (eds) Medicine and sports science, 4. Karger, Basel

Ulijaszek S J, Johnston F E, Preece M A 1998 The Cambridge encyclopedia of human growth and development. Cambridge University Press, Cambridge

Chapter 2

Interpreting performance in relation to body size

Joanne R. Welsman and Neil Armstrong

CHAPTER CONTENTS

LEARNING OBJECTIVES

After studying this chapter you should be able to:
1. describe why appropriate scaling is fundamental to the understanding of relationships between growth, maturation and exercise performance
2. understand the statistical limitations of conventional ratio scaling to remove body size effects from performance variables
3. discuss the merits and disadvantages of linear regression scaling
4. understand the non-linear nature and components of an allometric relationship
5. understand the theoretical and statistical reasons why models based on log-linear regression are better at partitioning size-related effects
6. interpret the results of studies that have reported allometric scaling results
7. discuss the limitations of ontogenetic allometry to analyse longitudinal performance data
8. interpret the results of a simple multilevel regression model.

INTRODUCTION

The journey from childhood, through adolescence and into adulthood is accompanied by marked changes in body size. Although the timing and tempo of the maturational processes vary considerably from individual to individual and between the sexes, between the ages of 8 and 16 years the body mass of a typical boy increases by approximately 160%, and that of an average girl by 125%. Stature increases by 40% and 30%, respectively. Not surprisingly, these changes in physical size are accompanied by parallel increases in absolute measures of exercise performance. For example, from similar starting points at 8 years by 16 years, peak oxygen uptake (peak $\dot{V}O_2$) increases by around 150% in boys and 80% in girls, peak short-term power (anaerobic power) increases by 110% in girls and 180% in boys, and grip strength by 150% and 225% in girls and boys, respectively.

These increases in body size and markers of exercise performance demonstrate a strong statistical relationship and studies have repeatedly reported Pearson product-moment correlation coefficients between them of around $r = 0.7–0.8$. Therefore, if we wish to unravel the influence of growth and maturation upon performance or quantify the effects of training or disease upon performance or simply identify sex differences in these measures, we need a means of removing or controlling for differences in body size. This process of removing the influence of body size is termed scaling.

To be more specific, in studies involving the interpretation of size-related performance measures the objective of scaling is to produce a variable that is demonstrably 'size free'. In other words, the scaled variable should appropriately account for body size without retaining any residual correlation with the original size variable. In this chapter, various statistical methods that may be used to scale both cross-sectional and longitudinal exercise performance for body size will be reviewed in detail. It should be emphasized from the outset that there is no universally 'correct' method of scaling, neither is any one of these methods necessarily 'incorrect' in all instances. All of the methods discussed are constrained by underlying statistical assumptions which if ignored may confound any interpretations based on them. Ultimately, the choice of scaling technique depends on the nature of the research question being addressed but it is important that its validity is verified within a given context. Furthermore, although the examples used to illustrate these techniques are drawn from a paediatric database, it is important to realize that the principles behind, and limitations of, these techniques are equally applicable to the interpretation of adult exercise data.

INTERPRETATION OF CROSS-SECTIONAL DATA

For clarity, a single data set will be used to provide a framework for the evaluation of three scaling techniques for cross-sectional data: ratio scaling, linear regression scaling and allometric scaling. Cross-sectional studies are those most frequently used in paediatric exercise sciences. Here, groups of participants are tested on one occasion only and statistical comparisons are made between groups to infer, for example, age, maturity or sex differences in performance. For each of the techniques the key underlying assumptions will be illustrated and methods for assessing whether or not they succeed, as means of removing the size effects, will be evaluated. In this data set, peak $\dot{V}O_2$ is the performance variable being considered, but the techniques illustrated are equally applicable to any size-related exercise performance measure such as strength, short-term power, cardiac output, ventilation, etc.

Ratio scaling (ratio standards)

The data presented in Figure 2.1 represent the peak $\dot{V}O_2$ responses of 106 boys and 106 girls aged 12 years. These children were taking part in a 7-year longitudinal study of aerobic fitness that commenced at age 11 years, but most of the discussion of scaling

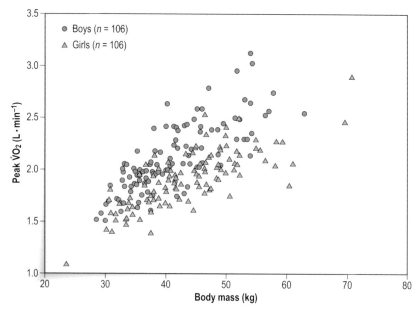

Figure 2.1   Peak oxygen uptake $(L \cdot min^{-1})$ versus body mass in 12-year-olds.

Table 2.1   Anthropometric data and peak oxygen uptake for the subject population presented in Figure 2.1

Variable	Boys ($n = 106$)	Girls ($n = 106$)
Age (years)	12.2 (0.04)	12.2 (0.04)
Stature (m)	1.51 (0.08)	1.52 (0.08)
Body mass (kg)	41.2 (7.5)	43.9 (8.4)
Peak $\dot{V}O_2$ $(L \cdot min^{-1})$	2.12 (0.34)	1.92 (0.29)
Peak $\dot{V}O_2$ $(mL \cdot kg^{-1} \cdot min^{-1})$	52 (6)	44 (5)
Adjusted peak $\dot{V}O_2$ – linear model $(L \cdot min^{-1})$	2.16	1.88
Adjusted peak $\dot{V}O_2$ – log-linear model $(L \cdot min^{-1})$	2.13	1.86
Peak $\dot{V}O_2$ $(mL \cdot kg^{-0.66} \cdot min^{-1})$	182 (17)	159 (14)

Values are mean (standard deviation).

techniques in this chapter is based on a cross-sectional analysis of the boys' and girls' data from the second test occasion. The descriptive statistics for these children are presented in Table 2.1.

Figure 2.1 is a simple scatterplot of the raw data for all children, with absolute peak $\dot{V}O_2$ (i.e. expressed in litres per minute $(L \cdot min^{-1})$) on the Y axis (dependent variable) plotted against body mass in kilograms (kg) on the X axis (independent variable). Data for boys and girls are differentiated by symbol. Producing such a scatterplot is an important first step in deciding on scaling method and much information about the data may be derived from this simple graph.

Firstly, the strong, positive relationship between peak $\dot{V}O_2$ and body mass is clearly evident. In these children a Pearson product-moment correlation coefficient of $r = 0.78$

was observed between peak $\dot{V}O_2$ and body mass in both the boys and the girls. Secondly, these data also highlight the extreme variability in body mass that exists even in a well-defined sample of children of the same chronological age – largely reflecting differences in biological age amongst these 12-year-olds. Thirdly, the individual data points can be seen to be more tightly clustered in the lighter children, becoming progressively more dispersed with increasing body mass. This 'fanning' of data points is very typical of size-related physiological measures. The correct statistical description of this feature is 'heteroscedasticity' and, as will be discussed in sections below, must be appropriately accommodated in any scaling technique applied.

The conventional method of scaling for differences in body mass is to simply divide the performance variable, in this case peak $\dot{V}O_2$ (in mL $\cdot$ min^{-1}), by body mass (in kg) to produce the simple ratio mL $\cdot$ kg^{-1} $\cdot$ min^{-1} (sometimes referred to as a ratio standard). The computation of this ratio standard assumes that the simple linear equation $Y = bX$ appropriately describes the performance–body mass relationship where Y = peak $\dot{V}O_2$ and X = body mass. As illustrated in Figure 2.2, this model represents a straight line that passes through zero and the intersection of the mean values for the dependent and independent variables for the boys and girls, respectively. The different values obtained for the b coefficient for boys ($b = 0.05$) and girls ($b = 0.04$) thus reflect the magnitude of the sex difference in peak $\dot{V}O_2$. Mean values of simple mass-related peak $\dot{V}O_2$ for the children are presented in Table 2.1 and are typical for values reported for untrained children of similar age in many other studies.

It is, in fact, remarkably simple to assess whether a given scaling technique has effectively eliminated the influence of body size from a performance measure. In an early paper to draw attention to the statistical and practical limitations of simple ratio scaling (Tanner 1949) it was demonstrated that the ratio standard would only remove

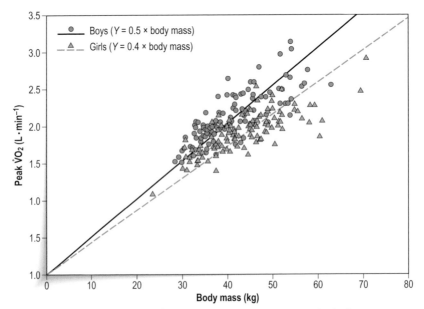

Figure 2.2 Ratio model ($Y = bX + \varepsilon$) describing the peak oxygen uptake–body mass relationship in 12-year-olds.

the influence of body size appropriately when: $CV_X/CV_Y = r_{XY}$, where CV = coefficient of variation and r = the Pearson product-moment correlation coefficient between the X and Y variables.

Albrecht et al (1983) have expanded upon these concerns, suggesting three objective tests for assessing the effectiveness of a simple ratio. Firstly, the statistical criterion states that the product-moment correlation coefficient between the mass-adjusted value (in our example peak $\dot{V}O_2$ in $mL \cdot kg^{-1} \cdot min^{-1}$) and body mass should not be significantly different from zero. The application of this criterion to the present data set is illustrated in Figure 2.3. The significant, negative coefficients of $r = -0.476$ and $r = -0.640$ obtained for boys and girls, respectively, demonstrate unequivocally the failure of simple ratio scaling to produce a size-free variable in this data set.

Secondly, the graphical criterion examines in more detail the exact nature of the relationship between the adjusted variable and body size. Ideally, the relationship between the adjusted variable and body size can be plotted as a horizontal line, i.e. the slope of the least squares regression line is not significantly different from zero. It is evident from the data presented in Figure 2.3 that mass-related peak $\dot{V}O_2$ remains size dependent with significant, linear regression slope coefficients of $b = -0.35$ and $b = -0.39$ in boys and girls, respectively.

Thirdly, the algebraic criterion states that the expected value of adjusted Y is algebraically equal to a constant, e.g. b. All three of these approaches are equivalent when assessing a linear relationship between two variables: i.e. a correlation coefficient of zero implies a horizontal regression line whose equation is equal to a constant (Albrecht et al 1993).

As illustrated in Figures 2.2 and 2.3, if ratio scaling is applied inappropriately the outcome results in larger individuals appearing less fit than lighter individuals. This causes problems when ratio-scaled variables are used subsequently in correlation or

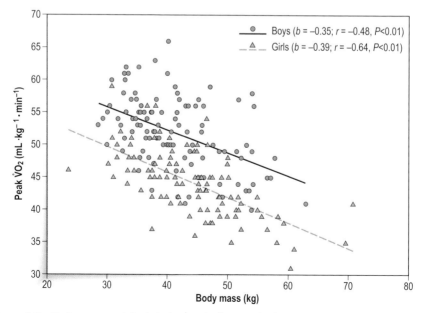

Figure 2.3   Peak oxygen uptake ($mL \cdot kg^{-1} \cdot min^{-1}$) versus body mass in 12-year-olds.

Table 2.2 Relationships between Wingate anaerobic test mean power and cycle ergometer peak oxygen uptake in 11- to 12-year-olds

	Boys (n = 28)	Girls (n = 28)
WAnT MP (W) vs. peak $\dot{V}O_2$ (L · min^{-1})	0.77*	0.88*
WAnT MP (W · kg^{-1}) vs. peak $\dot{V}O_2$ (mL · kg^{-1} · min^{-1})	0.48*	0.74*
WAnT MP (W · kg$^{-0.68}$) vs. peak $\dot{V}O_2$ (mL · kg$^{-0.65}$ · min^{-1})	0.37	0.58*

WAnT, Wingate anaerobic test; MP, mean power.
* Significant differences ($P < 0.01$).
Adapted from Bloxham et al (2005).

regression analyses yielding spurious results. To illustrate this consider the results of Bloxham et al (2005), who examined the effect of scaling technique upon the relationship between Wingate anaerobic test (WAnT) derived peak power in 1 s and cycle ergometer peak $\dot{V}O_2$ in 11- to 12-year-olds. When correlations were calculated on appropriately adjusted allometric exponents (see section below for explanation of allometry), the strength of the relationship was substantially reduced compared to the values obtained when simple ratio-adjusted values formed the basis of the correlations (Table 2.2).

This example demonstrates how ignoring this failure of the conventional ratio standard to produce a size-free variable can confound the interpretation of the influence of body size upon exercise performance measures during growth and maturation. As illustrated in the data presented here, unless a data set can be shown to conform to a simple linear model, and the derived ratio is uncorrelated with the original size variable, an alternative scaling method should be used.

Linear regression scaling (regression standards)

One alternative to ratio scaling is to adopt a scaling model based on least squares regression incorporating an intercept term. In Figure 2.4 least squares linear regression lines ($Y = a + bX$) have been fitted to the boys' and girls' data separately. The slope (b) and intercept (a) terms can be statistically compared using the standard statistical technique analysis of covariance (ANCOVA), a combination of regression and analysis of variance. The statistical comparison of the intercept terms (i.e. the values of the intersection of the regression lines on the Y axis) reflects any difference in the magnitude of peak $\dot{V}O_2$ between the sexes. However, in order for this comparison to be valid, the slopes of the regression lines must be constrained to be parallel. In other words, if the slope coefficients can be demonstrated to be not significantly different a common slope can be fitted. For the data illustrated in Figure 2.4 the slope coefficients for boys (0.035) and girls (0.026) were not significantly different ($P > 0.05$), with a common slope of 0.03 (SE 0.08) describing the peak $\dot{V}O_2$–body mass relationship in both sexes. Subsequent comparison of the intercept terms revealed a significant difference, confirming the higher peak $\dot{V}O_2$ of the boys. The 'adjusted means' derived from the ANCOVA are presented in Table 2.1. Although expressed in L · min^{-1} these values have been adjusted for the influence of the linear covariate – in this case body mass.

In the present example the results of ratio versus linear regression scaling did not differ, with boys' peak $\dot{V}O_2$ shown to be significantly higher than girls' in both

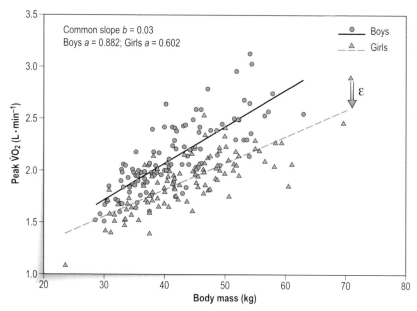

Figure 2.4   Linear regression relationship ($Y = a + bX + \varepsilon$) between peak oxygen uptake and body mass in 12-year-olds.

analyses, although the magnitude of the difference decreased slightly from 15.4% (ratio scaling) to 13.0% (linear regression scaling). In other comparisons, however, the interpretation of results may be markedly altered by the application of this alternative method. As an illustration, the graph presented in Figure 2.5 summarizes the peak $\dot{V}O_2$ data of two groups of boys aged 11 years and 17 years, respectively.

When fitness levels of the groups were compared using traditional mass-related ratio scaling, no significant age difference in aerobic fitness was identified, with mean values for the 11-year-olds of 49 mL · kg^{-1} · min^{-1} compared with 51 mL · kg^{-1} · min^{-1} for the older boys. This suggests the two groups share essentially the same simple linear relationship as indicated by the dotted line in Figure 2.5. However, when the same data were analysed using ANCOVA with separate linear regression lines fitted for each age group, the data were differentiated into two groups. The slopes of the regression lines were not significantly different and a common slope of $b = 0.034$ was derived. If the intercept terms are extrapolated back to the Y axis it is evident that the value of a is significantly ($P < 0.001$) higher in the older ($a = 1.131$) than the younger boys ($a = 0.534$), demonstrating that, in fact, they possess significantly higher fitness relative to their body mass than the younger children.

As mentioned previously, it is essential to verify that the statistical technique used to scale a particular data set provides an appropriate statistical fit for the data and does not violate any of the test's underlying assumptions. A key limitation shared by both simple ratio scaling and linear regression scaling centres on the nature of the error term (ε) assumed by both models. In both cases this is additive, i.e. $Y = aX + \varepsilon$; $Y = a + bX + \varepsilon$; thus the model assumes that the error term is consistent throughout the range of Y and X values measured.

Unfortunately, exercise performance data are frequently heteroscedastic, that is, the error term (i.e. the distance of the individual data point from the regression line)

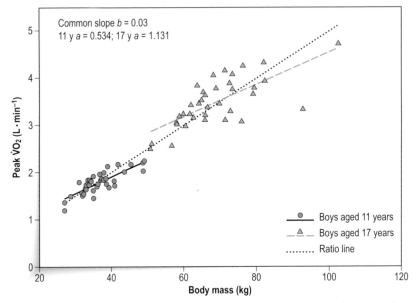

Figure 2.5 Linear regression relationship between peak oxygen uptake and body mass in 11-year-old versus 17-year-old boys.

increases as the values of Y and X increase. The data presented in Figure 2.4 clearly display this characteristic, with the size of the error (sometimes called a residual) increasing as body mass becomes greater. A simple way of checking for the presence of heteroscedasticity is to plot the absolute residuals from the regression equation against body mass. If a significant correlation is observed the data are confirmed as heteroscedastic. For the present data set this is illustrated in Figure 2.6 where $r = 0.240$, $P < 0.01$. In these circumstances, the simple linear regression model is inappropriate and an alternative scaling method is required.

One further problem with linear regression scaling is that, rather than regressing to zero, the relationship has a positive intercept. Thus if data are extrapolated beyond the bounds of the specific data set being modelled the situation arises where a peak $\dot{V}O_2$ is predicted for a body mass of zero. On this basis the model is clearly not physiologically plausible.

Allometric scaling/log–linear scaling

Allometric analyses have a long history of use in the biological sciences for describing and interpreting size-related changes in physiological function – for example, for understanding the relationship between size and resting metabolic rate in mammals (Schmidt-Nielsen 1984) but only recently have they become more widely applied to the understanding of paediatric exercise physiology. The allometric, or power function, model describes a proportional, curvilinear relationship between two variables summarized by the equation: $Y = aX^b$.

The value of the b exponent describes the curvature of the relationship as illustrated in Figure 2.7 for boys and girls separately. Where this is less than 1.0, as shown in this

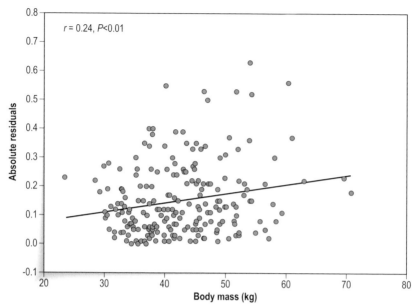

Figure 2.6 Residuals (absolute) from the linear analysis of covariance versus body mass in 12-year-olds.

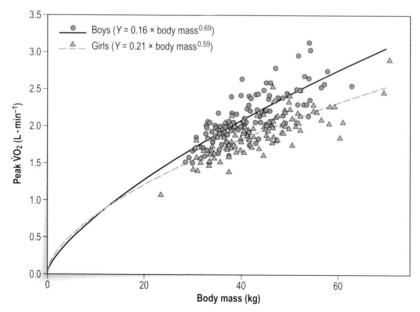

Figure 2.7 Allometric relationship ($Y = aX^b$) between peak oxygen uptake and body mass in 12-year-olds.

graph, the value of the independent variable is increasing at a slower rate than the dependent variable. Ratio scaling can be seen to be a special case of an allometric model where the exponent is observed to be $b = 1.0$ indicative of the directly proportional, linear relationship illustrated in Figure 2.2. Where the value of the b exponent exceeds 1.0, the independent variable is increasing at a faster rate than the dependent variable and the line curves upwards. For example, Armstrong et al. (2001) identified mass exponents for peak 1 s power of $b = 1.2$.

Allometric modelling is particularly useful for exercise data as it assumes a multiplicative, rather than an additive, error term, i.e. $Y = aX^b \cdot \varepsilon$, thus accommodating heteroscedastic data.

Identifying the numerical value of the parameters a and b is achieved by transforming the curvilinear allometric relationship model into a linear relationship which can then be solved using least squares regression. This transformation is achieved by taking the natural logarithms of both the X and Y variables. The allometric equation then becomes: $\log_e Y = \log_e a + b \cdot \log_e X + \log_e \varepsilon$. Once the model has been log-linearized, group comparisons are effectively achieved by applying ANCOVA exactly as described above for the simple linear regression model.

Figure 2.8 illustrates the log-linear relationship between peak $\dot{V}O_2$ and body mass in the 12-year-old boys and girls. As depicted in the legend, the regression slopes for the boys ($b = 0.70$) and girls ($b = 0.62$) were not significantly different, with a common slope of 0.66 (standard error 0.04) adequately describing the population. Incidentally, the 95% confidence intervals ($\pm 2 \times$ standard error) for this coefficient encompass the range 0.58 to 0.74, thus precluding the value 1.0 assumed by simple ratio scaling. As expected, the intercept terms and derived adjusted means (see Table 2.1) from the analysis confirmed the significantly higher peak $\dot{V}O_2$ of the boys.

Several lines of evidence confirm that this allometric model most appropriately normalized the data and represented a better statistical fit than the previous models investigated. A simple visual examination of the scatterplot in Figure 2.8 suggests that the log-linear model has successfully accommodated the heteroscedasticity with the

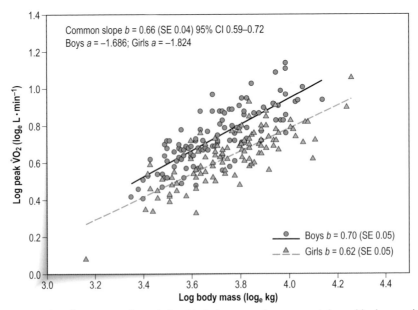

Figure 2.8 Log-linear regression relationship between peak oxygen uptake and body mass in 12-year-olds.

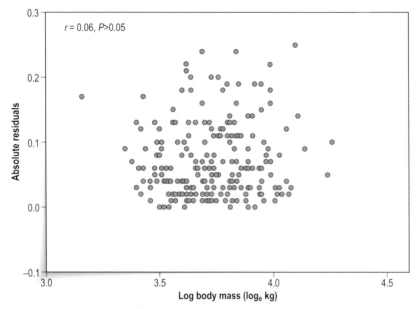

Figure 2.9   Residuals (absolute) from the log-linear analysis of covariance versus body mass.

data points more consistently spread around the regression lines. Further confirmation of this was obtained by examining the correlation between the residuals from the log-linear analysis and body mass as shown in Figure 2.9. No significant relationship was observed, with $r = 0.060$, $P > 0.05$.

Although not necessary where a simple comparison between groups is required, the derived common slope coefficient may be used to compute a power function ratio, Y/X^b, which provides an appropriately size-adjusted ratio for use in subsequent correlation or regression analyses. In Figure 2.3, the failure of simple ratio scaling to control for body size differences was evident, with significant, negative relationships retained between peak $\dot{V}O_2$ (mL kg^{-1} · min^{-1}) and body mass in both boys and girls. In Figure 2.10, the power function ratio mL · kg$^{-0.66}$ · min^{-1} is plotted against body mass. The absence of a negative relationship is apparent immediately and is confirmed by the non-significant ($P > 0.05$) correlation coefficients obtained for boys ($r = 0.075$) and girls ($r = -0.115$).

Theoretical exponents

There has been considerable debate in both the adult and paediatric literature concerning the numerical value of the mass exponent and whether there is a 'true' mass exponent that might provide a universal alternative to simple per body mass scaling at least for maximal power outputs. The two values most frequently discussed are 0.67 and 0.75. The value of 0.67 is derived from dimensionality theory (see Astrand & Rodahl 1986), which states that in geometrically similar individuals (i.e. where proportions of the body components are constant regardless of size), all linear measurements such as stature have the dimension L, all areas, including body surface area and muscle cross-sectional area, have the dimension L^2 and all body volumes, such as

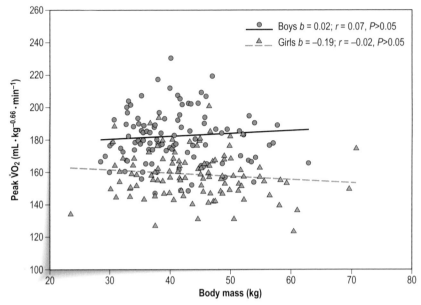

Figure 2.10   Peak oxygen uptake (mL · kg$^{-0.66}$ · min^{-1}) versus body mass in 12-year-olds.

the lungs and heart, have the dimension L^3. Time has the dimension L in physiological systems; therefore peak $\dot{V}O_2$ as a volume per unit time should scale to $L^3 \cdot L^{-1} = L^2$ (e.g. stature^2). In physiological systems, stature^2 is analogous to body mass$^{0.67}$.

The alternative theoretical mass exponent of 0.75 (analogous to stature$^{2.25}$) derives from empirical observations that metabolic rate in many animal species does not conform to the expected surface law, described above, but increases proportional to mass$^{0.75}$. A model of elastic similarity has been proposed to provide a rationale for this exponent whereby biological proportions and metabolic rates are limited by the elastic properties of the animal, properties which ensure that bending and buckling forces during locomotion do not impair the structural integrity of the limbs and joints. The validity of this theory has been questioned and debate remains as to the value of the true exponent for peak $\dot{V}O_2$.

In practice, the results of studies identifying allometric mass exponents for peak physiological variables do not support the indiscriminate application of either theoretical exponent. For example, reported mass exponents for peak $\dot{V}O_2$ have ranged from around 0.40 to values exceeding 1.0. A key contributory factor to this variation appears to be sample size. For example, in a large ($n = 164$) representative sample of prepubertal 11-year-olds Armstrong et al (1995) identified a mass exponent common to boys and girls of 0.66, but in a sample of only 32 similar aged children a value of 0.52 was obtained (Welsman et al 1997). Exponents approximating the theoretical values are only likely to be obtained when modelling large subject groups where the range of body mass is extensive. Even so, unless the group is homogeneous for other confounding covariates (e.g. training or physical activity status, body composition, etc.) the effect of these will distort the value of the mass exponent (Heil 1998). These factors suggest that it is unwise to extrapolate a mass exponent derived in a previous study to a different subject population, and that if power function ratios are required these should be computed using sample-specific mass exponents.

INTERPRETATION OF LONGITUDINAL DATA

Data from longitudinal studies have the potential to provide the most valuable insights into developmental changes in exercise performance measures. Their major advantage is that they offer the opportunity to investigate changes in a population based on measurements made within a genetic continuity. An ideal longitudinal analysis should also describe and understand individual growth trajectories and how these vary around underlying population trends. It is, therefore, critical that body size and, ideally, other confounding or explanatory effects are appropriately accounted for.

Traditional methods of analysing longitudinal (repeated measures) data lack sufficient flexibility to achieve these aims. As will be seen later, either the population response is described at the expense of interpreting individual responses or, alternatively, the individual forms the basis of the analysis with inadequate or incomplete description of how the subject group as a whole is changing.

The analysis and interpretation of longitudinal data within an allometric framework presents a major challenge to the researcher. Some commercial statistical packages may calculate a repeated measures analysis of covariance but this analysis describes responses at a group level and may not allow for varying covariates, i.e. accommodating changes in body mass at each measurement occasion. This type of analysis is also limited by restrictive data requirements including discrete measurement occasions and complete data sets for each individual.

Application of theoretical exponents

Several authors have analysed longitudinal changes in peak $\dot{V}O_2$ using one or both of the theoretically derived mass exponents, i.e. 0.67 or 0.75, or their stature analogues (e.g. Rowland et al 1997). Although large-scale cross-sectional studies have derived mass exponents approximating the theoretical predictions, as illustrated by the common b exponent of 0.66 in the data presented in Figure 2.8, the sample specificity of exponents and the sensitivity of exponents to the confounding influences of other covariates suggest that this may not be the most sensitive way of analysing valuable longitudinal data.

Ontogenetic allometry

One approach to analysing longitudinal growth in peak $\dot{V}O_2$ is to use an ontogenetic allometric approach. Ontogenetic allometry refers to body size–performance relationships at the individual level. So, for example, within a longitudinal study of peak $\dot{V}O_2$ with four annual measurement points, individual or ontogenetic mass exponents are computed by fitting a linear regression line to plots of log peak $\dot{V}O_2$ $L \cdot min^{-1}$ versus log body mass for each individual (Fig. 2.11). Exponents describing individual growth trajectories may then be averaged to describe different groups, for example by sex, chronological age or stage of maturity.

Not surprisingly, studies using this approach have reported wide inter-individual variability in the ontogenetic mass exponents for peak $\dot{V}O_2$. This variability largely reflects differences in individual rates of growth and maturation and is particularly pronounced where individuals are measured during the circumpubertal years.

As a means of interpreting growth-related exercise performance data, the ontogenetic approach has several limitations. This analysis focuses on describing

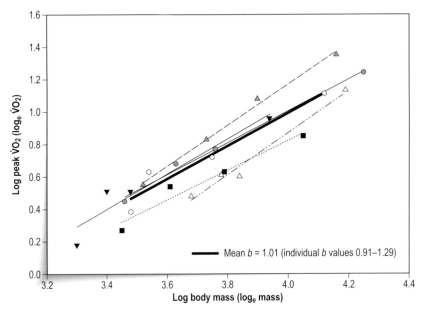

Figure 2.11   Longitudinal measurements of peak oxygen uptake in five individuals.

individual allometric relationships between the performance measure and a single body size indicator. Thus there is no overall quantification of the pattern or magnitude of change in exercise performance over time at either the group or individual level and it is similarly impossible to partition out or quantify any interactive effects of sex, maturity and body size or composition. Furthermore, within and between subject effects cannot be examined within the same statistical analysis but require an inefficient two-stage process in which individual slope and intercept parameters can only be partially accommodated.

Multilevel modelling

Multilevel modelling (Duncan et al 1996, Goldstein et al 2002) is essentially an extension of multiple regression appropriate for analysing multilevel or hierarchical data and can be applied within many study designs including cross-sectional, repeated measures and multivariate. The data obtained in longitudinal studies of children's growth or exercise performance may be viewed as a hierarchical structure, with most studies representing a simple two-level hierarchy. This is illustrated in Figure 2.11 where the set of measurement occasions for each individual represent the level 1 units that are clustered within the level 2 unit – the individual.

Multilevel modelling has several advantages over more traditional methods of analysing repeated measures data. Importantly, the method is not hindered by the requirement for balanced, complete data sets, i.e. both the number of measurement occasions and the timing between those occasions may vary between individuals. This is an important consideration for longitudinal exercise studies with children that almost inevitably incur some overall attrition and/or missed interim measurements due to illness or injury. In a multilevel analysis, all available data can be incorporated into the analysis.

As will be illustrated in more detail later, the multilevel modelling procedure enables the underlying population mean response to be described (referred to as the 'fixed' part of the analysis) whilst simultaneously summarizing how individual responses deviate from this mean response at both levels of the analysis (described as the 'random' elements of the model). For example, as illustrated in Figure 2.11, the slope and intercept terms describing individual growth rates vary randomly around the population mean response, denoted by the thick, solid regression line. This is defined as level 2 variation. Each individual's observed measurements also vary randomly around their own growth trajectory. This represents the level 1 variation. Thus multilevel modelling represents a flexible method of analysing longitudinal changes in exercise performance, allowing the effects and relative importance of a variety of explanatory variables or combinations of explanatory variables to be investigated and quantified (Duncan et al 1996). The procedure is statistically efficient, and if required, can be adapted to a multivariate approach. By analysing data at different levels of a hierarchy, the researcher is able to examine where and how different effects occur and can address more complex questions than are possible within a traditional analytical approach.

The recent literature reflects a steadily increasing number of publications in which a multilevel regression modelling approach has been used to analyse longitudinal changes in young people's peak $\dot{V}O_2$ (Armstrong & Welsman 2001), submaximal cardiovascular performance (Armstrong & Welsman 2002, Welsman & Armstrong 2000), isokinetic strength (De Ste Croix et al 2002), short-term power (Armstrong et al 2001, Santos et al 2003) and physical activity patterns (Armstrong et al 2000a).

In the same way as described for the use of regression techniques for modelling cross-sectional data, the researcher using multilevel regression modelling should use a log-linear (allometric) structure assuming multiplicative error. Table 2.3 illustrates the results of a simple multilevel regression analysis for WAnT-determined mean power (i.e. over the 30 s test) derived from a study of 97 boys and 100 girls tested on two occasions 1 year apart starting at the age of 12 years (Armstrong et al 2000b).

Two models are presented to demonstrate how the multilevel modelling process allows a parsimonious solution to be progressively formulated and highlights the effects of adding and removing various explanatory variables. The model initially explored (model 1) was based on that derived by Nevill & Holder (1994) following careful evaluation of several alternative model formulations and can be written as follows:

$$\text{Mean power } (Y) = \text{mass}^{k1} \cdot \text{stature}^{k2} \cdot \exp(\alpha_j + b_j \cdot \text{age}) \, \varepsilon_{ij}$$

Here all parameters are fixed with the exception of the constant (α, intercept term) and age parameters which are allowed to vary randomly at level 2 (between individuals), and the multiplicative error ratio ε_{ij} that varies randomly at level 1, describing the error variance between occasions. The subscripts i and j denote this random variation at levels 1 and 2, respectively. In all models age is centred on the group mean age of 12.7 years.

In order to allow the unknown parameters to be solved using multilevel regression the model is linearized by logarithmic transformation. Once transformed, the equation above becomes:

$$\text{Log}_e \text{ mean power } (\log_e y) = k_1 \cdot \log_e \text{mass} + k_2 \cdot \log_e \text{stature} + \alpha_j + b_j \cdot \text{age} + \log_e (\varepsilon_{ij})$$

Table 2.3   Multilevel regression analyses for mean power

Parameter	Model 1 estimate (SE)	Model 2 estimate (SE)
Fixed:		
Constant	3.131 (0.184)	2.162 (0.155)
Log_e mass	0.547 (0.056)	1.153 (0.048)
Log_e stature	1.357 (0.197)	ns
Log_e skinfolds	Not entered	−0.255 (0.022)
Age	0.146 (0.027)	0.132 (0.027)
Sex	−0.083 (0.017)	−0.054 (0.015)
Age · sex	−0.046 (0.017)	−0.031 (0.017)
Maturity 4	0.046 (0.016)	ns
Maturity 5	0.084 (0.031)	ns
Random:		
Level 2		
Constant	0.011 (0.001)	0.008 (0.001)
Age	0.003 (0.002)	0.003 (0.002)
Covariance	−0.004 (0.001)	−0.003 (0.001)
Level 1		
Constant	0.004 (0.001)	0.004 (0.001)
−2*log(like)	−500.067	−534.339

$N = 327$; ns, not significant.
Adapted from Armstrong et al (2001).

From this baseline model additional explanatory variables were investigated including sum of triceps and subscapular skinfold thicknesses, sex and stage of maturity (stages 2 to 5 for pubic hair development). The latter two variables were incorporated into the model as indicator variables (e.g. for sex, boys = 0, girls = 1). This sets the boys' constant as the baseline from which the girls' parameter is allowed to deviate. Interaction terms may also be constructed to investigate interactions between explanatory variables. In this example, the interaction term 'age by sex' was constructed to investigate differential growth in boys and girls.

For each model, fixed parameters are presented along with random effects specified at levels 1 and 2 of the analysis. The fixed effects describe the underlying population mean response. As age was centred on the group mean age, and sex and maturity were included as indicator variables, the intercept term represents the mean power for a prepubertal boy of average age. The remaining parameter estimates therefore represent deviations from this baseline. The statistical significance of a parameter estimate is judged by dividing the value of the parameter estimate by its standard error. If this ratio exceeds plus or minus 2.0, the estimate may be considered significantly different from zero at $P < 0.05$.

The results obtained in model 1 demonstrate that the longitudinal increase in mean power was related to the overall increase in body size, with both stature and mass making significant independent contributions. The negative sex difference reflects a lower mean power for girls once body size effects have been controlled for. The model also indicates a positive and incremental effect of maturity at stages four and five that is in addition to an independent effect of age. However, the age by sex interaction term, which should be deducted from the age term for girls only, indicates that the magnitude of this age effect is greater for boys than for girls. This model suggests, therefore, that increases in mean power cannot be simply explained by increases in overall body size as age and maturity exert additional independent effects for both boys and girls.

Model 2 summarizes the results of including sum of two skinfolds as an explanatory variable. This addition negated the independent effect of stature, completely explained the maturity effects identified in model 1 and reduced the magnitude of the sex difference. The positive effect for body mass combined with the negative effect for sum of skinfolds suggests that mean power increased in relation to lean body mass.

The value of the log-likelihood ($-2*$log-like), the deviance statistic, reflects the model's goodness of fit. In nested models, such as models 1 and 2, the smaller the number the better the model fit. The change in the deviance statistic must be considered relative to the change in the number of fitted parameters. Thus in model 2, there is a deviance of 34.272 for two fewer fitted parameters (which represent 2 degrees of freedom) compared with model 1. This exceeds the chi-squared critical value of 5.99 for significance at $P < 0.05$.

The random parameters reflect the error associated with specified terms at both levels of the analysis, i.e. they represent the part of the model unexplained by the fixed parameter estimates. The random structure of the models presented in Table 2.2 was comparatively simple. In models 1 and 2 the random variation associated with the intercept (constant) reflects the degree of variation from the mean intercept both between (level 2) and within (level 1) individuals. Age varied randomly at level 2 (between individuals), allowing each child to have their own growth trajectory. The variation associated with the slope parameter for age was not significant but the covariance between the slope and intercept parameters was (-0.004), indicating that the higher the mean power in year 1 the smaller the predicted increase with age.

As described above, in ontogenetic allometry body size exponents are derived for each individual in a sample population. Multilevel regression modelling is sufficiently flexible to allow the need for this to be examined whilst concurrently deriving a population exponent. This is achieved by allowing body mass to vary randomly at level 2. Although not shown in the models in Table 2.2, this was investigated in both of these. In neither case was a significant parameter estimate obtained, suggesting that once key covariates were controlled for, the fixed part mass exponent adequately described the proportional relationship between the performance measure and body mass for all subjects.

SUMMARY

Conventional ratio scaling rarely represents an appropriate means of enabling size-adjusted group comparisons in measures of exercise performance. As illustrated, simple per body mass ratios (e.g. $mL \cdot kg^{-1} \cdot min^{-1}$) often remain size dependent, thus confounding interpretations based on them. Although offering some advantages, linear regression scaling is limited by its assumption of an additive error term, as exercise performance data are typified by heteroscedastic error terms, and positive intercept. Cross-sectional group comparisons are most effectively achieved using allometric (log-linear) scaling techniques that not only control for heteroscedasticity but also facilitate the construction of appropriately size-adjusted ratios for use in subsequent analyses. The application of allometry to longitudinal data is more complex. Given the sample-specificity of the b exponent, the application of a theoretically derived value cannot be recommended. Ontogenetic allometry describes the individual growth process but cannot quantify changes in performance or adequately describe group or population responses. In this respect, multilevel regression modelling offers many advantages. Working within an allometric framework, under-lying group trends can be modelled whilst concurrently investigating individual growth trajectories. This process thus enables the effects of body size and other explanatory variables upon the performance measure to be examined in a sensitive and flexible manner.

KEY POINTS

1. Increases in body size during growth and maturation are strongly correlated with increases in physiological performance measures.
2. The key objective of any scaling technique is to produce a size-adjusted variable which retains no correlation with the original size variable.
3. Size-related performance data such as peak $\dot{V}O_2$ are commonly heteroscedastic, that is, data are clustered at low levels of body mass and become progressively dispersed at higher values of body mass.
4. Conventional ratio scaling assumes that the simple, linear relationship $Y = bX + \varepsilon$ appropriately describes the relationship between body mass and peak $\dot{V}O_2$. However, the scaled variable $mL \cdot kg^{-1} \cdot min^{-1}$ retains a significant, negative correlation with body mass (see key point 2 above).
5. If ratio scaling is inappropriately applied this will confound the interpretation of growth-related changes in performance measures and yield spurious results if used in regression or correlation analyses.
6. Linear regression scaling, $Y = a + bX + \varepsilon$, may provide a better statistical fit than ratio scaling and discriminate group differences that are masked when ratio scaling is applied. However, this technique is limited by its failure to accom-modate heteroscedastic data and does not regress through zero.
7. The allometric equation $Y = aX^b \cdot \varepsilon$ describes a curvilinear, proportional relationship between the size and performance variable which also accom-modates heteroscedastic data by virtue of a multiplicative error term.
8. Allometric relationships are simply resolved through log-linearization of the equation to $\log_e Y = \log_e a + b \cdot \log_e X + \log_e \varepsilon$. Analysis of covariance may be applied to examine group differences, as for simple linear regression, and the slope coefficients (b exponents) may be used to compute power function ratios which represent size-free variables for use in subsequent analyses.
9. Ontogenetic allometry describes the relationship between performance and body size in an individual through computation of individual allometric exponents. This approach to analysing longitudinal data is limited in that the magnitude of age-related increases in performance is not quantified.
10. Multilevel modelling represents a sensitive and flexible approach to modelling longitudinal data within an allometric framework. Individual growth trajectories are modelled while simultaneously describing and quantifying average growth in a given population. The effect of many explanatory variables and interactions between these variables can be modelled.

References

Albrecht G H, Gelvin B R, Hartman S E 1993 Ratios as a size adjustment in morphometrics. American Journal of Physical Anthropology 91:441–468

Armstrong N, Welsman J R 2001 Peak oxygen uptake in relation to growth and maturation in 11–17 year olds. European Journal of Applied Physiology 85:546–551

Armstrong N, Welsman J 2002 Cardiovascular responses to submaximal treadmill running in 11 to 13 year olds. Acta Pediatrica 91:125–131

Armstrong N, Kirby B, McManus A et al 1995 Aerobic fitness of pre-pubescent children. Annals of Human Biology 22:427–441

Armstrong N, Welsman J R, Kirby B J 2000a Longitudinal changes in 11–13 year olds' physical activity. Acta Paediatrica 89:775–780

Armstrong N, Welsman J R, Kirby B J et al 2000b Longitudinal changes in young people's short term power output. Medicine and Science in Sports and Exercise 32:1140–1145

Armstrong N, Welsman J R, Chia M Y H 2001 Short term power output in relation to growth and maturation. British Journal of Sports Medicine 35:118–124

Astrand P O, Rodahl K 1986 Textbook of work physiology. McGraw-Hill, New York

Bloxham S R, Welsman J R, Armstrong N 2005 Ergometer-specific relationships between peak oxygen uptake and peak power output in children. Pediatric Exercise Science 17:136–148

De Ste Croix M B A, Armstrong N, Welsman J R et al 2002 Longitudinal changes in isokinetic leg strength in 10–14 year olds. Annals of Human Biology 29:50–62

Duncan C, Jones K, Moon G 1996 Health-related behaviour in context: a multilevel modelling approach. Social Science in Medicine 42:817–830

Goldstein H, Browne W, Rasbash J 2002 Multilevel modelling of medical data. Statistics in Medicine 21:3291–3315

Heil D P 1998 Body mass scaling of peak oxygen uptake in 20- to 79-yr-old adults. Medicine and Science in Sports and Exercise 29:1602–1608

Nevill A M, Holder R L 1994 Modelling maximum oxygen uptake – a case-study in non-linear regression model formulation and comparison. Applied Statistics 43:653–666

Rowland T, Vanderburgh P, Cunningham L 1997 Body size and the growth of maximal aerobic power in children: a longitudinal analysis. Pediatric Exercise Science 9:262–274

Santos A M C, Armstrong N, De Ste Croix M B A et al 2003 Optimal peak power in relation to age, body size, gender and thigh muscle volume. Pediatric Exercise Science 15:405–417

Schmidt-Nielsen K 1984 Scaling: why is animal size so important? Cambridge University Press, Cambridge

Tanner J M 1949 Fallacy of per-weight and per-surface area standards and their relation to spurious correlation. Journal of Applied Physiology 2:1–15

Welsman J R, Armstrong N 2000 Longitudinal changes in submaximal oxygen uptake in 11–13 year olds. Journal of Sports Sciences 18:183–189

Welsman J R, Armstrong N, Kirby B J et al 1997 Exercise performance and MRI determined muscle volume in children. European Journal of Applied Physiology 76:92–97

Further reading

Armstrong N, Welsman J, Nevill A M et al 1997 Modeling, growth and maturation changes in peak oxygen uptake in 11–13-year-olds. Journal of Applied Physiology 87:2230–2236

Nevill A, Ramsbottom R, Williams C 1992 Scaling physiological measurements for individuals of different body size. European Journal of Applied Physiology 65:110–117

Nevill A M, Holder R L, Baxter-Jones A et al 1998 Modeling developmental changes in strength and aerobic power in children. Journal of Applied Physiology 84:963–970

Welsman J R, Armstrong N 2000 Statistical techniques for interpreting body size-related exercise performance during growth. Pediatric Exercise Science 12: 112–127

Welsman J R, Armstrong N, Kirby B et al 1996 Scaling peak oxygen uptake for differences in body size. Medicine and Science in Sports and Exercise 28:259–265

Chapter 3

Muscle strength

Mark B. A. De Ste Croix

CHAPTER CONTENTS

LEARNING OBJECTIVES

After studying this chapter you should be able to:

1. describe the mechanisms involved in muscle force production
2. evaluate the various methods available to determine muscle cross-sectional area
3. describe the age- and sex-associated development in muscle size
4. evaluate the factors that influence the reliability of strength testing in children
5. examine different methods of controlling for differences in body size in relation to paediatric strength data
6. use correct terminology in describing different types of muscle actions
7. explore age- and sex-associated differences in muscle strength
8. describe the influence of stature and mass on the development of strength
9. explore the role that maturation and testosterone have in age- and sex-associated differences in strength
11. discuss the relationship between muscle size and muscle strength
10. discuss the evidence that suggests that factors over and above muscle size contribute to the age- and sex-associated development in strength.

INTRODUCTION

Muscle strength is a multifaceted, performance-related fitness component that is underpinned by muscular, neural and mechanical factors. The complex interaction of these components makes the study of the increase in muscle strength during growth and maturation challenging. As strength is an essential component of most aspects of performance it is surprising that we know very little about the factors associated with strength development during childhood in comparison to other physiological variables. This may be attributed to the difficulty in measuring internal forces and the inherent methodological problems associated with determining external force. As there are no physiological markers to indicate that a maximal effort has been given, the methodology and assessment tools are critical in studies of muscle strength during growth and maturation.

MUSCLE GROWTH

The origins of the diversity in muscularity in adults occur early in fetal development, at approximately the fifth week of gestation when some mesodermal cells differentiate into myoblasts. Most of the myoblasts fuse to form myotubes containing multiple nuclei that attach to the developing skeleton to form primordial muscles. The primordia of most muscle groups are well defined by the end of the ninth week of gestation. The others stay as mononucleate cells that become the satellite cells of more mature muscle, responsible for muscle cell repair. Within the myotubes of primordial muscles a chain of central nuclei forms and soon after the contractile proteins actin and myosin, with their characteristic striations, are synthesized. From 11 to 18 weeks hypertrophy of the muscles occurs due to both the multiplication of myofibrils and the addition of sarcomeres onto the ends of the muscle. By 23 weeks the nuclei of mature myotubes have moved to the edges of the muscle cell.

At about 10 weeks of gestation outgrowths from the spinal motor neurons begin to innervate the developing muscle fibres. What initially begins with multiple synapses ends up with only one neuromuscular junction, usually in the centre of the fibre. The fibre type or the contractile and metabolic characteristics are determined at this early stage since muscle is a slave to its innervation or electrical frequency of stimulation. Generally about half of the developing fibres express slow myosin isoforms and the other half express fast isoforms. Muscle fibre differentiation usually occurs after about 32 weeks of gestation but is not fully complete until a few months after birth. The muscularity of an individual is reliant on the size and number of muscle fibres. The number of muscle fibres is due to the number of fetal myoblasts, with a significant genetic component. The question of whether increases in muscle size during growth are due to hypertrophy or hyperplasia has been difficult to answer in situ due to the ethics of muscle biopsy and also to the limitations of non-invasive imaging techniques. It is clear from cross-sectional studies of whole autopsied vastus lateralis muscle that despite wide inter-individual variation, the average total number of fibres remains stable across age groups. Therefore in normal growth and development, increases in muscle cross-sectional area are generally agreed to be due to increased fibre size or hypertrophy rather than cellular hyperplasia.

MUSCLE MECHANISM – SLIDING FILAMENT THEORY

Structurally the interior of the muscle fibre contains myofibrils that are surrounded by the smooth sarcoplasmic reticulum, which is involved in the growth, repair and development of muscle. The striated appearance of muscle fibres is attributed to the cross-banding arrangement of the myofibrils, with light I bands alternating with dark A bands. A sarcomere is the region between two Z lines and is the smallest functional unit of the muscle fibre. In essence each myofibril is a series of sarcomeres laid end to end. The thin filaments extend across the I band and part way into the A band and comprise the proteins actin, tropomyosin and troponin. The thick filament extends the entire length of the A band and contains the protein myosin.

When both adenosine triphosphate (ATP) and calcium are present in sufficient quantities the thick and thin filaments interact to form actomyosin and slide over one other, moving the Z bands closer together and reducing the size of the I band. When an action potential passes along the sarcolemma and down the T tubules, calcium is released from the sarcoplasmic reticulum into the sarcoplasm. Following this excitation by a nerve impulse the calcium ions bind to troponin C, causing the tropomyosin to physically move away from the myosin binding sites. This allows the activated myosin heads to bind to the actin by changing to a bent shape and pulling on the thin filament. This action is referred to as the power stroke and simultaneously inorganic phosphate (P_i) and adenosine diphosphate (ADP) are released from the myosin head. The myosin cross-bridge detaches itself from the actin as a new ATP molecule binds to the myosin head. Hydrolysis of the ATP provides the energy for the next cross-bridge attachment–power stroke sequence. Whilst the myosin head is in an activated state it will attach to another actin unit further along the thin filament and the cycle of attachment, power stroke, detachment and activation of myosin is repeated. As long as calcium is present this action will continue. Removal of the calcium by the calcium pump causes tropomyosin inhibition of cross-bridge formation and the muscle fibre relaxes.

DETERMINING MUSCLE SIZE

Measurement techniques

When measuring muscle cross-sectional area (mCSA) in children for research purposes the technique used should be non-invasive with no potential side effects. Many studies with children have used anthropometric techniques to estimate mCSA because they are low cost, not labour intensive, equipment is portable and easily accessible, and measurement protocols take little time to complete. Every effort should be made to ensure accuracy and standardization of techniques and measurements should always be made by the same trained observers, especially if measurements are to be taken over time, in order to safeguard the validity and usefulness of the data.

At the simplest level coaches have been known to take circumference measurements alone to estimate mCSA but circumference measurements ignore the fact that limb circumference is influenced by fat and bone cross-sections as well as muscle, such that a large circumference need not mean a large muscle. Efforts have been made to take into account the contribution of fatness to the circumference measurement by incorporating skinfold thickness into the equation (Jones & Pearson 1969).

The technique described by Jones & Pearson (1969) is the most widely used anthropometric technique for estimating thigh muscle volume plus bone in children, although more recent equations by Housh et al (1995) for determining total mCSA plus bone have also become popular. The main problem with both of these techniques is that the regression equations have been derived from adult data and therefore cannot be confidently applied to children. Work exploring the reliability of the Jones and Pearson technique in children, comparing the anthropometric technique to muscle volumes determined using magnetic resonance imaging (MRI), found that the anthropometric technique underestimates lean thigh volume by 31% (range 14–46%). Limits of agreement further support this conclusion by identifying a consistent bias towards an underestimation in total thigh volume. Therefore, while anthropometric estimates may be valid for a 'snapshot' of mCSA plus bone or for characterizing various populations, they are not acceptable for monitoring changes over time, particularly in studies examining changes during growth and maturation (Housh et al 1995).

Radiography is a technique that can potentially provide estimates of mCSA but due to the radiation exposure required to produce well-defined radiographs, ethical considerations mean this technique is generally unsuitable for use with healthy children. In any case, conventional radiographs depict a three-dimensional object as a two-dimensional image so that overlying and underlying tissues are superimposed on the image, which makes determination of mCSA difficult.

Computerized tomography (CT) overcomes this problem by scanning thin slices of the body with a narrow X-ray beam which rotates around the body, producing an image of each slice as a cross-section of the body and showing each of the tissues in a thin slice. Unlike conventional radiography, CT can distinguish well between muscle, bone and fat. However, children are particularly sensitive to radiation; therefore this technique is contraindicated in children.

Ikai & Fukunaga (1968) made the first measurement of strength per mCSA using ultrasonography with children. The technique has also been applied in studies concerned with fibre pennation of the quadriceps muscle after training, mCSA of the calf of the dominant leg of junior soccer players and the effect of strength training on upper arm mCSA of children. One of the major issues of ultrasonography is the difficulty in distinguishing tissue boundaries and the difficulty in determining individual muscles/muscle groups.

Magnetic resonance imaging (MRI) is an ethically acceptable technique that in recent years has offered exciting opportunities for the study of gross structure and metabolism of healthy and diseased muscle. Anatomical mCSA can be accurately measured by MRI, distinct muscle groups can be differentiated and it appears to be more suitable than other imaging techniques used for the examination of mCSA. With unparalleled picture clarity (Fig. 3.1) it is possible to differentiate individual muscle/muscle groups and identify both intramuscular fat and blood vessels.

By using an infrared mouse on a gridded mouse mat it is possible to trace around relevant areas of interest to determine the CSA of different tissues. Despite the financial limitations numerous studies have recently used MRI with children and adolescents to determine muscle volume and mCSA.

Site of mCSA measurement

A methodological problem with many previous studies of force or torque per mCSA with growth and maturation is that the optimal site for the measurement of maximum mCSA within and between subjects has not been clearly identified. Instead, an arbitrary location on the limb has been used for mCSA determination of mid-femur in

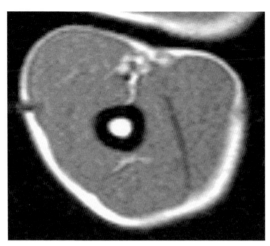

Figure 3.1   Mid-upper arm MRI scan of a 16-year-old male.

the case of thigh muscles and mid-humerus in the case of elbow flexors and extensors. Adult data suggest that for the knee extensors two-thirds femur height and for the knee flexors one-third femur height should be used as the site of maximal mCSA. De Ste Croix et al (2002) measured the maximal mCSA of each individual subject using MRI and found maximal thigh mCSA to occur between 51% and 69% of ascending femur length in 10- to 14-year-olds. Deighan et al (2006) used MRI-determined thigh and arm mCSA in 9-year-olds, 16-year-olds and adults and demonstrated that there are age differences in the location of maximal mCSA of the elbow extensors. In order for age, sex and muscle group comparisons to be made, an optimal site of mCSA needs to be individually determined for the paediatric population. Therefore the site chosen to determine mCSA should be taken into account when interpreting the age- and sex-associated development in mCSA.

AGE- AND SEX-ASSOCIATED DEVELOPMENT IN mCSA

The CSAs of muscle fibres reach their maximal adult size by 10 years of age in girls and 14 years of age in boys. Although muscle fibres appear to reach their maximal CSA early in childhood this does not mean that muscle has reached its maximal length as muscle will continue to grow in length simultaneously with growth in limb length segments. It has been suggested that the increase of tension on the muscle from bone growth will in turn provide a stimulus for the muscle fibre to increase in size.

The Harpenden Growth study examined age and sex differences in radiographically determined upper arm and calf widths of British children from infancy to age 18 years (Tanner 1962). Boys' muscle widths appeared greater than those of girls during childhood but the difference was small. MRI studies have also found no significant sex difference in knee and elbow mCSA up until 13/14 years. The Harpenden study suggested that girls exhibited their adolescent spurt before the boys at age 11 years, at which time they had a temporary size advantage in calf muscle width. Arm muscle width demonstrated less of a growth spurt in the girls so that the sex difference was only temporarily reduced. The sex difference was magnified when the boys underwent their adolescent spurt at the age of approximately 13 years. Boys'

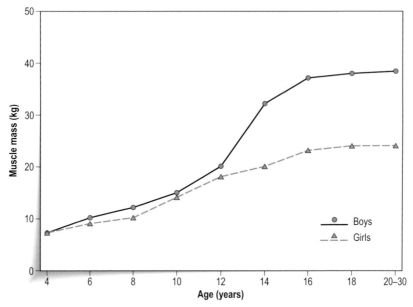

Figure 3.2 Changes in muscle mass with chronological age in relation to sex (redrawn from data in Malina & Bouchard 1991).

calf width eventually overtook that of the girls at around 15 years and both arm and calf width were still rising but at a slower rate at 18 years. In girls, both muscle widths peaked at 17 years and began to show a slight decrease by 18 years. The sex differences in muscle widths persisted into adulthood and were more apparent for musculature of the upper extremity. Deighan et al (2006) used MRI to measure mCSA and demonstrated a significant age effect in elbow mCSA up until 24 years. These data indicate that from 9 to 24 years elbow extensor and flexor mCSA increase by 207% and 210% in males and 65% and 78% in females, respectively. By adulthood, CT-determined muscle size showed that the mCSA of the arm and thigh of adult females was around 57% and 73%, respectively, that of adult males. Changes in muscle mass with age are illustrated in Figure 3.2.

DEFINING MUSCLE STRENGTH

There are various definitions of muscle strength, probably attributable to the numerous factors that interact to form the expression of strength. Jargon has permeated the strength literature and scientists have failed to agree on a single definition of strength. One of the more appropriate definitions is: 'the maximum force, torque or moment developed by a muscle or muscle groups during one maximal voluntary or evoked action of unlimited duration, at a specified velocity of movement' (Blimkie & Macauley 2001, p. 23). Strength can be thought of in terms of a variety of muscle actions: (1) maximal voluntary isometric, (2) electrically evoked isometric twitch, (3) electrically evoked isometric tetanus and (4) maximal voluntary isokinetic muscle actions. Electrically evoked stimulation of muscle provides a clearer indication of the internal forces that a muscle or muscle group has the potential to generate, although the force is still measured externally. Most laboratory and field-based tests only

Table 3.1 Types of muscle actions

Concentric action	The muscle shortens whilst developing tension
Eccentric action	The muscle lengthens while developing tension
Isotonic action	The muscle develops tension against a resistance that remains constant throughout a range of motion
Isometric action	There is no change in the muscle length while developing tension (static)
Isokinetic action	The muscle shortens or lengthens at a constant velocity while developing tension

measure the external development of force. Additionally, there are few paediatric studies that have examined muscle strength under electrically evoked conditions, probably due to the ethical issues associated with the technique. Therefore, unless otherwise stated, any subsequent mention of strength shall be referred to as the measurement of voluntary external force. It is also inappropriate to refer to all muscle strength movements as being under 'contraction'. It is more relevant to refer to strength movements as a muscle 'action' or 'moment' (the rotational effect of force). The term 'action' is favoured throughout this chapter as it refers to the state of the muscle, which is dependent upon the external force that is applied to that muscle via the skeletal system. The five major types of muscle action are described in Table 3.1.

During concentric muscle actions the muscle force exceeds the external force and the muscle shortens. In eccentric actions the musculotendinous unit lengthens because the external force exceeds the force exerted by the muscle. It is beyond the scope of this chapter to explore the differences associated with varying muscle actions. However, the reader should note that there are neuromuscular and mechanical differences between static and dynamic actions, as well as concentric and eccentric actions. Given the significance of both concentric and eccentric actions in everyday life, investigations of age- and sex-associated strength development should consider concurrently the ability of the individual to perform both types of action. Underpinning the choice of muscle action to examine must be the activity- or sport-specific component under investigation. For example, in sports where maximal strength is an important component it may be wise to assess children's strength at very slow velocities, based on the force–velocity relationship. However, during activities where fast velocity movements are common it may be prudent to assess functional strength at faster velocities rather than maximal strength.

The muscular force therefore is the product of the forces exerted by the contractile components and the stretch of the connective tissue. It is evident that the maximal force that a muscle can produce is influenced by a number of factors. In order to examine the influence of growth and maturation on the development of muscle strength from childhood through adolescence into adulthood all of these factors need to be considered. Throughout this chapter these elements will be categorized as neural, muscular and mechanical, and can be seen in Figure 3.3.

ASSESSMENT OF MUSCLE STRENGTH

Assessment of isotonic exercise has been popular in terms of the maximal amount lifted during one repetition (1 RM) and where the external load remains constant.

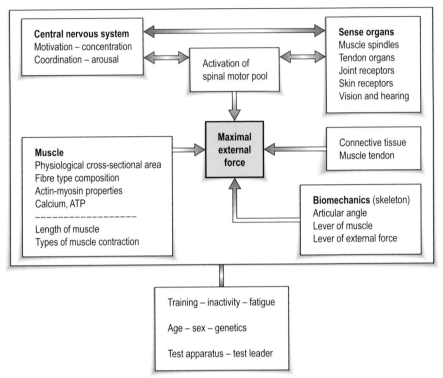

Figure 3.3 Factors that influence the generation of maximal external force (adapted from Reilly et al 1990).

Assessment using free weights is appealing as it examines both the concentric and eccentric portion of the muscle. However, with children the unstable external loads may cause injury as well as the load not accommodating the full joint range of motion (ROM). For example, at the extremities of joint ROM the elastic component of muscle is inefficient at producing force.

Most early strength development studies examined isometric forces generated from handgrip data. It has been suggested that strength measured as isometric or dynamic force reflects the same relative strength between individuals regardless of the type of test method. However, dynamic actions are far more reflective of dynamic muscle properties, themselves a function of neuromuscular factors and fibre type composition, more so than isometric actions. It would also appear logical that if the strength of the arm, and in particular the leg muscles, is to be determined then dynamic tests should be advocated since their everyday functions are dynamic and not static. Force, work and power are not easily measured if angular velocity is not kept constant because the changing mechanical advantage of the limb-lever system alters the force applied to the muscle through the range of motion, i.e. the load applied to the muscle is highest at the point of least mechanical advantage of the muscle at the extremes of the range of motion. Due to the increased accessibility to isokinetic dynamometers in sports science laboratories there has been an increase in paediatric studies that have examined the age- and sex-associated changes in muscle strength under dynamic conditions and during varying velocities.

Choice of testing protocol with children and adolescents may be influenced by subjects, test equipment availability, cost and specificity of testing. Previous authors have suggested that the key issues relating to testing protocols should include the muscle group to be tested, joint angle, type of muscle action, velocity of muscle action and movement pattern. There are numerous generic protocol considerations when undertaking strength testing which are beyond the scope of this chapter. However, there are some that are specific to paediatric groups which will be addressed here. In particular, adaptation to equipment, stabilization and technique, habituation and learning effects, and safety will be examined.

Modifications to most strength testing equipment are required when examining young people in order to isolate the target muscle group. This is especially critical where the axis of rotation of the dynamometer needs to be aligned with the axis of rotation of the joint. Some dynamometers can now be purchased with paediatric attachments which accommodate the short limbs of young subjects. Where this is not possible some researchers have used attachments that are designed for upper limb assessment in adults to test the lower limbs of children.

Reliability

In order for any strength measurement to be used as an objective and accurate measure of maximum strength it must be demonstrated to be a reliable measurement tool. Poor reliability may lead to erroneous conclusions about the strength parameter being measured. Experimental error can be minimized effectively by standardization of test protocols which will provide greater sensitivity to detect biological sources of variation in a child's ability to exert maximum muscular effort.

An habituation period is critical for paediatric strength testing as this essential period of learning facilitates a phase in which the specific movements, neuromuscular patterns and demands of the test become familiar to the individual. Previous studies have reported good reliability in repeated isokinetic actions of the knee in 6- to 8-year-olds (extension $r = 0.95$; flexion $r = 0.85$); isokinetic actions of the elbow in 9- to 10-year-olds (extension $r = 0.97$; flexion $r = 0.87$) and isometric handgrip data in 8-11-year-olds ($r = 0.92$). Others have reported limits of agreement showing no systematic difference in knee and elbow peak torque measured on two separate occasions. It would appear that strength testing in children, irrespective of muscle action or muscle joint assessed, has a test–retest variation of around 5–10%.

It is difficult to compare results across studies as different statistical methods, many of which are questionable, have been used to assess reliability, which is also protocol, measured parameter and dynamometer specific. However, the available literature currently supports the reliability of strength testing with children but suggests that extension movements are more reliable than flexion movements and that concentric actions are more reliable than eccentric actions.

Interpretation of data

It has become common in the literature to express strength in absolute terms, with isometric data expressed in newtons (N) and isokinetic data expressed in newton metres (Nm). In the study of muscle strength in relation to growth and maturation comparisons are made between individuals of different sizes. It is therefore important that a size-free strength variable is used for interpretive purposes. Current methods used for scaling for differences in body size are discussed in detail in Chapter 2. From a strength perspective the key issues to be addressed when scaling for body size differences are the body size variable with which to scale and the method to be employed.

The most commonly used technique in the strength literature to partition out differences in size is the ratio standard with body mass as the most widely used denominator. However, stature and fat-free mass have also featured as covariates. Others have used allometric scaling techniques to examine the theory that mCSA and strength are a function of the second power of stature. The b exponents identified in the study of Kanehisa et al (1995) ranged from 2.4 to 3.6, which were significantly higher than the predicted 2.0, and the authors concluded that strength should be scaled to stature$^{3.0}$, or body mass.

Three longitudinal studies have used multilevel modelling to examine a number of known covariates to determine their influence on the age- and sex-associated changes in muscle strength (De Ste Croix et al 2002, Round et al 1999, Wood et al 2004). Most authors currently support the view that suitable scaling factors should be derived from careful modelling of individual data sets, and therefore be sample specific rather than adopting assumed scaling indices.

DEVELOPMENT OF MUSCLE STRENGTH

Most of our early understanding of the age- and sex-associated development in strength was restricted to physical performance tests.

Historically, field tests have been advocated as a measure of muscle strength. However, they must be viewed with caution as they frequently measure endurance rather than strength. Field tests tend to lack measurement sensitivity and often result in a high percentage of zero scores. As strength testing is dependent upon motivation, field tests may not be sensitive enough to detect the more generalized gains in strength. A good example of this is the data presented in the National Children and Youth Fitness Study (1985) in which 60% of girls aged 10–18 years failed to do one pull-up. As field tests require the resistance or movement of the individual's body mass it follows that children with a larger mass will be disadvantaged. Studies that have used pull-ups as the criterion measure for determining sex differences in muscle strength have clouded our understanding of strength development during growth and maturation. It is hardly surprising therefore that correlations between strength measurements using field tests and dynamometers are often non-significant in paediatric populations.

It is important to bear in mind that our understanding of the development of strength with age will be influenced by the nuances of the testing procedures used, such as subject positioning, degree of practice, level of motivation, lateral dominance and level of understanding about the purpose and nature of the test.

When examining data relating to changes in strength due to growth and maturation it is important to remember that the majority of data have been derived from isometric testing. Children may not produce maximal force during isometric actions, and this has been attributed to inhibitory mechanisms that preclude children from giving a maximal effort due to a feeling of discomfort caused by the rapid development of force during isometric actions. Therefore, the whole motor pool may not be activated due to a reduction in the neural drive under high tension loading conditions.

In a comprehensive review, Blimkie (1989) noted that while there are a number of studies examining strength development, few studies show commonality in age ranges assessed, muscle groups tested, methodology used, muscle action studied and physiological condition under which muscles were tested. The literature on strength during childhood has been derived largely from cross-sectional studies as there are few longitudinal studies available.

Data from isometric actions indicate that in both boys and girls strength increases in a fairly linear fashion from early childhood up until the onset of puberty in boys and until about the end of the pubertal period in girls. The marked difference seen between boys and girls is due to a strength spurt in boys during the pubertal period, which is not evident in girls. Girls' strength appears to increase during puberty at a similar rate to that seen during the prepubertal phase and then appears to plateau after puberty. There is some disagreement about the age at which sex differences become evident (this will be discussed in more detail later). However, although conflicting evidence is available it is generally agreed that before the male adolescent growth spurt there are considerable overlaps in strength values between boys and girls. By the age of 16/17 years very few girls outperform boys in strength tests, with boys demonstrating 54% more strength on average than girls (Figs 3.4 and 3.5).

Throughout childhood and puberty, particularly in males, isometric elbow flexor and knee extensor strength are highly correlated with chronological age. Although there are some data on the age-related changes in the knee extensors and flexors for children, the trends affecting these muscle groups are limited. In line with isometric data most cross-sectional studies of changes in dynamic strength have demonstrated a significant increase with age. For example, an increase in males' and females' absolute knee extensor (314% and 143%) and flexor (285% and 131%) strength have been noted from the ages of 9 to 21 years (De Ste Croix et al 1999).

Some studies have suggested that age exerts an independent effect on strength development over and above maturation and stature (Maffulli et al 1994). Others have indicated that even when mCSA is accounted for using a multilevel modelling

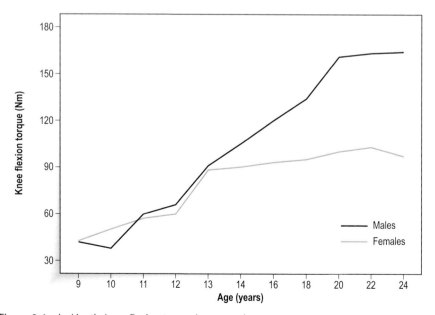

Figure 3.4   Isokinetic knee flexion torque by age and sex.

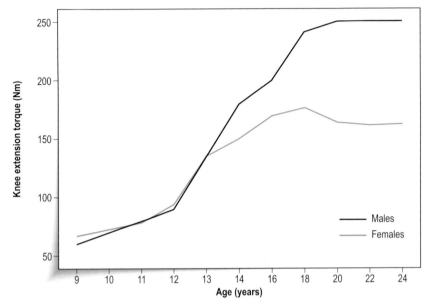

Figure 3.5 Isokinetic knee extension torque by age and sex.

procedure, age explains a significant amount of the additional variance for isometric elbow extensors (Wood et al 2004). It was suggested that this positive age term may be explained by the shared variance with maturation as maturation was not included in the model. However, another longitudinal data set, using multilevel modelling, suggested that age is a non-significant explanatory variable of isokinetic knee torque once stature and mass are accounted for (De Ste Croix et al 2002). This is probably attributable to differing rates of anatomical growth and maturation, which vary independently, and thus their effects on strength do not correlate simply with chronological age. It would appear that although there is a strong correlation between strength and age, a large portion of this association is probably attributable to the shared factors of biological and morphological growth rather than age itself.

There is little consensus about when sex differences in muscle strength become apparent. Some authors have suggested that sex differences in muscle strength are evident from as early as 3 years of age. Other studies have shown clear sex differences by 13–14 years of age. A recent longitudinal study using multilevel modelling to control for known covariates suggested that there are no sex differences in dynamic strength up until the age of 14 years (De Ste Croix et al 2002). After 14 years of age boys outperform girls in muscle strength irrespective of the muscle action examined even with body size accounted for.

Isometric data suggest that sex differences in strength are relatively greater in muscles of the upper compared to the lower body in children. Gilliam et al (1979) reported no significant sex difference in 15- to 17-year-olds' knee extension peak torque but sex differences were apparent for the elbow extensors. This has been attributed to the weight-bearing role of the leg muscle. It has also been suggested that during growth and maturation boys use their upper body more than girls through habitual physical activities (such as climbing). This sociocultural explanation has recently been brought into doubt as there is no overlap in strength between sexes as would be expected with physically active girls and sedentary boys if this contention was true (Round et al 1999).

Determinants of strength development

Many factors have been associated with the age- and sex-associated development in muscle strength (see Fig. 3.2) but the complex interaction of these factors remains challenging to identify. There are few longitudinal studies of strength development that have spanned early childhood to adulthood and examined these variables concurrently using appropriate scaling methods. The following sections focus on the role played by the factors associated with the development of muscle strength.

Stature, mass and strength development

The influence of gross body size on strength development has been examined in several studies. Stature and mass are traditionally the size variables of choice because they can be quickly and easily measured. Early longitudinal studies demonstrated that isometric strength per body mass varied only slightly during childhood and through puberty in girls. In contrast, around the time of boys' peak height velocity (PHV), i.e. age 14 years, there was an increase in strength per body mass in boys which was still continuing by age 18 years.

Body mass has been found to be highly correlated with maximal voluntary isometric strength of elbow flexors and knee extensors in males aged 9 to 18 years (Blimkie 1989). Figure 3.6 demonstrates the strong positive correlation between

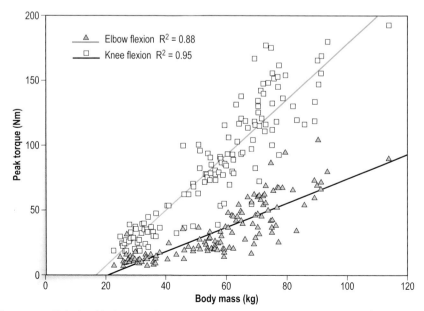

Figure 3.6 Relationship between knee and elbow flexion torque and body mass (data from Deighan et al 2002).

isokinetic knee and elbow flexion torque and body mass in 9- to 24-year-old males and females.

However, age-specific correlation coefficients between strength and body mass for males are generally low to moderate during the mid-childhood years, increase then peak during puberty, and abate in the late teens. Data on this relationship are sparse for females but moderate positive coefficients between strength and body mass for females during the prepubertal years and at the onset of puberty and low correlations at the end of puberty and during puberty have been reported. Others have found the relationship between female strength and body mass to be high during the teen years and to decline during young adulthood. When related to shorter periods of growth (in which the range of the anthropometric variable in question is small), correlations become weaker. This reliance of the correlation coefficient on the characteristics of the sample shows that comparison of correlation coefficients between studies should be done cautiously. It is worth noting here that when isokinetic knee extension and flexion torque were adjusted for body mass using the ratio standard the rate of change in strength between 9 and 21 years of age was underestimated compared to mass-adjusted data using allometric techniques (De Ste Croix et al 1999).

It is well recognized that peak strength velocity occurs about a year after PHV (11.4–12.2 years in girls and 13.4–14.4 years in boys). It has been suggested that the difference in attainment of PHV and subsequent peak strength gains account for the lack of a significant sex difference in strength at 14 years. Girls will be in the phase of peak strength gains at 14 years whereas many boys will not have experienced the strength spurt.

Three recent longitudinal studies, one examining isometric strength and two examining isokinetic strength, have used multilevel modelling to examine the factors related to strength development. Round et al (1999) reported that isometric knee extensor strength in girls increased in proportion to the increase in stature and mass in 8- to 13-year-olds. De Ste Croix et al (2002) also demonstrated that stature and mass are significant explanatory variables of isokinetic knee extension and flexion torque in 10- to 14-year-olds. This was further reinforced by Wood et al (2004), who demonstrated a significant influence exerted by stature on the development of isometric and isokinetic elbow flexion and extension in 13- to 15-year-olds. Conflicting data are available and the study of Round et al (1999) suggested that in boys the strength of the knee extensors was disproportionate to the increase in body size. This difference was explained once testosterone was added to the multilevel model.

Although simple body dimensions appear to be important in the development of strength with age, only between 40–70% of the variance in strength scores of 5- to 17-year-old children could be accounted for by age, sex, stature and body mass, which leaves a large portion of the variance unexplained.

Maturation and hormonal influences

Early studies indicated that maturation, determined using the indices of pubic hair development described by Tanner (1962), was a better predictor of 1 RM isotonic knee extension and flexion strength than simple chronological age. A recent longitudinal study of 10- to 14-year-olds indicated that maturation was a non-significant explanatory variable in the development of isokinetic knee extension and flexion, once stature and mass were accounted for, using multilevel modelling procedures (De Ste Croix et al 2002). However, the authors did acknowledge that their sample consisted of a narrow range of maturational stages. Supporting data are available, with previous studies indicating that maturation does not exert an independent effect upon isometric strength development in 10- to 18-year-old athletes (Maffulli et al 1994) and 12- to 14-year-old football players (Hansen et al 1997) once age and body size have been controlled for.

An important consideration regarding the development of muscle function is the effect of endocrine adaptations typical of sexual maturation such as increased levels of testosterone and growth hormone (GH). There is both direct and indirect evidence to demonstrate the association between testosterone and strength development during puberty.

Testosterone levels accelerate from a modest fourfold increase during the early stages of puberty to a rapid 20-fold increase in mid–late puberty in boys (around Tanner stage 3). It is not surprising that testosterone levels appear to coincide with the divergence of strength between boys and girls as circulating testosterone begins to rise 1 year before PHV, increasing steadily and reaching adult levels about 3 years after PHV. Testosterone has been shown to stimulate anabolic processes in skeletal muscle and appears to be the principal hormone responsible for the development of strength. This effect is mediated by androgen receptors in the myofibres. As well as increasing protein synthesis, other ways in which testosterone could augment strength include promoting transition of type IIa motor units to a more glycolytic profile of type IIX motor units, increasing the production of insulin-like growth factor 1 (IGF-1), influencing the amplitude of GH pulses and regulating neurotransmitter release thereby enhancing force. Round et al (1999) suggested that testosterone accounts for the sex difference that exists in isometric strength even after making allowances for body size. Detailed analysis of their data showed that there was an increase of 0.7% in isometric knee extension strength for every unit of circulating testosterone (nmol $\cdot$ L^{-1}). The analysis showed that the young men in the sample were 15–20% stronger as a result of testosterone than might be expected from their overall body stature. In contrast, the same analysis for biceps showed that sex differences could not be fully accounted for by the effects of testosterone in teenage boys. These authors speculated that the linear measure inserted into the model for biceps should be humerus length as opposed to stature. Their plausible suggestion was based on the well-known increase in the upper limb girdle dimensions in boys during puberty that provides an additional stimulus for muscle growth with the direct action of testosterone in the muscle. Jones & Round (2000) indicated that increasing levels of oestrogen in girls causes inhibition of muscle growth as a result of a speedier skeletal maturation which removes the lengthening stimulus for muscle growth.

Ramos et al (1998) also reported that body mass did not eliminate the age effect in isokinetic peak torque in boys and that testosterone increased with age in boys but not in girls. This increase in testosterone preceded the gains in muscle strength but perhaps more importantly there was a moderate positive correlation ($r = 0.64$) between serum testosterone and isokinetic angle specific torque.

Fat-free mass and strength development

Typically, during childhood and puberty, strength increases coincide with changes in fat-free mass (FFM). Moderate to strong correlations have been found for knee extension and flexion torque versus FFM in 8- to 13-year-old wrestlers (Housh et al 1996). However, further studies have reported age-related increases in torque per FFM for knee extensors and elbow extensors and flexors that could not be accounted for by changes in FFM. The age effect for increases in strength independent of FFM may be attributable to an increase in muscle mass per unit of FFM or neural maturation which allows for a greater expression of strength. The proportion of FFM that is skeletal muscle has been suggested to increase with age. In addition, the proportion of muscle mass that is distributed at various sites is thought to vary and at birth approximately 40% of total muscle mass is located in the lower extremities, increasing to approximately 55% at sexual maturity in both boys and girls.

Studies that have used anthropometric estimations of total body muscle mass have reported that estimated total body muscle mass cannot account for the age-related increase in strength and that non-significant correlations exist between age and estimated muscle mass covaried for FFM (Housh et al 1996). This suggests that there are nearly proportional increases in total body muscle mass and FFM across age and that age-related increases in strength are not due to an increase in muscle mass per unit of FFM. It is possible that the anthropometric equations in these studies were not sensitive enough to detect a change across age in the contribution of muscle mass to FFM.

If conclusions are made about the factors affecting strength development based on age- or sex-related differences in strength per FFM, then the assumption must be that a muscle or muscle group mCSA is always the same proportion of FFM across ages and between sexes. It may be that regional mCSA increases from prepuberty to postpuberty at the same rate as FFM and not that total muscle mass increases at the same rate as FFM.

Strength development and mCSA

According to Blimkie (1989, p. 127) 'It is likely that quantitative differences in muscle width account for a large proportion of the observed age and sex differences in strength development during childhood and adolescence'. It is important at this point to reconsider that there have been variations in the methods used to measure both strength and muscle size. The relationship between muscle size and strength during growth has been examined by measuring muscle widths, muscle volume and mCSA. It is also important to note that most studies have reported anatomical mCSA due to the difficulties in determining physiological mCSA.

There are numerous data that support the contention that differences in muscle size account for differences in muscle strength during growth. One of the earliest studies examined the relationship between isometric elbow flexion strength and mCSA determined by ultrasonography in 12- to 29-year-olds (Ikai & Fukunaga 1968). Although correlation coefficients were not given, the authors indicated that strength 'is fairly proportional' to elbow flexor mCSA regardless of age or training status. The relationship appeared weaker for girls than boys. Others have reported a strong positive correlation between muscle size, and isometric knee strength ($r = 0.87$), isokinetic knee strength ($r = 0.73$), isokinetic elbow strength ($r = 0.82$) and isokinetic triceps surae strength ($r = 0.91$). In addition, based on grip strength data from children, the sex-related growth curve patterns for body muscle are virtually identical to those for strength, suggesting a strong association between muscle growth and gains in strength. Numerous longitudinal studies have shown that as an independent covariate mCSA is a significant explanatory variable in the age-associated development in strength. However, as we will go on to discuss, it appears that when additional variables are examined concurrently alongside mCSA its influence is reduced or disappears.

Age differences in strength per mCSA

There is still some debate about whether strength per mCSA increases with age. Early studies demonstrated increasing strength per mCSA from 7 to 13 years of age. Also, Kanehisa et al (1995) suggested that isokinetic strength per mCSA, measured using ultrasonography, was greater in older age groups (18 years) than younger age groups (7 years) in every muscle group measured. It was hypothesized that children in the early stages of puberty may not develop strength in proportion to their muscle anatomical CSA. It is likely that the deficiency of strength per mCSA in the younger age groups might be related to a lack of the ability to mobilize the muscle voluntarily. The same group of authors found that the isometric strength of the ankle dorsiflexors and plantarflexors per mCSA measured by ultrasonography in boys and girls aged 7 to 18 years was significantly greater only for plantar flexion in 16- to 18-year-old boys compared to the other groups. In a comprehensive cross-sectional study others have reported a significant increase in isokinetic knee and elbow torque per MRI-determined mCSA from 9 to 16 years but no significant difference from 16 to 24 years (Deighan et al 2002, 2003). Further investigation is required to establish whether these differences in torque per mCSA are due to biomechanical or neuromuscular factors. What these data do suggest is that torque per mCSA of the elbow and knee extensors and flexors are at adult levels by 16 years of age. Conflicting data are available indicating that, despite smaller MRI-determined triceps surae mCSA, early pubertal boys' torque scaled to muscle size is not different from that of adult males. These conflicting data emphasize the need to measure the strength per mCSA in a variety of muscles as the strength development characteristics of one muscle or group of muscles may not be the same as another, even within the same joint.

Sex differences in strength per mCSA

Whether sex differences exist in strength per mCSA is debatable. Early work reported that absolute isometric strength differences between sexes disappeared when data were normalized to anthropometric muscle (plus bone) CSA in 9- to 12-year-olds. Sunnegardh et al (1988) showed that boys had significantly greater torque per CSA than girls at 13 years. Deighan et al (2002) recently reported significant sex differences in isokinetic elbow flexion per mCSA in 9- to 10-year-olds and 16- to 17-year-olds. These studies are in contrast to others that have demonstrated similar strength to mCSA ratios between sexes (Deighan et al 2003, Ikai & Fukunaga 1968, Wood et al 2004). Deighan et al (2003) reported no significant sex differences in isokinetic torque per mCSA of the knee extensors and flexors and elbow flexors in 9- to 10-year-olds, 16- to 17-year-olds and adults. Using multilevel modelling procedures on longitudinal data, Wood et al (2004) also reported that sex effects for isokinetic elbow extensors and flexors became non-significant once mCSA was controlled for. The majority of recent studies would lead us therefore to the conclusion that there is no significant sex difference in strength per mCSA irrespective of the muscle joint or action examined. It would appear that factors in addition to mCSA may account for the age- and sex-associated development in strength.

For example, the peak gain in muscle strength in boys occurs more often after peak stature and mCSA velocity but there is no such trend for girls. Therefore, particularly in boys there may be factors other than mCSA that affect strength expression during puberty. It has been shown that the sex differences that occur in the strength of boys and girls of the same stature cannot be accounted for by muscle size alone. A longitudinal study of upper arm area and elbow flexor strength has shown that boys have muscles roughly 5% greater in area but which produce approximately 12% more strength. Others have indicated that mCSA is a non-significant explanatory variable once stature and mass are accounted for (De Ste Croix et al 2002).

Peak muscle mass velocity has been shown to occur at an average age of 14.3 years, whereas peak strength velocity occurs at age 14.7 years. This supports the view that muscle tissue increases first in mass, then in functional strength. Consequently, this would seem to suggest a qualitative change in muscle tissue as puberty progresses and perhaps a neuromuscular maturation affecting the volitional demonstration of strength.

Biomechanical factors and strength development

The mechanical advantage of the musculoskeletal system is variable across different muscle groups and is considered unfavourable because the measured force or torque is somewhat smaller than the corresponding tension developed in the muscle tendon. Another unfavourable biomechanical influence on the measured force lies in the internal muscle architecture, i.e. the greater the angle of pennation to the long axis of the muscle the smaller proportion of force in the muscle fibres that is transmitted to the muscle tendon. The age-associated relationships between these factors have not yet been extensively investigated in children.

It is probable that small differences between subjects in the location of the centre of rotation of the joint or in the length of the lower limb could contribute to the observed variability in the ratio of muscle strength to mCSA. It is difficult to account for biomechanical factors but some authors have divided strength values by the product of mCSA and stature ($Nm \cdot cm^{-3}$), i.e. the product of mCSA and possible differences in moment arm length or mechanical advantage which they assumed to be proportional to stature. There are few published data on the relationship between strength per mCSA and mechanical advantage covering different age groups, both sexes and different muscle groups but it seems sensible to correct strength for possible differences in mechanical advantage, especially if comparing children of different sizes, by normalizing to mCSA × limb length (LL) (Blimkie & Macauley 2001). One of the major assumptions with using this method is that muscle moment arm and limb length are proportional to one another.

Numerous authors have demonstrated moderately strong, positive correlations ($r = 0.57$ to 0.85) between stature and isometric torque per mCSA for the elbow flexors and knee extensors, isokinetic knee extensors and flexors, and isokinetic elbow extensors and flexors. Kanehisa et al. (1994) found that isokinetic torque was significantly correlated to mCSA × thigh length ($r = 0.72$ to 0.83). These data suggest that at least part of the age-associated variability in voluntary strength may be attributed to differences in mechanical advantage that occur with growth.

Blimkie (1989) reported that age effects were the same whether dividing torque by the product of mCSA and stature or just mCSA. Young adults have been found to have significantly higher ratios of isokinetic knee extension torque per unit of mCSA × thigh length than children, with the difference becoming greater with increasing velocity of movement. Deighan et al (2002) suggested that the influence of mechanical advantage on the development of isokinetic strength may be muscle group specific. Data showed a non-significant age effect for the elbow extensors and flexors but a significant difference between 9- to 10-year-olds and 16- to 17-year-olds in knee extension and flexion torque per mCSA × LL. The knee data suggested that mCSA × LL alone cannot account for the age differences in strength. It is difficult to attribute physiological reasons to the muscle group differences but it is possible that part of the explanation may lie in the differing function of the arms and legs. For example, there is some evidence to suggest that the extent of motor unit activation of the arm muscles remains essentially unchanged with growth but increases in the muscles of the thigh.

Early work indicated that sex differences in absolute torque remain statistically significant, although diminished, when expressed per unit mCSA × thigh length. Kanehisa et al (1994) reported no significant sex differences in young children but that sex differences became apparent in adulthood when expressing torque per mCSA × LL. Deighan et al (2002) reported non-significant sex differences for the knee and elbow extensors and flexors in torque per mCSA × LL in 9- to 10-year-olds, 16- to 17-year-olds and adults. Recent data therefore suggest that sex differences, at least for dynamic strength, can be accounted for by the product of mCSA and limb length. Further investigation is needed to examine if this pattern remains in relation to isometric strength.

There has been speculation that the angle of muscle pennation plays a role in the group differences in strength per mCSA (Blimkie 1989). Conventional scanning techniques all measure mCSA at right angles to the limb, i.e. anatomical mCSA. However, the maximum force a whole muscle or muscle group can produce is a function of the tension generated by each individual fibre in the direction of the muscle's line of pull. Most muscle groups that are tested in humans are pennate (with the exception of the biceps brachii). By design, the total capacity for tension development is enhanced in pennate muscle by having more sarcomeres arranged in parallel and fewer in series within a given volume of muscle. In other words fibres are not orientated in true parallel to the long axis of the muscle. This can affect measurements of in vivo strength per anatomical mCSA in two opposing ways. Firstly, the shortening force transferred to the tendon at the muscle's insertion is less than that generated along the axis of the muscle fibres. Secondly, individual fibres do not span the whole length of the muscle, so anatomical mCSA will not include all fibres contributing to the force. Therefore, physiological mCSA is thought to be a better predictor of force-producing capacity than anatomical mCSA. However, true physiological mCSA cannot easily be determined in vivo and to date there are no paediatric studies that have examined physiological mCSA.

Neuromuscular factors and strength development

Measured voluntary strength depends highly on the degree of percentage motor unit activation (%MUA). Both the level of voluntary neural drive or motor unit recruitment and the level of activation or frequency of stimulation govern %MUA. The ideal way to measure the contractile capacity of a muscle is to record the force developed during supramaximal electrical stimulation of the nerve innervating the muscle. When an electrical stimulus is applied to a motor nerve near the muscle, the resultant muscle force is free of any inhibitory influence from above the point of stimulation. On the other hand, force or torque measured during a voluntary action is the result of neuromuscular influences from the brain and inhibitory reflex influences from the spinal cord in addition to the maximum force-producing capacity of the muscle. The results of tetanic electrical stimulation may not be comparable to voluntary muscle actions, since in the former method synergistic muscles may not be excited and the procedure is very painful, leading to reduced compliance and, with child subjects, ethical concerns.

Due to these problems with tetanic stimuli of children's muscles, most studies that have investigated maximum force-producing capacity in children have used twitch stimuli because various properties of an electrically evoked twitch reveal information about intrinsic muscle properties and %MUA. Assuming that %MUA stays constant with age, then the ratio of evoked twitch force to voluntary force should stay constant with age. Based on this assumption, Davis (1985) measured both evoked twitch force and maximum voluntary force in groups of 9-, 11-, 14- and 21-year-old males and females. The twitch torque/voluntary torque ratio of the triceps surae was similar in boys and girls aged 9 years but it gradually decreased with age in the males. However, no conclusion of a greater %MUA with increasing age in boys could be made because there was also a change in the twitch to evoked tetanus ratio with increasing age. On examination of the tetanic/voluntary ratio it appeared that %MUA may vary with age but not sex. The possibility that an inability to fully recruit the available motor unit pool may be reflected in smaller strength per mCSA values in children than in adults has not been extensively investigated.

The interpolated twitch technique (ITT) has been used to provide an answer to the painful tetanic stimuli method and to allow %MUA to be calculated more directly. Blimkie (1989) used the ITT on maximum voluntary isometric actions of the elbow extensors and knee flexors. He found that %MUA of the knee extensors increased with age in boys from 77.7% at 10 years to 95.3% at 16 years, an increase in %MUA of 17.6%. A different pattern was found for the elbow flexors whose respective values were 89.4% and 89.9%, indicating no change in the %MUA of elbow flexors. No studies have investigated this phenomenon in females. However, it appears that boys at least are unable to fully activate the available motor units during maximum voluntary muscle actions of the knee extensors but not the elbow flexors. In support of this others have reported that %MUA in prepubertal boys was 78% of the intrinsic force-producing capacity during maximum voluntary knee extension. Also, the maximum rate of force production, being largely dependent on the amount and rate of neural activation, has been found to be lower in children aged 8 to 11 years compared to college-age men and women.

In adults, a sex difference has been demonstrated in the rate of force development, which is an important quality for dynamic muscle actions in which there is limited time to generate force. Recent data examining isokinetic time to reach peak torque suggest that there are non-significant sex differences in the knee and elbow extensor and flexor muscles (De Ste Croix et al 2004). In the same study age-related changes in time to peak torque were muscle group and muscle action specific, leading the authors to the conclusion that care must be taken when making assumptions on differing muscle groups and actions.

Time to peak twitch torque and twitch relaxation indices can be used as measures of rate of energy turnover and fibre type composition. Twitch relaxation times have been shown to be similar in boys and girls and are not influenced by age. Also, it has been found that time to peak twitch force and relaxation times were the same regardless of age during childhood. Likewise, similar time to peak twitch tension was demonstrated in 3-year-olds as in 25-year-olds. These data suggest that muscle fibre composition and muscle activation speed are similar between these age groups and that there is no difference in the fibre type distribution from the age of around 7 years. Previous authors have suggested that the neuromuscular system is still maturing with respect to the myelination of the nerves in younger children. Also muscle fibre conduction velocity has been seen to increase with age in children. The influence that neuromuscular factors have on the development of muscle strength, concurrently with other known variables, remains to be established.

SUMMARY

There is still a clear need for further longitudinal investigation into the static and dynamic development of muscle strength through childhood and adolescence into adulthood. It is clear that many of the factors discussed in this chapter play a role in this development when examined as independent variables. The challenge is to elucidate the factors that contribute to the age- and sex-associated development in strength concurrently with other known explanatory variables. The major difficulty in describing the age- and sex-associated development in strength is that much of the current data reveal muscle group and muscle action specific differences in the relationships described. For example, the factors responsible for the development of isokinetic eccentric elbow flexion may be different from isometric knee extension.

It would appear that, for dynamic muscle actions in particular, mechanical factors may play a large role in the development of muscle torque and accurate investigation of the muscle moment arm, employing MRI techniques, would provide us with a clearer picture of the age- and sex-associated development.

KEY POINTS

1. Measurement of muscle size in children using anthropometric techniques underestimates muscle volume by about 30%.
2. There are overlaps in muscle size in boys and girls up until the ages of 13–14 years when boys demonstrate a spurt in muscle size. Girls' muscle size increases at a slower rate up until about 17 years when it reaches a plateau. Boys' muscle growth continues into their mid-twenties.
3. There are distinct differences in static and dynamic strength characteristics in children which must be acknowledged when examining age- and sex-associated changes in strength.
4. Without appropriate adaptations to equipment and protocols strength testing in children is unreliable.
5. Children do not produce maximal force during isometric actions and functional strength may be as important as maximal strength in sport performance.
6. The age-associated development in strength is attributable to the shared variance in growth and maturation. Sex differences appear at around 14 years of age and very few girls outperform boys in strength tests at 18 years.
7. Stature and mass appear to be important explanatory variables in the development of muscle strength. PHV is a particularly important time for maximal gains in strength during childhood.
8. Sexual maturation has not been shown to exert an influence on strength development once body size is controlled for but circulating hormones, such as testosterone, stimulate development in muscle size.
9. Muscle CSA exerts an independent effect on strength development but is a non-significant explanatory variable once body size is accounted for.
10. Neuromuscular maturation is poorly understood and may contribute to the improvement in motor unit activation with age.
11. The muscle moment arm is possibly the most important factor in the development of muscle strength with age but further longitudinal studies are needed to elucidate this hypothesis.

12. The age- and sex-associated development in muscle strength combined with the factors that contribute to this development appear to be muscle group and muscle action specific.

References

Blimkie C J R 1989 Age and sex-associated variation in strength during childhood: anthropometric, morphologic, neurologic, biomechanical, endocrinologic, genetic and physical activity correlates. In: Gisolf C V, Lamb D R (eds) Perspectives in exercise science and sports medicine. Vol 2. Youth, exercise and sport. Benchmark Press, Indianapolis, p 99–163

Blimkie C J R, Macauley D 2001 Muscle strength. In: Armstrong N, Van-Mechelen W (eds) Pediatric exercise science and medicine. Oxford University Press, Oxford, p 23–36

Davies C T M 1985 Strength and mechanical properties of muscle in children and young adults. Scandinavian Journal of Sport Sciences 7:11–15

Deighan M A, Armstrong N, De Ste Croix M B A et al 2002 Peak torque per arm muscle cross-sectional area during growth. In: Koskolou M, Geladas N, Klissouras V (eds) Proceedings of the 7th Annual Congress of the European College of Sport Science. Pashalidis Medical Publisher, Athens, p 47

Deighan M A, Armstrong N, De Ste Croix M B A et al 2003 Peak torque per MRI-determined cross-sectional area of knee extensors and flexors in children, teenagers and adults. Journal of Sports Sciences 21:236

Deighan M, De Ste Croix M B A, Grant C et al 2006 Measurement of maximal cross-sectional area of elbow extensors and flexors in children, teenagers and adults. Journal of Sports Sciences 24:543–546

De Ste Croix M B A, Armstrong N, Welsman J R 1999 Concentric isokinetic leg strength in pre-teen, teenage and adult males and females. Biology of Sport 16:75–86

De Ste Croix M B A, Armstrong N, Welsman J R et al 2002 Longitudinal changes in isokinetic leg strength in 10–14 year olds. Annals of Human Biology 29:50–62

De Ste Croix M B A, Deighan M A, Armstrong N 2004 Time to peak torque for knee and elbow extensors and flexors in children, teenagers and adults. Isokinetic and Exercise Science 12:143–148

Gilliam T B, Villanacci J F, Freedson P S et al 1979 Isokinetic torque in boys and girls ages 7 to 13: effect of age, height and weight. Research Quarterly 50:599–609

Hansen L, Klausen K, Muller J 1997 Assessment of maturity status and its relation to strength measurements. In: Armstrong N, Kirby B J, Welsman J (eds) Children and exercise. XIX: Promoting health and well-being. E&FN Spon, London

Housh D J, Housh T J, Weir J P et al 1995 Anthropometric estimation of thigh muscle cross-section. Medicine and Science in Sports and Exercise 27:784–791

Housh T J, Johnson G O, Housh D J et al 1996 Isokinetic peak torque in young wrestlers. Pediatric Exercise Science 8:143–155

Ikai M, Fukunaga T 1968 Calculation of muscle strength per unit cross-sectional area of human muscle by means of ultrasonic measurement. Arbeitsphysiologie 26:26–32

Jones P R M, Pearson J 1969 Anthropometric determination of leg fat and muscle plus bone volumes in young male and female adults. Journal of Physiology 240:63–66

Jones D A, Round J M 2000 Strength and muscle growth. In: Armstrong N, Van-Mechelen W (eds) Pediatric exercise science and medicine. Oxford University Press, Oxford, p 133–142

Kanehisa H, Ikegawa S, Tsunoda N et al 1994 Strength and cross-sectional area of knee extensor muscles in children. European Journal of Applied Physiology 68:402–405

Kanehisa H, Ikegawa S, Tsunoda N et al 1995 Strength and cross-sectional areas of reciprocal muscle groups in the upper arm and thigh during adolescence. International Journal of Sports Medicine 16:54–60

Maffulli N, King J B, Helms P 1994 Training in elite youth athletes: injuries, flexibility and isometric strength. British Journal of Sports Medicine 28:123–136

Malina R M, Bouchard C 1991 Growth, maturation and physical activity. Human Kinetics, Champaign, IL

National Children and Youth Fitness Study 1985 Journal of Physical Education, Recreation and Dance 56:45–50

Ramos E, Frontera W R, Llopart A et al 1998 Muscle strength and hormonal levels in adolescents: gender related differences. International Journal of Sports Medicine 19:526–531

Reilly T, Secher N, Snell P et al 1990 Physiology of sports. E&FN Spon, London

Round J M, Jones D A, Honour J W et al 1999 Hormonal factors in the development of differences in strength between boys and girls during adolescence: a longitudinal study. Annals of Human Biology 26:49–62

Sunnegardh J, Bratteby L E, Nordesjo L O et al 1988 Isometric and isokinetic muscle strength, anthropometry and physical activity in 8 and 13 year old Swedish children. European Journal of Applied Physiology 58:291–297

Tanner J M 1962 Growth at adolescence, 2nd edn. Blackwell Scientific, Oxford

Wood L E, Dixon S, Grant C et al 2004 Elbow flexion and extension strength relative to body size or muscle size in children. Medicine and Science in Sports and Exercise 36:1977–1984

Further reading

Backman E, Henriksson K G 1988 Skeletal muscle characteristics in children 9–15 years old: force, relaxation rate and contraction time. Clinical Physiology 8:521–527

Carron A V, Bailey D A 1974 Strength development in boys from 10 through 16 years. Monographs of the Society for Research in Child Development 39:1–37

Froberg K, Lammert O 1996 Development of muscle strength during childhood. In: Bar-Or O (ed) The child and adolescent athlete. Blackwell Scientific, London, p 25–41

Gaul CA 1996 Muscular strength and endurance. In: Docherty D (ed) Measurement in pediatric exercise science. Human Kinetics, Champaign, IL, p 225–258

Herzog W 2000 Force production in human skeletal muscle. In: Nigg B, MacIntosh B, Mester J (eds) Biomechanics and biology of movement. Human Kinetics, Champaign, IL, p 269–281

Jaric S 2002 Muscle strength testing: use of normalisation for body size. Sports Medicine 32:615–631

Kellis E, Unnithan V B 1999 Co-activation of vastus lateralis and biceps femoris muscles in pubertal children and adults. European Journal of Applied Physiology 79:504–511

Parker D F, Round J M, Sacco P et al 1990 A cross-sectional survey of upper and lower limb strength in boys and girls during childhood and adolescence. Annals of Human Biology 17:199–211

Chapter 4

Exercise metabolism

Neil Armstrong and Joanne R. Welsman

LEARNING OBJECTIVES

After studying this chapter you should be able to:

1. describe the hydrolysis of adenosine triphosphate (ATP) and its resynthesis from phosphocreatine
2. describe the resynthesis of ATP by glycolysis and glycogenolysis
3. describe the resynthesis of ATP by the tricarboxylic acid cycle
4. explain the interplay between anaerobic and aerobic metabolism in the resynthesis of ATP during exercise of different intensities and durations
5. describe muscle fibre types in terms of their metabolic characteristics
6. evaluate the outcomes of muscle biopsy studies of children and adolescents
7. discuss blood-borne indicators of adult–child differences in exercise metabolism
8. discuss respiratory indicators of adult–child differences in exercise metabolism
9. evaluate the role of magnetic resonance spectroscopy in elucidating age-dependent changes in exercise metabolism
10. synthesize the evidence suggesting that exercise metabolism is age-dependent.

INTRODUCTION

Children's exercise performance steadily improves with age even in athletic events that require moving their increasing body mass over set distances in the minimum time period. This can be illustrated by considering athletic records and Figures 4.1 to 4.3 show the average speed attained in relation to age in world-best performances at 100 m, 400 m and 1500 m. These data are cross-sectional and take no account of individual differences in body size, body composition or training status but they do show clearly the age-related increase in performance over a range of distances.

The contribution of anaerobic and aerobic sources to the total energy production in 100 m, 400 m and 1500 m events has been estimated in adults (Table 4.1) but few data on the interplay of anaerobic and aerobic sources during childhood and adolescence are available. Adult athletes who train and compete for specific events are highly specialized. For example, the sprinter and the distance runner may be distinguished both morphologically and physiologically and do not excel in each other's disciplines.

In children, the ability to demonstrate extreme specialization is less apparent than in adults and those who sprint the fastest often also excel in aerobic endurance tasks, an observation which led Bar-Or (Bar-Or & Rowland 2004) to suggest that children might be considered 'metabolic non-specialists' with regard to sports performance.

Several studies of young and prepubertal children have identified significant relationships between the results of aerobic and anaerobic performance tests and interpreted them as reflecting metabolic non-specialization (Bar-Or & Rowland 2004). The biological significance of these relationships, however, remains to be established. Children's growth and maturation are associated with increases in many physiological performance measures including anaerobic and aerobic power and it could be argued that prepubertal and early pubertal children are unlikely to demonstrate the specialization seen in adults' exercise performance partly because of their immaturity. Changes

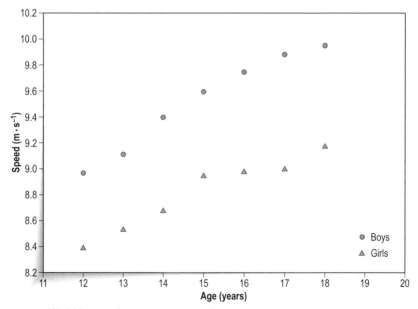

Figure 4.1   World best performances at 100 m by age.

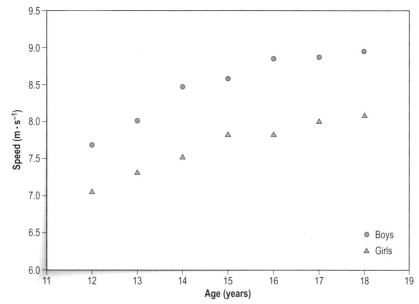

Figure 4.2   World best performances at 400 m by age.

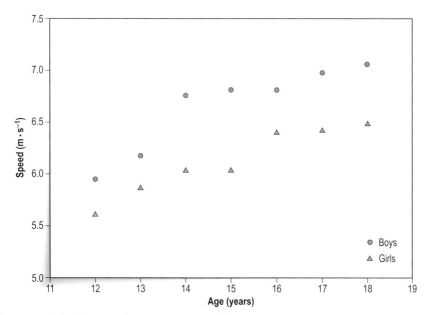

Figure 4.3   World best performances at 1500 m by age.

in body shape, size and muscularity during maturation undoubtedly influence the nature of the relationships between measures of anaerobic and aerobic power.

Direct measures of young people's maximal anaerobic fitness (or power) are not available and research has focused on the assessment of short-term power output. The Wingate anaerobic test (WAnT), which allows the determination of cycling peak

Table 4.1 Contribution of anaerobic and aerobic energy sources in adults to events of different durations

Distance	% Anaerobic	% Aerobic
100 m	90	10
400 m	70	30
1500 m	20	80

power (PP) usually over a 1 s or 5 s period and mean power (MP) over the 30 s test period, is the most popular test of short-term power. Much of the available data from young people has been derived from the WAnT but for methodological reasons discussed in Chapter 5 the extant literature must be interpreted cautiously. Cross-sectional data are conflicting and longitudinal data sparse. However, a consistent finding is that both PP and MP increase with age. Sex differences are minimal until about 12 years of age, with boys generally outscoring girls thereafter. Both sexes benefit from an enhanced non-linear increase in PP and MP during the early and mid teen years, with the effect being more marked in boys. Body mass, body composition and thigh muscle volume are strongly correlated with short-term power output but age exerts an additional positive effect on both PP and MP independent of these factors. There is no strong evidence to suggest that maturation exerts an independent effect on PP and MP once age, body size and body composition have been controlled for (see Chapter 5 for further details).

Aerobic fitness during growth and maturation is extensively documented. Peak oxygen uptake (peak $\dot{V}O_2$) is widely recognized as the criterion measure of maximal aerobic fitness (or power) and its direct determination is a well-established technique in paediatric exercise physiology (see Chapter 8 for further details). Cross-sectional and longitudinal data are consistent and show that peak $\dot{V}O_2$ increases with age in both sexes. Peak $\dot{V}O_2$ is strongly correlated with body size, and inappropriate methods of partialling out body size have clouded our understanding of the independent contributions of age and maturation to the growth of peak $\dot{V}O_2$ (see Chapter 2). With body size appropriately accounted for, boys' peak $\dot{V}O_2$ increases through childhood and adolescence and into adulthood whereas girls' values tend to level off as they approach young adulthood. Maturation induces increases in peak $\dot{V}O_2$ in both sexes independent of those explained by body size, body composition and age. Boys' peak $\dot{V}O_2$ is higher than girls', at least from 8 years of age, and sex differences progressively increase with age (see Chapter 8 for further details).

Bar-Or & Rowland (2004) proposed the ratio of peak anaerobic power to peak aerobic power as an index of young people's performance. Based on a combination of cross-sectional and longitudinal data from several studies, they reported the ratio to be less than 2 at age 8 years, increasing to almost 3 by age 13 to 14 years in girls and age 14 to 15 years in boys (Fig. 4.4). Comparative anaerobic and aerobic data are available in a single longitudinal study where the PP, MP and peak $\dot{V}O_2$ of the same participants were measured at ages 12, 13 and 17 years. PP and MP increased by 121% and 113% in boys and by 66% and 60% in girls. The increases in peak $\dot{V}O_2$ over the same period were somewhat less at 70% and 50% for boys and girls, respectively (Armstrong et al 2001).

The age-related rise in anaerobic and aerobic fitness (or power) is therefore not synchronous and untrained children experience a more marked increase in anaerobic fitness than in aerobic fitness during adolescence. Although the expression of both

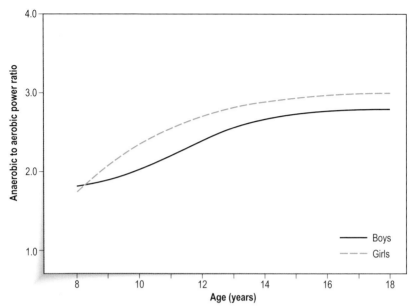

Figure 4.4   Changes with age in the anaerobic-to-aerobic power ratio of children and adolescents. (From Bar-Or O and Rowland T W, *Pediatric Exercise Medicine: From Physiologic Principles to Health Care Application*, page 18, figure 1.21. (© 2004 by Oded Bar-Or and Thomas W Rowland. Reprinted with permission from Human Kinetics (Champaign, IL).)

anaerobic and aerobic fitness is dependent on body size and composition, anaerobic and aerobic performance potential is reflected in the metabolic characteristics of the muscles. It is the muscles that display the fibre type and biochemical profile necessary to support the energetic demands of various performances or athletic events. In this chapter we explore what we know of exercise metabolism during growth and maturation.

EXERCISE METABOLISM

Our understanding of the metabolic processes within children's skeletal muscle is limited and to place the relatively few paediatric data into context we will initially review metabolic activity during exercise as determined principally by studies of adults.

Adenosine triphosphate and phosphocreatine

Muscle contraction and a myriad of other energy-requiring processes in the muscle are driven by the energy released during the sequential hydrolysis of the two terminal phosphate bonds of adenosine triphosphate (ATP). The degradation of ATP to adenosine diphosphate (ADP), adenosine monophosphate (AMP) and inorganic phosphate (Pi) is catalysed by enzymes generically known as ATPases:

$$ATP + H_2O \rightarrow ADP + Pi + H^+ + energy$$

$$ADP + H_2O \rightarrow AMP + Pi + H^+ + energy$$

To prevent accumulation of the products during maximal exercise, if AMP rises it is deaminated (loss of ammonia, NH_3) to inosine monophosphate (IMP) or, to a lesser extent, dephosphorylated to adenosine.

Muscles can perform up to 24 kJ of work for each mole of ATP hydrolysed but the intramuscular stores of ATP are limited to about 5 mmol · kg^{-1} wet weight of muscle, sufficient to support maximal exercise for no more than 2 s. However, muscle ATP stores never become completely depleted because during exercise ATP is efficiently resynthesized from ADP and AMP. At the onset of exercise, the momentary rise in ADP concentration stimulates the hydrolysis of phosphocreatine (PCr), another intramuscular store of high energy phosphate. The free energy of PCr hydrolysis is greater than that of ATP, resulting in a much higher probability of free energy transfer from PCr to ADP. In a reaction catalysed by creatine kinase (CK) one molecule of ATP is regenerated for each molecule of PCr degraded:

$$PCr + ADP + H^+ \rightarrow ATP + Cr$$

The PCr content of skeletal muscle is about four times that of ATP but ATP resynthesis from PCr occurs almost instantaneously once exercise commences and it is depleted rapidly during very heavy intensity exercise. PCr production of ATP reaches its zenith within 2 s and declines thereafter so that during the last 10 s of a 30 s WAnT the contribution of PCr to ATP resynthesis is only about 2% of that within the first 2 s. For high intensity exercise to be sustained beyond a few seconds ATP supply must be maintained and this is ensured, at least in the short term, by glycogenolysis and glycolysis.

Glycogenolysis and glycolysis

Carbohydrates are stored in the muscles and in the liver as glycogen. Adult skeletal muscle contains about 75–80 mmol · kg^{-1} wet weight of glycogen which is immediately available to resynthesize ATP during exercise. About 90–100 g of glycogen resides in the liver. Here it can be broken down and released into the blood as glucose where it is available to all tissues as an energy substrate.

Glycolysis is the anaerobic degradation of glucose to pyruvate whereas glycogenolysis begins with glycogen but shares a common pathway with glycolysis once the glycogen has been converted into glucose 6-phosphate (G6P). Hereafter we will refer to the energy-generating degradation of G6P to pyruvate simply as glycolysis. Glycogenolysis and glycolysis take place in the cytoplasm and are stimulated by the presence of calcium and the accumulation of products of ATP hydrolysis such as ADP, AMP, IMP, Pi and NH_3. Despite the number of reactions involved (Fig. 4.5) the glycolytic system responds very quickly to exercise, with a time constant of about 1.5 s. Peak production of ATP is therefore reached within 5 s and the glycolytic pathway becomes the major provider of ATP within 10 s of the onset of maximal exercise. At its peak glycolysis resynthesizes ATP at about half the rate of resynthesis from PCr.

The first reaction of glycogenolysis is the splitting off of a single glucose molecule. This is catalysed by the enzyme phosphorylase with a product of glucose 1-phosphate (G1P) and a glycogen molecule which is one glucose residue shorter than the original. The enzyme phosphoglucomutase rapidly converts the G1P to G6P, which then proceeds down the glycolytic pathway.

The passage of blood glucose into the muscle cell requires a specific transporter protein (GLUT 4) but once it is inside the cell it is phosphorylated to G6P. This step is irreversible in skeletal muscle, therefore trapping the glucose in the cell. It is catalysed

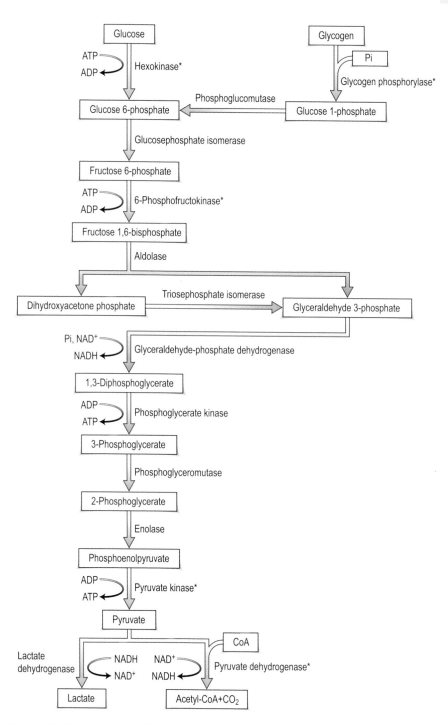

Figure 4.5 The reactions of glycogenolysis and glycolysis; *irreversible reactions. (From Maughan et al 1997, by permission of Oxford University Press.)

by the enzyme hexokinase (HK) but this is an energy-consuming reaction requiring the hydrolysis of one molecule of ATP for each molecule of phosphorylated glucose. During heavy exercise G6P accumulates and inhibits the action of HK, thus limiting the blood glucose contribution to glycolysis and emphasizing the role of glycogenolysis.

Glucose 6-phosphate is converted to fructose 6-phosphate, which is subsequently phosphorylated to fructose 1,6-diphosphate (FDP). The phosphate group is donated by ATP and the reaction is catalysed by phosphofructokinase (PFK). This is a key reaction in the glycolytic pathway as it normally determines the overall rate at which glycolysis can proceed. At this point, two molecules of ATP have been invested in glycolysis with no immediate return.

Aldolase splits FDP into two interconvertible three carbon molecules and each of the subsequent steps in glycolysis can be considered to occur in duplicate. Further metabolism occurs only through glyceraldehyde 3-phosphate, which is converted to 1,3-diphosphoglyceric acid (1,3-DPG) in a reaction involving the conversion of the oxidized form of nicotinamide adenine dinucleotide (NAD^+) to its reduced form NADH and the release of a hydrogen ion (H^+). A phosphate group is transferred from 1,3-DPG to ADP and a molecule of ATP is resynthesized. 1,3-DPG is converted to 3-phosphoglycerate which is internally reorganized and then dehydrated to form phosphoenolpyruvate (PEP) catalysed by enolase. In the presence of pyruvate kinase (PK) the phosphate group from PEP is transferred to ADP, forming ATP and pyruvate. The end product of glycolysis is therefore the conversion of one molecule of glucose to two molecules of pyruvate with the formation of two molecules of ATP. With glycogen as the starting point, three molecules of ATP are resynthesized for each molecule of glucose degraded.

The conversion of glyceraldehyde 3-phosphate to 1,3-DPG relies on the reduction of NAD^+ to NADH and the release of H^+. However, the amount of NAD^+ in the muscle cell is limited and if NADH is not reoxidized to NAD^+ at an equal rate to its production glycolysis will be unable to proceed. One mechanism to replenish NAD^+ involves the transport of pyruvate across the mitochondrial membrane where it is converted to acetyl coenzyme A (acetyl CoA) in a reaction catalysed by pyruvate dehydrogenase (PDH). Subsequent oxidative metabolism to carbon dioxide and water regenerates NAD^+, which is transported by substrate shuttles from the mitochondria to the cytoplasm to support glycolysis.

When the demand for energy is high, the rate of glycolysis and therefore the rate of production of NADH exceeds the maximum rate at which the oxidative system can supply NAD^+, and an anaerobic mechanism is required. This is provided by the reduction of pyruvate (CH_3COCOO^-) to lactate ($CH_3CH(OH)COO^-$), catalysed by lactate dehydrogenase (LDH), which regenerates NAD^+ and enables the continuation of glycolysis:

$$CH_3COCOO^- + NADH + H^+ \rightarrow CH_3CH(OH)COO^- + NAD^+$$

As glycolysis proceeds, lactate accumulates within the muscle and some will diffuse into the extracellular space and into the blood where it is often measured and used as an index of glycolytic activity. Blood lactate concentration does not, however, directly reflect muscle lactate as it is a function of several processes including muscle production, muscle consumption, rate of diffusion into the blood and rate of removal from the blood. In the muscle, the build-up of lactate is accompanied by an increasing acidosis (reduction in pH) which inhibits the activity of PFK, interferes with the muscle contractile mechanism, and stimulates the free nerve endings in the muscle giving rise to the painful sensations that accompany high intensity exercise of long duration.

Regulation of glycogenolysis and glycolysis

The energy supply within each muscle cell must be matched exactly to the energy demand and this requires precise regulation of the rate of glycolysis. The mechanisms are complex but the control of glycolysis is achieved through the coordination of factors which affect the activity of key enzymes.

At the entry points of glycogenolysis and glycolysis lie the enzymes phosphorylase and HK. Phosphorylase exists in two forms which are designated phosphorylase *a* and phosphorylase *b*. Phosphorylase *a* is the active form of the enzyme and its activity is enhanced in the presence of adrenaline. However, phosphorylase *a* will only result in a high rate of glycogenolysis if the intracellular concentration of calcium is above a certain threshold. As calcium is also necessary to initiate muscle contraction this ensures a close coupling between muscle activity and energy supply. It enables a rapid increase in anaerobic glycogenolysis when required but prevents a wasteful breakdown of glycogen when it is not needed. Hexokinase is stimulated by Pi but inhibited by G6P. When glycogen degradation is rapid, G6P concentration rises, inhibits HK and slows the entry of blood glucose into the glycolytic pathway. On the other hand, following carbohydrate feeding, insulin levels rise, inhibit the activity of phosphorylase and promote glycogen storage.

The reaction catalysed by PFK is the rate-limiting reaction in the glycolytic pathway and central to the regulation of glycolysis. Phosphofructokinase activity is stimulated by the high levels of ADP and AMP and inhibited by high levels of ATP and PCr. Citrate accumulation inhibits PFK and provides a means of integrating anaerobic glycolysis and oxidative metabolism. Other potential PFK activators include Pi and NH_3 and this stimulation may help to overcome the inhibitory effects of acidosis (H^+) on PFK. Phosphofructokinase inhibition causes the accumulation of G6P, which in turn inhibits HK activity and reduces the entry of glucose into the muscle cell. The factors that affect PFK, particularly levels of ATP, PCr and ADP, also regulate PK.

Pyruvate dehydrogenase is a complex of three enzymes which exist in active and inactive forms and control mechanisms are not fully understood. It appears, however, that increases in the concentration of pyruvate and of calcium, a rise in the NADH/NAD^+ ratio, a decrease in the ATP/ADP ratio and a decrease in the acetyl CoA/free CoA ratio all increase the activity of the PDH complex.

Oxidative metabolism

Oxidative metabolism is relatively slow to adapt to the demands of exercise and the time constant of the response to heavy exercise is about 25 s. The rate at which ATP can be resynthesized is aerobically much slower than that of anaerobic ATP resynthesis but oxidative metabolism can use carbohydrates, free fatty acids (FFAs) and even amino acids as substrates, although protein catabolism contributes less than 5% of energy provision during exercise. Oxidative metabolism therefore has a much greater capacity for energy generation than anaerobic pathways and although it makes a relatively minor contribution during short-term high intensity exercise the contribution to ATP provision gradually increases with time and the oxidative contribution is dominant during exercise of longer than 90 s duration. Adults' lipid stores are sufficiently large to fuel 30 marathons.

Substrate utilization during submaximal exercise is dependent on a number of factors including exercise duration, diet, level of conditioning and the relative intensity of the exercise. In general, muscle glycogen is the principal fuel during the early stages of submaximal exercise but as time progresses FFAs become the main energy source for exercise below the lactate threshold (T_{LAC}). If the relative intensity of the exercise increases, the contribution of FFAs falls and carbohydrates become the dominant energy substrate.

Several hormones influence the interplay between carbohydrate and lipid availability and utilization. The catecholamines (adrenaline and noradrenaline), growth hormone and cortisol promote lipolysis and increase the availability of blood FFAs, whereas insulin inhibits lipolysis and increases lipid synthesis. Insulin increases the uptake of glucose from the blood, inhibits the release of glucose from the liver, and promotes the synthesis of glycogen in both liver and muscle. Glucagon antagonizes the actions of insulin and raises the blood glucose level by increasing the rate of glycogenolysis in the liver and promoting the formation of glucose from non-carbohydrate precursors in the liver. The catecholamines stimulate glycogenolysis in the liver and the increase in adrenaline in response to exercise plays a major role in activating phosphorylase and stimulating glycogenolysis in skeletal muscles.

Oxidative carbohydrate metabolism

The initial step of oxidative carbohydrate metabolism is the entry of pyruvate into the mitochondria. During a reaction which reduces NAD^+ to NADH in the presence of PDH, each pyruvate molecule is attached to a molecule of CoA and, at the same time, one of the carbon atoms is lost as carbon dioxide (CO_2), creating acetyl CoA. Acetyl CoA then enters the tricarboxylic acid cycle (TCA), where it combines with a four carbon molecule, oxaloacetate, to form citrate, a six carbon tricarboxylic acid. A series of reactions, described in Figure 4.6, lead to the sequential loss of H^+ and CO_2 and the regeneration of oxaloacetate.

Citrate is converted via its isomer isocitrate to α-ketoglutarate and during this reaction, catalysed by isocitrate dehydrogenase (ICDH), NAD^+ is reduced to NADH and a molecule of CO_2 is released. α-Ketoglutarate undergoes oxidative decarboxylation to form succinyl CoA another NADH molecule is formed and a further molecule of CO_2 is released. Succinyl CoA forms succinate and in the process guanosine diphosphate (GDP) is phosphorylated to guanosine triphosphate (GTP). Nucleotide diphosphate kinase catalyses the resynthesis of a molecule of ATP by transferring the terminal phosphate group of GTP to ADP. Succinate is oxidized to fumarate by succinic dehydrogenase (SDH) and in the process flavin adenine dinucleotide (FAD) is reduced to $FADH_2$. The enzyme fumarase catalyses the hydration of fumarate to form malate, which is subsequently oxidized by the enzyme malate dehydrogenase to form oxaloacetate with the reduction of another molecule of NAD^+ to NADH.

One complete turn of the TCA cycle therefore produces one molecule of ATP, three molecules of NADH and one molecule of $FADH_2$ but remember that each molecule of glucose generates two molecules of acetyl CoA.

NADH and $FADH_2$ are energy-rich molecules because they each contain a pair of electrons that have a high energy transfer potential. These electrons are transferred to O_2 via a series of carriers located on the inner mitochondrial membrane and known as the electron transport chain (ETC). The energy liberated during the process is used to phosphorylate ADP to ATP. Each molecule of NADH that enters the ETC generates three molecules of ATP and, as $FADH_2$ exists at a lower energy state than NADH, each molecule of $FADH_2$ generates two molecules of ATP. At the end of the ETC H^+ combines with O_2 to form water and prevent acidification.

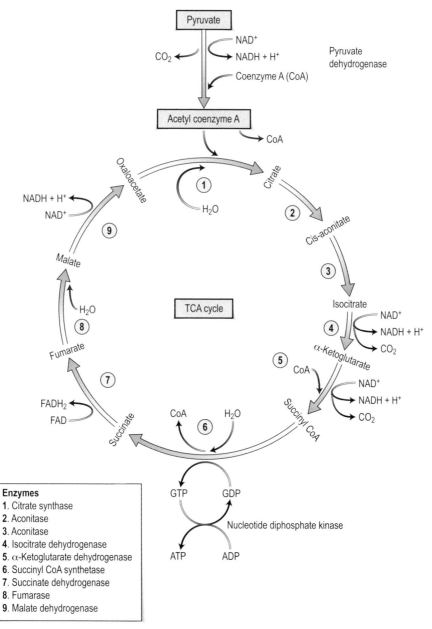

Figure 4.6 The reactions of the tricarboxylic acid cycle. (From Maughan et al 1997, by permission of Oxford University Press.)

The ATP yield from the aerobic catabolism of glucose is described in Table 4.2 but it can be summarized as follows:

Glucose + $6O_2$ + 38ADP + 38Pi → $6CO_2$ + $6H_2O$ + 38ATP

Table 4.2   The ATP yield from the aerobic catabolism of glucose

Glycolysis		Glycogenolysis
−1 ATP	(hexokinase reaction)	
−1 ATP	(phosphofructokinase reaction)	−1 ATP
+2 ATP	(phosphoglycerate kinase reaction)	+2 ATP
+2 ATP	(pyruvate kinase reaction)	+2 ATP
	Tricarboxylic acid cycle	
+6 ATP	(mitochondrial oxidation of cytoplasmic NADH)	+6 ATP
+24 ATP	(mitochondrial oxidation of mitochondrial NADH)	+24 ATP
+4 ATP	(mitochondrial oxidation of mitochondrial $FADH_2$)	+4 ATP
+2 ATP	(nucleotide diphosphate kinase reaction)	+2 ATP
Total		*Total*
+38 ATP		+39 ATP

Regulation of the tricarboxylic acid cycle

The rate of flux through the TCA cycle is regulated by substrate availability, inhibition by accumulating products and feedback inhibition of early enzymes by late intermediates in the cycle so that optimal concentrations of ATP and NADH are sustained.

It appears that there are three key regulatory enzymes. The CS reaction is inhibited by low levels of acetyl CoA and oxaloacetate. An increase in the $NADH/NAD^+$ ratio inhibits the reactions catalysed by ICDH and α-ketoglutarate dehydrogenase. Product accumulation inhibits all three rate-limiting steps in the cycle. Succinyl CoA inhibits α-ketoglutarate dehydrogenase and CS, citrate blocks CS, and ATP inhibits both CS and ICDH. Adenosine triphosphate inhibition is relieved by ADP and calcium activates both ICDH and α-ketoglutarate dehydrogenase.

Lipid metabolism

Lipids are stored in the body as triglycerides and provide a much larger reservoir of energy-generating substrate than carbohydrates. The vast majority of triglyceride is stored in adipose tissue although a small amount is contained in skeletal muscles. Triglyceride is mobilized as an energy source through lipolysis catalysed by lipase. Each molecule of trigyceride is broken down into three molecules of free fatty acids (FFAs) and one molecule of glycerol. Both FFAs and glycerol are transported in the blood and the uptake of FFA by skeletal muscle is directly related to the plasma FFA concentration.

Free fatty acids are transported into the muscle cell by facilitated diffusion which only occurs if the intracellular FFA concentration is less than that in solution in the extracellular fluid. On entry into the muscle cell the FFAs are converted to fatty acyl CoA molecules through the action of ATP-linked fatty acyl CoA synthetase. The fatty acyl CoA molecules move across the mitochondrial outer and inner membrane through the action of carnitine acyltransferase. Once released into the mitochondria, fatty acyl CoA undergoes a series of reactions called β-oxidation. At each reaction the fatty acid chain experiences the removal of a molecule of acetyl CoA and two pairs of hydrogen atoms. The acetyl CoA enters the TCA cycle and the pairs of hydrogen atoms enter the ETC.

lactate. The reduction of pyruvate to lactate results in an accumulation of lactate in muscle although, as lactate may be produced in some muscle fibres whilst being simultaneously consumed in others, the net lactate output of muscle does not directly reflect muscle production. Eriksson & Saltin (1974) reported muscle lactate concentrations following a peak $\dot{V}O_2$ test as 8.8, 10.7, 11.3 and 15.3 mmol · kg^{-1} wet weight for boys aged 11.6, 12.6, 13.5 and 15.5 years, respectively, suggesting an age-dependency of lactate production.

Lactate diffuses into the blood, where it is removed by oxidation in the heart or skeletal muscles or is converted to glucose through gluconeogenesis in the liver. The lactate measured in blood therefore reflects all those processes by which lactate is produced and eliminated. Consequently, blood lactate provides only a qualitative indication of the degree of stress placed on anaerobic metabolism by a bout of exercise, not a precise measure of glycolytic activity. Nevertheless, due to ethical restraints paediatric exercise physiologists have looked to blood lactate accumulation to provide a window into muscle lactate production.

The assessment and interpretation of blood lactate accumulation as a measure of aerobic fitness is considered in detail in Chapter 8 and the blood lactate response to exercise will only be summarized here.

At the onset of moderate exercise, there are minimal changes in blood lactate with rate of diffusion into blood being matched by rate of removal from blood. As exercise intensity progressively increases, a point is reached where blood lactate levels begin to rise rapidly with a subsequent steep rise until exhaustion (see Fig. 8.3). The point at which blood lactate increases non-linearly is referred to as the lactate threshold (T_{LAC}). The maximal lactate steady state (MLSS) defines the exercise intensity that can be maintained without incurring a further accumulation of blood lactate and it therefore represents the highest point at which diffusion of lactate into the blood and removal from the blood are in equilibrium. Exercise above the MLSS results in a steady increase in blood lactate until terminated by exhaustion.

Young people accumulate less blood lactate than adults during submaximal exercise. There is a negative correlation between T_{LAC} as a percentage of peak $\dot{V}O_2$ and age from childhood to adulthood and but there is no convincing evidence to relate MLSS to age. Blood lactate concentrations following maximal 'aerobic' tests (peak $\dot{V}O_2$) and maximal 'anaerobic' tests (e.g. WAnT) are consistently higher in adults than in children. Several studies have examined specific relationships between measures of maturity and blood lactate accumulation but there is no strong evidence to support an independent effect of maturity on exercise-driven blood lactate concentration (Welsman & Armstrong 1998). Children's lower blood lactates are, however, in accord with the lower levels of LDH that have been reported (Berg & Keul 1988, Kaczor et al 2005).

Pianosi and colleagues (1995) monitored blood pyruvate and lactate concentrations at rest, immediately after 6 min of cycling exercise at one third and at two thirds of maximal work capacity, and 20 min post-exercise. Twenty-eight volunteers were divided into three groups: 7- to 10-year-olds ($n = 6$), 11 to 14-year-olds ($n = 12$) and 15- to 17-year-olds ($n = 10$). Post-exercise blood lactate concentration and the lactate/pyruvate ratio were correlated with age but there was no relationship between age and pyruvate concentration. Following exercise at two thirds of maximum, blood lactate concentration increased out of proportion to that of pyruvate such that the lactate/pyruvate ratio rose in an age-related manner. This suggests that the greater increase in exercise-driven blood lactate in the older subjects is related more to a better glycolytic function than a compromised oxidative capacity.

Substrate utilization

The relative contribution of lipid and carbohydrate as energy substrates can be estimated from the ratio $\dot{V}CO_2/\dot{V}O_2$ (the respiratory exchange ratio, R) measured at the mouth, during submaximal exercise. An R of 1.00 indicates that the fuel is exclusively carbohydrate and a value of 0.7 indicates 100% lipid utilization. Research findings are equivocal and interpretation is often difficult due to the different modes of exercise employed. For example, Rowland & Rimany (1995) observed no significant differences in R between 9- to 13-year-old girls and 20- to 31-year-old women during 40 min cycling at 63% peak $\dot{V}O_2$, whereas Martinez & Haymes (1992) reported significantly lower R values in 8- to 10-year-old girls than in 20- to 32-year-old women during 30 min treadmill running at 70% peak $\dot{V}O_2$. Boisseau & Delamarche (2000) extensively reviewed published studies and concluded that, despite conflicting reports, the data indicate greater lipid utilization during submaximal exercise in young people than in adults.

Other studies have been founded on blood concentrations of glucose, FFAs and glycerol. No clear blood glucose concentration differences with age have been reported during exercise. Data comparing blood FFA and glycerol concentrations between children and adults are equivocal but the work of Delamarche, Berg and their collaborators suggests that, on balance, there exists an age-dependent preference for lipid utilization, with children having higher FFA oxidation than adults during exercise (Berg & Keul 1988, Boisseau & Delamarche 2000).

Timmons et al (2003) used ^{13}C stable isotope methodology to compare substrate utilization between twelve 9-year-old boys and ten 22-year-old men during cycling exercise at a similar relative exercise intensity (70% peak $\dot{V}O_2$). They observed that compared to the men, the boys utilized about 70% more fat and about 23% less carbohydrate and commented that the higher fat oxidation in boys may be a default mechanism due to an underdeveloped glycogenolytic and/or glycolytic system.

Hormonal responses

Insulin increases the uptake of glucose by the muscles, promotes the synthesis of glycogen, inhibits lipolysis and increases lipid synthesis; therefore it has been speculated that age-dependent changes in blood insulin concentration might influence metabolic characteristics. Supporting data are, however, not convincing. In one of the most comprehensive studies, Wirth et al (1978) determined the blood insulin, FFA and glucose concentrations of prepubertal, pubertal and postpubertal boys and girls at rest and in the 15 min of an exercise test at 70% peak $\dot{V}O_2$ on a cycle ergometer. They observed that insulin levels increased during exercise in the prepubertal children, remained constant in pubertal individuals and decreased in the postpubertal groups. However, neither glucose nor FFA concentrations changed during exercise and differences between sexes or stages of maturity were not present.

The catecholamines stimulate glycogenolysis, glycolysis and lipolysis and any developmental differences would be expected to affect the rate of glycolytic and TCA cycle activity. Few data are available and they are both inconsistent and confounded by the wide intra-individual variability of circulating catecholamine levels. Resting levels of adrenaline have been reported to fall with age and stage of maturation in some studies, whereas others have reported no differences between children and adults (Berg & Keul 1988). During intense exercise catecholamine levels rise in both children and adults and the balance of evidence suggests that exhaustive exercise induces a lower sympathetic response in young people than in adults. The evidence is too scant to permit firm conclusions but, following their review of the literature, Berg & Keul (1988) suggested that reduced maximum sympathetic activity causes a reduced maximum anaerobic capacity in children.

^{31}P magnetic resonance spectroscopy

Magnetic resonance spectroscopy (MRS) holds the potential to revolutionize our understanding of children's exercise metabolism as it provides, in real time and in vivo, a non-invasive window into muscle metabolism during exercise. The safety of the technique for human research is well documented and as no ionizing radiation or injected labelling agents are involved it represents an ideal technique for quantifying aspects of bioenergetics in children.

Magnetic resonance spectroscopy studies are, however, constrained by the need to exercise within a small-bore tube and the requirement that the acquisition of data be synchronized with the rate of muscle contraction. With young children this can be problematic and the construction of a to-scale replica scanner which allows the children to overcome any fears of exercising within a tube is a useful tool in studies of this type. The children can practise matching the up–down movement of the leg to moving vertical bars thrown onto a visual display without using expensive magnet time. In a typical MR scanner, the software driving the rhythmic movement incorporates signals from a non-magnetic ergometer to record changes in work done, power output, leg stroke frequency and stroke height during exercise. With the subject lying either prone or supine within the magnet the field is activated. The nuclei of atoms align with the magnetic field, then an additional oscillating magnetic field is applied and the subsequent nuclear transitions allow spectral analysis of the interrogated muscle(s). Different molecules produce their own spectra and once the molecules have been identified any changes in the spectral lines can be interpreted. The nucleus used most extensively for metabolic studies is ^{31}P, the naturally occurring phosphorus nucleus. ^{31}P magnetic resonance spectroscopy enables ATP, PCr and Pi, the metabolites which play a central role in bioenergetics, to be monitored. Typical ^{31}P MRS spectra obtained during rest, exercise and recovery are illustrated in Figure 4.7 where, from left to right, the peaks represent free inorganic phosphate (Pi), the single phosphorus of PCr and the three phosphorus nuclei of ATP. The decline in PCr and the corresponding rise in Pi with incremental exercise are clearly evident. The shift in the Pi peak towards the PCr reflects the acidification of the muscle, and the change in pH which can be calculated reflects muscle glycolytic activity although it is not a direct measure of glycolysis.

The spectra can be analysed to show changes in metabolites and acidity during incremental exercise and the intracellular thresholds (ITs) can be determined from plots of the ratio of Pi/PCr against power output and pH against power output as shown in Figure 4.8. Intracellular thresholds for Pi/PCr show good reliability during thigh muscle exercise with typical errors across three trials of 10% with prepubertal children.

Few studies have used ^{31}P MRS techniques to compare the exercise metabolism of young people and adults (Kuno et al 1995, Taylor et al 1997, Zanconato et al 1993). The data have provided valuable insights but must be interpreted in the light of methodological concerns regarding small, mixed age and/or sex participant groups, varying exercise protocols, no measures of maturation and, in some studies, inappropriate

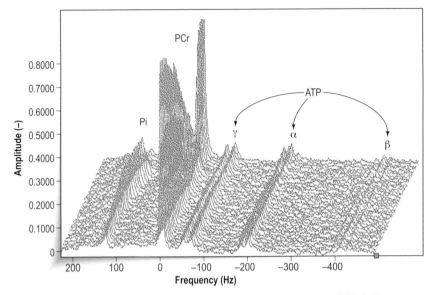

Figure 4.7   ³¹P magnetic resonance spectra obtained from a 9-year-old child during rest, exercise and recovery. From left to right the peaks represent free organic phosphate, phosphocreatine and the three phosphorus nuclei of adenosine triphosphate.

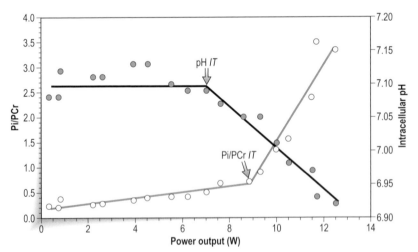

Figure 4.8   pH and Pi/PCr ratio in relation to power output determined in the quadriceps muscle of a 9-year-old child during exercise in the magnet. The intracellular threshold (IT) is indicated.

data normalization techniques. Taylor and Zanconato and their colleagues used a treadle ergometer to exercise the calf muscles and this technique has some method-ological limitations when applied to children. The small size of the calf muscles in children leads to a lower signal to noise ratio and hence more difficulty in curve fitting the spectra. In combination with the small size, the known heterogeneous metabolic composition of the gastrocnemius and the soleus muscles represents a potential source of error in any studies comparing individuals of different size. The soleus is composed mainly of type I and the gastrocnemius of type II fibres so if there are varying amounts of soleus and gastrocnemius in the area of muscle being interrogated this may bias the interpretation of metabolic responses.

The first ^{31}P MRS exercise study to include children was carried out by Zanconato et al (1993) with 8 boys and 2 girls, aged 7 to 10 years, and 5 men and 3 women, aged 20 to 42 years, who underwent a supine, progressive exercise to volitional fatigue. A slow phase and a fast phase of Pi/PCr increase and pH decrease (as illustrated in Fig. 4.8) were detected in 75% of the adults and 50% of the children. The characteristics of the initial slopes in Pi/PCr and pH were similar in children and adults, but following the intracellular threshold, the incline in Pi/PCr and decline in pH were both steeper in adults than in children. The final pH observed in adults was significantly lower than in children, whose end-exercise Pi/PCr was only 27% of adult values.

These findings suggest a similar rate of mitochondrial oxidative metabolism during low intensity exercise but the different responses in Pi/PCr ratio and pH during high intensity exercise strongly indicate superior glycolytic activity in adults. The data were subsequently supported by a study of 14 trained and 23 untrained 12- to 17-year-olds and 6 adults which reported lower values of pH and higher Pi/PCr ratio in adults at exhaustion but no significant difference between the trained and untrained adolescents (Kuno et al 1995).

As part of a study of ageing effects on skeletal muscle function, Taylor et al (1997) compared the ^{31}P MRS spectra of fifteen 6- to 12-year-olds with twenty 20- to 29-year-olds at rest, during and following exercise. They found, in accordance with Eriksson's (1980) biopsy studies, a lower ratio of PCr/ATP in the children at rest. The children had a higher pH during exercise, indicating a lower glycolytic contribution to metabolism and a faster resynthesis of PCr during recovery than adults. As PCr resynthesis is O_2 dependent they concluded that oxidative capacity is higher during childhood than in young adulthood.

Peterson and co-workers (1998) focused on maturational differences in exercise metabolism and compared the responses to 2 min of submaximal (40% maximal work capacity, MWC) followed by 2 min of supramaximal (140% MWC) exercise of nine prepubertal 10-year-old girls and nine pubertal 15-year-old girls. All the girls were trained swimmers. At the end of exercise, muscle pH was lower and the Pi/PCr ratio was 66% higher in the pubertal girls but the differences were not found to be statistically significant. The results indicate that glycolytic metabolism is not maturity dependent but the magnitude of the difference in the Pi/PCr ratio and the small sample sizes suggest that the difference between the two groups may have biological meaning and might have been significant with larger sample sizes.

Oxygen uptake kinetics

A high degree of rigour is required to elucidate $\dot{V}O_2$ kinetics in children and these methodological issues are considered in detail in Chapter 9. Here we will briefly summarize the characteristics of $\dot{V}O_2$ kinetics and focus specifically on insights into paediatric exercise metabolism which have been provided by recent studies of young people's $\dot{V}O_2$ kinetic responses to moderate and heavy exercise (Barstow & Schuermann 2004, Fawkner & Armstrong 2004a, 2004b).

Moderate exercise

The moderate exercise domain encompasses all exercise intensities below T_{LAC} and is characterized by three phases (see Fig. 9.2). At the onset of constant intensity exercise there is an almost immediate increase in cardiac output which occurs prior to the arrival at the lungs of venous blood from the exercising muscles. Phase 1 is therefore independent of O_2 consumption at the muscles and is predominantly a reflection of the increase in pulmonary blood flow with exercise. Phase 2, the primary component, is a rapid exponential increase in $\dot{V}O_2$ that develops as a result of an additional effect of the increased O_2 extraction in the blood perfusing the exercising muscles. The speed of the phase 2 $\dot{V}O_2$ kinetics is described by the time constant (τ) which is the time taken to reach 63% of the change in $\dot{V}O_2$. The subsequent steady state which occurs within about 2 min is phase 3. During cycling exercise, $\dot{V}O_2$ increases to the steady-state value with a gain of about $10 \text{ mL} \cdot \text{min}^{-1} \cdot \text{W}^{-1}$ above that found during unloaded pedalling. This is the O_2 cost of the exercise.

During phases 1 and 2, ATP resynthesis cannot be met fully by the $\dot{V}O_2$ and the additional requirements of the exercise are met primarily by recycling of ATP from PCr with minor contributions from O_2 stores and glycolysis. The O_2 equivalent of these energy sources is known as the O_2 deficit and the faster the τ the smaller the O_2 deficit.

The $\dot{V}O_2$ kinetic response to moderate exercise is significantly faster in children compared with adults, resulting in a smaller absolute and relative O_2 deficit. Age-related effects on the phase 2 gain are equivocal but the balance of evidence indicates that a greater O_2 cost of exercise is found in children than in adults. There are no sex differences in children's $\dot{V}O_2$ kinetic responses to moderate exercise.

Children's faster τ and therefore lower contribution to ATP resynthesis from anaerobic sources during the non-steady state may be due to a more efficient O_2 delivery system, a greater relative capacity for O_2 utilization or both. There is no strong evidence to suggest that delivery of O_2 to the mitochondria is enhanced in children compared with adults or that increased availability of O_2 to the working muscles speeds $\dot{V}O_2$ kinetics during moderate exercise. The faster τ and smaller relative O_2 deficit therefore suggest that children have better mitochondrial capacity for oxidative phosphorylation than adults.

Heavy exercise

The heavy exercise domain falls between T_{LAC} and MLSS although some investigators prefer to use critical power as the upper criterion of heavy exercise (see Chapter 9). During heavy exercise, glycolysis makes a larger contribution to the O_2 deficit than during moderate exercise but over time blood lactate accumulation is stable. The phase 2 gain is similar to that observed during moderate exercise but within 2–3 min of the beginning of exercise a slow component of $\dot{V}O_2$ kinetics is superimposed upon the primary $\dot{V}O_2$ response and the achievement of a steady state might be delayed by 10 to 15 min (see Fig. 9.2). The mechanisms underlying the slow component $\dot{V}O_2$ are elusive but it appears that over 80% of the additional $\dot{V}O_2$ originates from the exercising muscle. Some aspect of either fibre type recruitment patterns (e.g. less efficient type II fibres) and/or fatigue processes within select fibre populations is thought to underlie this phenomenon.

Children have a significantly faster phase 2 τ, smaller O_2 deficit and higher O_2 cost of exercise during the primary component than adults. Even prepubertal children exhibit a slow component of $\dot{V}O_2$ but it is smaller than that of adults and increases with age. In contrast to moderate exercise, boys have a faster phase 2 τ than girls during exercise above T_{LAC} and the slow component contribution to the total change in $\dot{V}O_2$ amplitude during exercise is greater in girls.

The greater O_2 cost of the exercise during phase 2 and faster τ of children during exercise above T_{LAC} suggest an enhanced oxidative function during childhood. The higher O_2 cost of exercise during the primary component may be indicative of a higher percentage of type I fibres in children as, in adults, the ratio of type I/type II muscle fibres has been demonstrated to be positively related to the O_2 cost of exercise. Preferential recruitment of type I fibres by children would also help to explain the increase in amplitude of the slow component of $\dot{V}O_2$ with age.

Why there are sex differences in the primary τ above but not below T_{LAC} is not readily apparent. At exercise intensities above T_{LAC} O_2 delivery may play a more prominent role in limiting $\dot{V}O_2$ kinetics and boys may have a faster cardiac output response than girls at the onset of exercise. Alternatively, some studies with adults have reported negative correlations between percentage of type I fibres and the primary τ and slow component of $\dot{V}O_2$ during heavy exercise but no relationship between τ and percentage of type I fibres during moderate exercise. If boys have a greater percentage of type I fibres than girls this would be consistent with the extant literature.

Recovery studies

Recovery from high intensity exercise is addressed in the following chapter but the model of intermittent dynamic exercise with limited recovery periods has provided some relevant indicators of adult–child differences in metabolic responses which we will address here.

Ratel and his colleagues (2002, 2004) have published a series of studies of high intensity, intermittent exercise in which they have consistently demonstrated that during this type of activity short-term power output and/or running velocity is dependent on age, mode of exercise and time allowed for recovery. For example, during 10 maximal 10 s cycling sprints 10-year-old boys were able to sustain their PP with only 30 s recovery intervals. In contrast, 15-year-old boys and 20-year-old men required a 5 min recovery period. When 11-year-old boys and 22-year-old men performed 10 consecutive maximal 10 s sprints with 15 s recovery intervals on both a cycle ergometer and a non-motorized treadmill, the adults displayed a significantly greater decrement in power output compared to the boys on both ergometers. In all exercise models the men experienced a greater increase in blood lactate than the boys.

Research with females is less comprehensive but Chia (2001) has reported a lower decrement in power output in 13-year-old girls than in adult women over a series of three 15 s maximal cycling exercises separated by 45 s.

The factors underlying the greater ability of children to resist fatigue are not understood fully but potential mechanisms include muscle mass, muscle morphology, energy metabolism and neuromuscular activation. Here we will focus on muscle fibre type and energy metabolism.

At high glycolytic rates, muscle lactate content rises to high levels and the associated increase in acidity is often implicated as a cause of fatigue. If children place a lower reliance on glycolysis during very heavy exercise this would offer a distinct advantage in resisting fatigue. Similarly, if children have a higher percentage of type I fibres than adolescents or adults this would partly explain age differences in fatigability.

However, in exercise protocols involving repeated short bouts of high intensity exercise interspersed with limited rest periods, the key factor in maintaining short-term power output is likely to be the resynthesis of PCr. PCr is resynthesized by oxidative phosphorylation and the initial rate of PCr recovery is controlled by the rate of mitochondrial ATP synthesis. Following this fast stage of recovery of PCr is a slower phase which can be inhibited by increased acidity and may have a τ of up to 240 s. The initial stage of PCr recovery is therefore a measure of oxidative capacity whereas the slow component is affected by the build-up of H^+ ions. In a ^{31}P MRS study, Taylor et al (1997) reported the τ of the fast component of PCr resynthesis to be 17 s in 6- to 12-year-olds compared with 39 s in young adults.

SUMMARY

The view we have of young people's exercise metabolism is limited by ethical and methodological constraints but evidence from several methodologies provides a consistent, but incomplete, picture:

- Muscle biopsy studies (fibre types): indicate that the percentage of type I fibres in the vastus lateralis decrease in sedentary to moderately active individuals between the ages of 10 and 35 years.
- Muscle biopsy studies (energy stores): demonstrate that resting ATP stores are invariant with age but PCr and glycogen stores progressively increase from childhood into adolescence.
- Muscle biopsy studies (enzyme activity): suggest that prepubertal children have higher oxidative enzyme activity and lower glycolytic enzyme activity than adolescents. The evidence indicating that the glycolytic activity of adolescents is less than that of adults is equivocal but data showing that the ratio of PFK/ICDH activity is 1.633 in adults and 0.844 in adolescents suggest that the TCA as compared to glycolysis functions at a higher rate in adolescents than in adults.
- Lactate production: sparse data show muscle lactate production following maximal exercise to increase with age. In accord with their lower LDH activity, young people accumulate less blood lactate than adults during both submaximal and maximal exercise. The blood lactate/pyruvate ratio has been reported to rise with exercise in an age-related manner, indicating greater glycolytic activity in adults.
- Substrate utilization: data collected across several methodologies show an age-dependent preference for lipid utilization, with children demonstrating greater FFA oxidation than adults during submaximal exercise.
- Hormonal responses: exhaustive exercise induces a lower sympathetic response in young people than adults, supporting a reduced anaerobic capacity in children.
- ^{31}P MRS studies: monitoring the Pi/PCr ratio and pH during progressive exercise to voluntary exhaustion shows a similar rate of mitochondrial oxidative metabolism between children and adults during low intensity exercise but superior glycolytic activity in adults during heavy exercise. A significantly faster resynthesis of PCr following maximal exercise demonstrates a higher oxidative capacity during childhood than in young adulthood.
- $\dot{V}O_2$ kinetics studies: children's faster primary time constant, greater O_2 cost of exercise and smaller slow component of $\dot{V}O_2$ suggest the presence of an enhanced oxidative function and/or a greater percentage of type I muscle fibres during childhood.

- Recovery studies: demonstrate the greater ability of children than adults to resist fatigue during bouts of intermittent high intensity exercise interspersed with limited recovery periods. This phenomenon can be partly explained by children's ability to resynthesize PCr during recovery periods faster than adults. As the initial phase of PCr resynthesis is O_2 dependent, a higher oxidative capacity in young people is indicated.

The weight of evidence clearly indicates an interplay of anaerobic and aerobic exercise metabolism in which children have a relatively higher oxidative capacity than adolescents or adults. There is a progressive increase in glycolytic activity with age at least into adolescence and possibly into young adulthood.

KEY POINTS

1. The age-related increase in anaerobic and aerobic fitness is not synchronous and untrained children experience a more marked increase in anaerobic fitness than aerobic fitness during adolescence.
2. For exercise to be sustained for more than a few seconds ATP must be resynthesized. The resynthesis of ATP is brought about by an interplay of anaerobic and aerobic metabolism.
3. The energy-providing systems are finely regulated so that they can rapidly respond to the demands of exercise of different intensities and durations.
4. Muscle biopsy data from children are sparse but they have provided valuable insights into age-related changes in the proportion of type I muscle fibres, stores of ATP, PCr and glycogen, and the activity of key anaerobic and aerobic enzymes. It appears that the percentage of type I fibres decreases with age, PCr and glycogen stores increase with age, and the TCA cycle as compared to glycolysis functions at a higher rate in children and adolescents than in adults.
5. Blood lactate provides a qualitative indication of the degree of stress placed on anaerobic metabolism by a bout of exercise, not a precise measure of glycolytic activity. Young people accumulate less blood lactate than adults during both submaximal and maximal exercise. Lower blood lactates during youth are in accord with young people's lower levels of LDH.
6. Studies investigating substrate utilization during exercise have employed a range of methodologies including monitoring stable isotopes, respiratory exchange ratios, and blood concentrations of metabolites. Data are equivocal but the balance of evidence indicates an age-dependent preference for lipid utilization, with children having higher FFA oxidation than adults during exercise.
7. ^{31}P MRS has the potential to revolutionize our understanding of young people's exercise metabolism but studies are constrained by the need to exercise within a small-bore tube. Data are sparse but show superior glycolytic activity in adults and a higher oxidative capacity in children.
8. Oxygen uptake kinetics provide a non-invasive window into the muscle. Few studies have investigated children's $\dot{V}O_2$ kinetics but their faster τ and smaller O_2 deficits during the primary phase of both moderate and heavy exercise suggest that children have better mitochondrial capacity for oxidative phosphorylation than adults. This is supported by children's greater O_2 cost of exercise during phase 2 of the $\dot{V}O_2$ kinetic response.
9. During a series of repeated short-duration, high intensity exercises interspersed with limited recovery periods children have a greater ability to resist fatigue than

adults. Potential explanatory mechanisms include muscle mass, muscle morphology, energy metabolism and neuromuscular activation. From an energy metabolism perspective, the faster PCr resynthesis by the children suggests that they have a greater oxidative capacity.

10. Evidence from a range of sources strongly suggests that children have a relatively higher oxidative capacity than adolescents or adults and that there is a progressive increase in glycolytic activity during exercise at least into adolescence and possibly into young adulthood.

References

Armstrong N, Welsman J R, Chia M 2001 Short-term power output in relation to growth and maturation. British Journal of Sports Medicine 35:118–125

Bar-Or O, Rowland T W 2004 Pediatric exercise medicine: from physiologic principles to health care application. Human Kinetics, Champaign, IL

Barstow T J, Schuermann B 2004 $\dot{V}O_2$ kinetics effects of maturation and aging. In Jones A M, Poole D C (eds) Oxygen uptake kinetics in sport, exercise and medicine. Routledge, London, p 331–352

Berg A, Keul J 1988 Biochemical changes during exercise in children. In: Malina R M (ed) Young athletes. Human Kinetics Publishers, Champaign, IL, p 61–78

Boisseau N, Delamarche P 2000 Metabolic and hormonal responses to exercise in children and adolescents. Sports Medicine 30:405–422

Chia M 2001 Power recovery in the Wingate anaerobic test in girls and women following prior sprints of short duration. Biology of Sport 18:45–53

du Plessis M P, Smit P J, du Plessis L A et al 1985 The composition of muscle fibers in a group of adolescents. In: Binkhorst R A, Kemper H C G, Saris W H M (eds) Children and exercise XI. University Park Press, Baltimore, p 323–328

Eriksson B O 1980 Muscle metabolism in children – a review. Acta Physiologica Scandinavica 283:20–28

Eriksson B O, Saltin B 1974 Muscle metabolism during exercise in boys aged 11 to 16 years compared to adults. Acta Paediatrica Belgica 28:257–265

Fawkner S G, Armstrong N 2004a Longitudinal changes in the kinetic response to heavy intensity exercise. Journal of Applied Physiology 97:460–466

Fawkner S G, Armstrong N 2004b Sex differences in the oxygen uptake kinetic response to heavy intensity exercise in prepubertal children. European Journal of Applied Physiology 93:210–216

Glenmark B, Hedberg C, Jansson E 1992 Changes in muscle fibre type from adolescence to adulthood in women and men. Acta Physiologica Scandinavica 146:251–259

Haralambie G 1982 Enzyme activities in skeletal muscle of 13–15 year old adolescents. Bulletin Européen de Physiopathologie Respiratoire 18:65–74

Jansson E 1996 Age-related fiber type changes in human skeletal muscle. In: Maughan R J, Shirreffs S M (eds) Biochemistry of exercise IX. Human Kinetics, Champaign, IL, p 297–307

Kaczor J J, Ziolkowski W, Popinigis J, Tarnopolsky M A 2005 Anaerobic and aerobic enzyme activities in human skeletal muscle from children and adults. Pediatric Research 57:331–335

Kuno S, Takahashi H, Fujimoto K et al 1995 Muscle metabolism during exercise using phosphorus-31 nuclear magnetic resonance spectroscopy in adolescents. European Journal of Applied Physiology 70:301–304

Lexell J, Sjostrom M, Nordlund A-S et al 1992 Growth and development of human muscle: a quantitative morphological study of whole vastus lateralis from childhood to adult age. Muscle and Nerve 15:404–409

Martinez L R, Haymes E M 1992 Substrate utilization during treadmill running in prepubertal girls and women. Medicine and Science in Sports and Exercise 24:975–983

Maughan R, Gleeson M, Greenhaff P L 1997 Biochemistry of exercise and training. Oxford University Press, Oxford

Oertel G 1988 Morphometric analysis of normal skeletal muscles in infancy, childhood and adolescence. An autopsy study. Journal of the Neurological Sciences 88:303–313

Peterson S R, Gaul C A, Stanton M M et al 1998 Skeletal muscle metabolism during short-term high intensity exercise in prepubertal and pubertal girls. Journal of Applied Physiology 87:2151–2156

Pianosi P, Seargeant L, Hayworth J C 1995 Blood lactate and pyruvate concentrations, and their ratio during exercise in healthy children: developmental perspective. European Journal of Applied Physiology 71:518–522

Ratel S, Bedu M, Hennegrave A et al 2002 Effects of age and recovery duration on peak power output during repeated cycling sprints. International Journal of Sports Medicine 23:397–402

Ratel S, Williams C A, Oliver J et al 2004 Effects of age and mode of exercise on power output profiles during repeated sprints. European Journal of Applied Physiology 92:204–210

Rowland T W, Rimany T A 1995 Physiological responses to prolonged exercise in premenarcheal and adult females. Pediatric Exercise Science 7:183–191

Taylor D J, Kemp G J, Thompson C H et al 1997 Ageing: effects on oxidative function of skeletal muscle in vivo. Molecular and Cellular Biochemistry 174:321–324

Timmons B W, Bar-Or O, Riddell M C 2003 Oxidation rate of exogenous carbohydrate during exercise is higher in boys than in men. Journal of Applied Physiology 94:278–284

Welsman J, Armstrong N 1998 Assessing post-exercise lactates in children and adolescents. In: Van Praagh E (ed) Pediatric anaerobic performance. Human Kinetics, Champaign, IL, p 137–154

Wirth A, Trager E, Scheele K et al 1978 Cardiopulmonary adjustment and metabolic response to maximal and submaximal physical exercise of boys and girls at different stages of maturity. European Journal of Applied Physiology 39:229–240

Zanconato S, Buchthal S, Barstow T J et al 1993 ^{31}P-magnetic resonance spectroscopy of leg muscle metabolism during exercise in children and adults. Journal of Applied Physiology 74:2214–2218

Further reading

Armstrong N, Welsman J R 1997 Young people and physical activity. Oxford University Press, Oxford

Cooper D M, Barstow T J 1996 Magnetic resonance imaging and spectroscopy in studying exercise in children. Exercise and Sports Sciences Reviews 24:475–499

Fawkner S G, Armstrong N 2003 Oxygen uptake kinetic response to exercise in children. Sports Medicine 33:651–669

Maughan R, Gleeson M, Greenhaff P L 1997 Biochemistry of exercise and training. Oxford University Press, Oxford

Ratel S, Lazaar N, Williams C A et al 2003 Age differences in human skeletal muscle fatigue during high intensity intermittent exercise. Acta Paediatrica 92:1248–1254

Chapter 5

Maximal intensity exercise

Michael Chia and Neil Armstrong

LEARNING OBJECTIVES

After studying this chapter you should be able to:
1. define the principal nomenclature used to describe maximal intensity exercise
2. evaluate laboratory tests used for assessing maximal intensity exercise in children and adolescents
3. clarify the determinants of maximal intensity exercise during growth and maturation
4. discuss the development of anaerobic fitness in relation to sex, age, growth and maturation
5. compare and contrast the recovery in power of adults and adolescents during a series of maximal intensity exercises interspersed with short recovery periods
6. highlight future research directions in the study of maximal intensity exercise during growth and maturation.

INTRODUCTION

Children and adolescents derive their energy for exercise from both aerobic and anaerobic metabolism. The relative energy contributions in fuelling exercise are dependent on the intensity and duration of the physical exertion. For reasons outlined in Table 5.1,

Table 5.1 Why less is known about anaerobic fitness than aerobic fitness

No gold standard for anaerobic fitness comparable to peak oxygen uptake for aerobic fitness

The association between aerobic fitness and health is more apparent

The contribution of aerobic fitness to sport performance is better understood

Measuring anaerobic fitness is more complex than assessing aerobic fitness

Maximal intensity exercise is more strenuous than exercise at peak oxygen uptake

less is known about anaerobic fitness than aerobic fitness of young people but there are merits in studying maximal intensity exercise. First, brief maximal intensity exercise has greater relevance and resemblance to the activity and play patterns of children and adolescents; second, maximal intensity tests are brief and the motivation and attention spans of young people might be better harnessed during assessment; and third, knowledge of the interplay between anaerobic and aerobic fitness during growth and maturation provides a composite picture of the exercising young person.

Alactacid power, lactacid power, anaerobic power, anaerobic capacity, anaerobic work capacity, instantaneous power, peak power, mean power and short-term power are terms commonly and often indiscriminately used to describe non-identical aspects of maximal intensity exercise. Maximal intensity exercise should not be confused with 'maximal exercise' as referred to in a peak $\dot{V}O_2$ test, since the mechanical power elicited during the former is two to four times that elicited during the latter when using cycle ergometry. To differentiate between the two types of exercise, the terms 'maximal intensity exercise' and 'maximal aerobic exercise' will be used in this chapter. Maximal intensity exercise refers to the accomplishment of all-out intensity exercise, where the predominant, though not necessarily exclusive, source of energy is from anaerobic metabolism. Anaerobic fitness is defined as the capability to perform maximal intensity exercise. In essence, the competence to generate the highest mechanical power output over a few seconds (usually less than 5 s) and to sustain high power output over a short period of time (usually less than 60 s) are considered as indicators of anaerobic fitness.

Invasive procedures such as muscle biopsies are necessary for the direct determination of energy turnover during rest and exercise but the procedures are unethical with healthy young people. Non-invasive estimations of energy yield such as those using magnetic resonance spectroscopy are now available but, as discussed in Chapter 4, they are very expensive, not accessible to most researchers, and only limited types of exercise can be performed because of the size limitations of the apparatus. Consequently, researchers are reliant on laboratory tests using apparatus such as cycle ergometers, treadmills and isokinetic dynamometers. These tests usually last between 5 s and 60 s, and participants are verbally encouraged to give a maximal exercise effort throughout the duration of the test. Inevitably, considerations for selecting the appropriate test include the research question being addressed, the characteristics of the participants, and what modifications or customizations of the test protocol are necessary. The next section provides a general overview of maximal intensity exercise tests commonly used in paediatric exercise physiology laboratories.

CYCLE ERGOMETER TESTS

Wingate anaerobic test

The Wingate anaerobic test (WAnT) is the most established and researched test of maximal intensity exercise and the versatility of the test is affirmed by the large base of WAnT data on children and adolescents who are untrained, trained, healthy and diseased (see Inbar et al 1996). In healthy young people, at least two practice trials, using an abbreviated WAnT (i.e. of 15 s duration) and standardized warm-up routine are necessary to minimize any learning effects but the discretion of the researcher is necessary in deciding the amount of test familiarization required before testing is commenced. During the test, participants sprint cycle or arm crank at maximal intensity for 30 s against an applied resistance that is set at a percentage of body mass (usually 0.74 $N \cdot kg^{-1}$ for sprint cycling and 0.49 $N \cdot kg^{-1}$ for arm cranking).

Three indicators of WAnT performance are usually reported:

1. Peak power (PP) in watts (W) – the highest mechanical power output achieved during the test (usually within 5–6 s).
2. Mean mechanical power (MP) – the average mechanical power accomplished during the test (usually over 30 s), which can also be expressed as the total work done in joules (J).
3. A measure of power decline or fatigue index (FI) in %, the difference between the PP and the final power output, expressed as a percentage of PP. The FI, which is less often reported than PP or MP, may be associated with the percentage of muscle fibre type distribution but in young people, this has not been established.

Peak power and MP are generally expressed in absolute terms (W) and/or in relation to body mass or other estimates of body, muscle or limb size using the ratio standard ($W \cdot kg^{-1}$) but recently, WAnT power has been modelled in relation to estimates of body size using allometric techniques. The merits, assumptions and limitations of using these scaling techniques to account for body size in performance during growth and maturation are discussed in Chapter 2.

Data on the reliability and validity of the WAnT using intra- and interclass correlation coefficients are available and there is some consensus that the reproducibility of test results is higher in trained than in untrained young people. However, correlations measure the strength of associations between two data sets and are sensitive to sample heterogeneity or the spread of data. Recent arguments suggest that the typical error in repeated test measurements and/or level of agreement between different tests of maximal intensity exercise should be reported in preference to correlation coefficients but very few studies of young people's anaerobic fitness have adopted this methodology (see Bland & Altman 1995, Hopkins et al 2001). With 10-year-olds, Sutton et al (2000) reported mean (standard deviation) values of 256.8 (88.2) W and 226.1 (77.8) W for PP and MP with repeatability coefficients of 44.5 W and 42.1 W, respectively.

Criticisms

Test results are affected by the following factors:

1. The nature of the warm-up, the use of toe-clips and heel straps and whether the test is commenced from a stationary or rolling start.

2. The periods over which the PP and MP are averaged. For example, PPs that are averaged over 1 s are significantly greater than PPs averaged over 5 s, but PPs averaged over 3 s or 5 s tend to be not significantly different from one another.
3. Inclusion of the inertia of the flywheel and internal resistance in power computations. Chia et al (1997) demonstrated that PPs and MPs of 9-year-olds adjusted for the inertia of the cycle ergometer are 10–20% higher than PP and MP without this correction.
4. The aerobic contribution to energy metabolism in performing maximal intensity exercise in the WAnT is greater in young people as oxygen uptake kinetics slow with age in response to high intensity exercise (see Chapters 4 and 9).
5. The use of a fixed applied force, normally 7.5% of body mass for sprint cycling, is not optimal for eliciting both PP and MP in one test throughout childhood and adolescence, particularly as body composition (i.e. percent of muscle and fat in relation to body mass) varies during growth and maturation. Welsman et al (1997) showed that the use of a single applied force of $0.74 \, N \cdot kg^{-1}$ body mass for sprint cycling with children is not appropriate when comparing the PP and MP of boys and girls because the relative applied force used in the WAnT, when expressed in relation to thigh muscle volume (TMV), is markedly higher in girls than in boys.

Force–velocity cycling test

Force–velocity cycle tests (FVT) were developed because of the need to optimize power outputs in maximal intensity cycle tests. For example, the FVT protocol described by Santos et al (2002), involves a series of four to six maximal intensity cycle sprints against several applied forces (range 0.29 to $0.99 \, N \cdot kg^{-1}$ body mass), with an initial applied force of $0.74 \, N \cdot kg^{-1}$ body mass and subsequent applied forces selected randomly. The cycle sprint commences from a rolling start (at 60 rpm with a minimal applied force) and is terminated when the optical sensor of the ergometer detects three consecutive declines in pedal revolutions. Each completed sprint is followed by 60 s of active recovery (60 rpm with a minimal applied force) and another 4 min of passive rest before the next sprint is conducted. Some FVT protocols commence from a stationary start rather than from a rolling start and these protocol differences confound comparisons of results across different studies. Reproducibility data as indicated by the coefficient of variation (CV) range from 3.5% to 11.9% in adolescent subjects but validation data in young people using limits of agreement between tests modes are not available.

Optimized pedal velocity (Vopt), optimized applied force (Fopt) and optimized peak power (PPopt) are the prime variables of interest in the FVT. There is evidence that Vopt obtained on the test apparatus is affected by the type of cycle ergometer used. For instance, Williams et al (2003) reported mean (standard deviation) Vopts of 118 (10), 111 (10) and 98 (10) rpm, on the Monark (using an applied force of $0.49 \, N \cdot kg^{-1}$ body mass), SRM isokinetic and Ergomeca cycle ergometers (using an applied force of $0.49 \, N \cdot kg^{-1}$ body mass), respectively, when PPopt is attained. Santos et al (2002) observed that Vopt in preteen boys and girls is significantly lower than in teen and adult groups (82–90 vs. 100–109 vs. 105–116 rpm).

Criticisms

Limitations of FVTs include the following:

1. The longer time necessary for each subject to complete the test compared to the time taken to accomplish a single 30 s cycle test.

2. A warm-up or fatigue effect because of the repeated sprints. This can affect the force–velocity relationships of contracting muscles, which affect the resultant PPopt.
3. The inertia of the flywheel during acceleration and the internal resistance of the cycle ergometer might influence PPopt but no studies with children have addressed these factors.
4. Muscle lactate may be significantly elevated above pretest concentrations after multiple sprints. The accumulation of hydrogen ions can have adverse consequences for muscle force generation and can negatively affect the generation of PPopt (see Chapter 4).

Inertial load force–velocity test

The inertial load force–velocity test (iFVT) allows for the concomitant measurement of optimized force, velocity and power during the acceleration phase of a single maximal intensity cycle sprint of 5–8 s with the flywheel inertia of the cycle ergometer taken into account. Doré et al (2003) reported that the standard error of the test, as an indicator of test reproducibility in young people, is 2.8% for cycling peak power (CPP). The use of this test to monitor maximal intensity exercise with children and adolescents shows promise but despite large numbers of young people tested in some laboratories, the test has yet to gain prominence because of the technical expertise required for its instrumentation. Commercial models of the apparatus with the necessary computer software are currently not available.

Isokinetic cycling test

Maximal cycling power at preset velocities is measured and the test apparatus is more expensive than isoinertial friction-braked cycle ergometers because an electrical system is required for the maintenance of a constant velocity during testing. Testing using isokinetic cycling is attractive because there is no need to consider the optimal applied resistance and the resultant power generated is not affected by the acceleration of the ergometer flywheel. Williams & Keen (2001) have reported the test–retest reliability (CV) of isokinetic power in male adolescents as 5.4% for MP and 5.8% for optimal pedal cadence.

Maximal intensity exercise assessments using the isokinetic cycle ergometer are useful for rehabilitative purposes but the application of the test to sporting situations is more contentious as isokinetic muscle contractions are rare outside of the laboratory.

Accumulated oxygen deficit test

The accumulated oxygen deficit (AOD) test is used to estimate the anaerobic capacity of young people using mainly cycle ergometers, although treadmills have been used. Accumulated oxygen deficit can be achieved in 60–90 s by using exercise intensities of 110%, 130% and 150% of peak $\dot{V}O_2$. The predicted oxygen demand at 110%, 130% and 150% of peak $\dot{V}O_2$ is obtained by using four to five exercise bouts that are below peak $\dot{V}O_2$ intensity (e.g. 50, 70, 80, 90, 100 W using cycle ergometry) for each subject, to establish a linear relationship between exercise intensity and $\dot{V}O_2$. Up to 15 laboratory visits may be necessary to quantify AOD in young people and Carlson & Naughton (1998) reported the estimated aerobic contributions to the test at 110%, 130% and 150%

peak $\dot{V}O_2$ as 62%, 49% and 41%, respectively. Appropriate reliability and validity indicators with young people are not available for the AOD test.

The AOD is estimated by computing the predicted oxygen demand for a fixed period of exercise at an exercise intensity that is predetermined before the test commences (e.g. 110%, 130% or 150% of peak $\dot{V}O_2$) minus the actual $\dot{V}O_2$ for the same time period. The AOD is usually expressed in absolute (L) or relative terms (L · kg^{-1} body mass).

Criticisms

The AOD test has been criticized for the following reasons:

1. The validity of the assumption that the $\dot{V}O_2$ below peak $\dot{V}O_2$ intensity can be accurately extrapolated to an exercise intensity that is above peak $\dot{V}O_2$ intensity.
2. The inability to achieve a steady state $\dot{V}O_2$ at an exercise intensity above that required to elicit peak $\dot{V}O_2$.
3. The considerable aerobic contribution to energy metabolism during the AOD test which challenges the validity of the test as an estimate of anaerobic capacity.
4. The multiple laboratory visits and relatively long testing periods that are required to quantify the AOD.

Summary of cycle ergometry methodology

The results of cycle ergometer tests used to assess the anaerobic fitness of young people are affected by many protocol issues. These include:

• the quality and quantity of practice trials
• the nature of the pretest warm-up and whether the test uses a stationary or rolling start
• the duration of the test
• the applied force(s) used
• the outcome variable(s) of choice (i.e. PP, PPopt, CCP, MP, FI or AOD)
• the time period or pedal revolutions used to calculate power
• whether the resultant power includes adjustment for flywheel inertia during acceleration or deceleration during sprint cycling
• the generalizability of the results to non-cycling sports and exercise performances.

NON-MOTORIZED TREADMILL TEST

To measure horizontal sprinting power in the laboratory is difficult but several studies have used a non-motorized treadmill (NMT) with children and adolescents. In the most comprehensively documented study Sutton et al (2000) described the use of a tethered sprint test for assessing PP and MP in a self-powered 30 s sprint on an NMT. Peak power and MP were calculated from the product of the horizontal force measured using a strain gauge, and the treadmill belt velocity. Unique features of the NMT test described by Sutton et al (2000) include a special safety harness to prevent tripping and also a visual computer display set at eye level to help the child to stay upright during maximal sprint running (Fig. 5.1). With 8-year-old children they reported average PP over two tests conducted on separate days of 207.9 W and average MP of 143.6 W. The repeatability coefficients were 24.8 W and 14.1 W for PP and MP, respectively. Compare these values, which were from the same children, with those stated in the section on the WAnT.

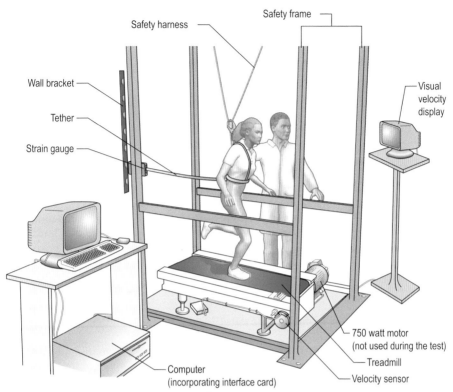

Figure 5.1   Non-motorized treadmill test. (Picture reproduced with permission from Children's Health and Exercise Research Centre, University of Exeter.)

Some data but not all, show that PP and MP achieved in the 30 s NMT test are lower than those attained in the 30 s WAnT despite blood lactate concentration being higher after the NMT test than after the WAnT in the same group of young people.

Criticisms

Limitations of the NMT test include:

1. It is not known if the body mass of the participant is optimal for the generation of PP and MP.
2. In most cases, PP and MP are computed without taking into account the vertical component of the forces exerted during sprinting, or the inertia of the treadmill belt plus body mass of the subject.
3. The aerobic contribution to energy metabolism during treadmill sprinting in young people has not been addressed.

In summary, the NMT test is a feasible alternative to cycle ergometer tests as many sports and games require sprinting with the full carriage of body mass. Adequate habituation or practice trials are necessary to minimize any significant learning effects, and to imbue confidence in young people to maximally exert themselves whilst sprinting on the NMT, as are standardized procedures for warming up and cooling down.

Also, the duration of the NMT test must be sufficiently short to maximize the anaerobic energy contribution to the test and yet be sufficiently long to yield meaningful data on power endurance and fatigue.

ISOKINETIC MONOARTICULAR TEST

Isokinetic assessments in young people are primarily focused on strength assessments as maximal force generated by the subject is sustained throughout the movement at a constant velocity. Importantly, these assessments yield various muscle function indices such as peak and average torque and joint angle of peak torque at a range of angular velocities (0.22–5.4 rad $\cdot$ s^{-1}). Peak power and MP in isokinetic assessments in lower limb and upper limb extension and flexion, though possible, are seldom reported since peak torque usually occurs at a low angular velocity while PP usually occurs at a high angular velocity when torque is no longer maximal. There are numerous contentious issues in the assessment and interpretation of young people's isokinetic muscle performance, such as protocol modifications, gravity correction factors and angular velocities used (see Chapter 3 for further details).

Criticisms

Criticisms of isokinetic monoarticular tests (IMTs) include:

1. Assessing muscle actions that are not common in normal exercise tasks because muscle actions occur at variable velocities throughout the range of motion rather than at a fixed velocity.
2. The high cost of the apparatus and the need to modify it for young people.
3. The inability of several isokinetic dynamometers to assess power at angular velocities that are greater than 5.2 rad $\cdot$ s^{-1}. The maximum angular velocity that the isokinetic apparatus can assess is significantly below the maximum speed of the lower limbs that children attain during maximal sprint running. Moreover, torques generated isometrically, isoinertially and isokinetically in the lower limbs by the same young people are likely to be distinctly different.

In summary, these tests are more useful for the assessment of peak and mean torques than PP and MP. Isokinetic actions in daily exercise tasks are rare and therefore IMTs are more useful for studying force–velocity characteristics of different muscle groups and for rehabilitative purposes than for assessing anaerobic fitness.

POST–EXERCISE BLOOD LACTATE CONCENTRATION

Post-exercise blood lactate is routinely sampled following maximal intensity exercise tests to provide an indication of the extent to which glycolysis has been stressed. The interpretation of post-exercise blood lactates is, however, complicated by the theoretical and methodological factors which are discussed in detail in Chapters 4 and 8.

During a test such as the WAnT, blood lactate concentration progressively rises as lactate diffuses from skeletal muscles into the blood but when the test terminates lactate continues to diffuse into the blood and accumulates until the rate of removal from the blood exceeds the rate of diffusion. Chia et al (1997) demonstrated the dynamics of post-exercise blood lactate by sampling blood from 25 boys and 25 girls aged 9 years every

30 s for 3 min following a WAnT. They observed the blood lactate concentration to rise, in boys, from a baseline value of 2.0 mmol · L^{-1} to 3.2 mmol · L^{-1} after 30 s, peak 2 min post-exercise at 3.6 mmol · L^{-1} and then fall to 3.1 mmol · L^{-1} after 3 min. The corresponding concentrations in girls were 1.6, 3.7, 4.9 and 4.7 mmol · L^{-1}, respectively. As serial blood sampling is not always possible, a single sample taken 2 min post-exercise can be assumed to reflect peak values in children but, in adults, peak values occur about 5 min post-exercise and this must be taken into account in child–adult comparisons.

Following a maximal intensity exercise test, the peak blood lactate concentration is not just specific to the individual but also dependent on the mode of exercise and test protocol. With children, cycling against relatively heavy resistances will induce anaerobic metabolism and lactate production during part of the pedal revolution and blood lactates should not be directly compared to blood lactate accumulated during a running test. The length of the test is important as a cycling test lasting 60 s will produce greater post-exercise blood lactate accumulation than a standard 30 s WAnT due to the longer period of glycolytic stress. Post-exercise peak blood lactate is therefore not a well-defined variable and comparisons across studies should be carried out with extreme caution and only when identical methodologies have been used.

Post-exercise blood lactate concentration following a maximal intensity exercise test provides only a qualitative indication of glycolytic stress not a measure of anaerobic fitness. However, data consistently show that adults exhibit higher blood lactate concentrations than children following tests of anaerobic fitness. It could of course be argued that this is a function of children's faster rate of lactate removal from the blood, through oxidation in the heart or skeletal muscles or through conversion to glucose in the liver and kidneys, rather than lower intramuscular production of lactate. Several threads of evidence suggest a relationship between maturation and post-exercise blood lactate concentration (see Chapter 4) but the empirical evidence is, at best, equivocal and not convincing. Sex differences in post-exercise blood lactate accumulation during childhood and adolescence remain to be proven.

DEVELOPMENT OF ANAEROBIC FITNESS

Anaerobic fitness data on boys are more abundant than those on girls and more data are derived from cross-sectional studies than from longitudinal studies. This is because subject compliance, logistics and costs incurred in longitudinal studies continue to pose serious research challenges (see Chapter 1).

The balance of evidence suggests that the anaerobic fitness of young people continues to develop from childhood through adolescence and into early to middle adulthood and the exercise capability of the lower limbs peaks during the third decade in men and during the second decade in women. As illustrated in Chapter 4, the world's best performances in 100 m sprints improve with age. Best performances in long jump, high jump, field throws and sprint swimming times (exercise exertions that depend predominantly on anaerobic metabolism) by children and adolescents are also inferior to those of adult subjects.

Cross-sectional studies

Table 5.2 provides examples of cross-sectional studies of the anaerobic fitness of young people compared to adults using cycle ergometer tests. Differences in subject characteristics and test protocols used preclude any direct comparisons across the studies.

Table 5.2   Anaerobic fitness of children and adolescents in comparison to adults

Study	Performance indicator 1 (absolute values)	Performance indicator 2 (absolute values)
Hebestreit et al 1993 WAnT Males aged 10.6 and 21.6 years	Peak power 62% of adult value	Work done 68% of adult value
Chia 2001 15 s WAnT Females aged 13.6 and 25.1 years	Peak power 81% of adult value	Mean power 96% of adult value
Armstrong et al 2001 WAnT Males aged 12.2 and 17.0 years	Peak power 45% of adult value	Mean power 47% of adult value
Williams & Keen 2001 5 s ICT Males aged 14.7 and 28.8 years		Mean power 66% of adult value
Doré et al 2001 iFVT Females aged 9.5, 14.4 and 18.2 years	Cycling peak power at 9.5 years, 44% of adult value	Cycling peak power at 14.4 years, 81% of adult value
Santos et al 2002 FVT Males aged 10.1, 14.8 and 21.2 years	Optimized peak power at 10.1 years, 21% of adult value	Optimized peak power at 14.8 years, 66% of adult value
Females aged 10.1, 14.8 and 21.2 years	Optimized peak power at 10.1 years, 33% of adult values	Optimized peak power at 14.8 years, 71% of adult value

WAnT, Wingate anaerobic test; ICT, isokinetic cycle test; iFVT, inertia-accounted force–velocity cycle test; FVT, force velocity cycle test.

However, within study data provide insights as they show that maximal power derived from a range of cycling tests during childhood and adolescence is significantly lower than that measured in young adulthood. The difference in anaerobic fitness between boys and men is greater than the difference in anaerobic fitness between girls and women but data on females are sparse.

Figures 5.2 and 5.3 show the relationship between CPP and age in males and females, from iFVT sprints lasting less than 10 s. The data represent more than 1000 participants aged between 7 and 21 years. Results show a significant increase in CPP with age, albeit with a smaller variance in performance observed in male subjects than in female subjects throughout the age span. Additionally, for both males and females, the CPP data are heteroscedastic, that is the spread of scores for maximal power widens with increasing age. Between the ages of 10 and 18 years, the timing and tempo of changes in anaerobic fitness are sex-specific.

Much of what is known about the anaerobic fitness of children and adolescents is based upon PP and MP derived from the WAnT. For instance, in a study of 306 males aged 8–45 years, PP and MP, expressed in absolute terms (W), for the upper and lower limbs was shown to increase from age 10 years to 25–35 years, with the highest WAnT

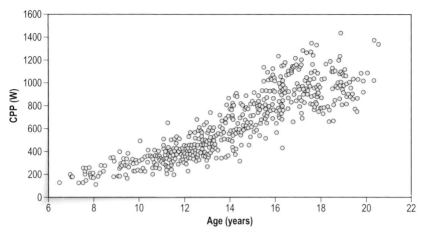

Figure 5.2   Relationship between cycling peak power (CPP) and age in male subjects. (From Van Praagh E 2000 *Pediatric Exercise Science* 12(2):154, with permission of Human Kinetics, Champaign, IL.)

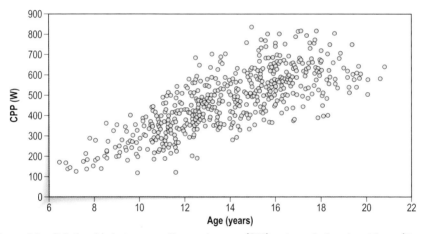

Figure 5.3   Relationship between cycling peak power (CPP) and age in female subjects. (From Van Praagh E 2000 *Pediatric Exercise Science* 12(2):154, with permission of Human Kinetics, Champaign, IL.)

power values for sprint arm cranking attained in the middle of the second decade (Inbar et al 1996). The typical WAnT-determined PP and MP of the lower limbs of boys (age 10–12 years) are about 43% and 47% respectively that of adult males (25–35 years). The PP and MP values of girls (age 10–12 years) are 44% and 55% respectively that of female adults (18–25 years). In both sexes, the maximal power generated by the upper limbs is 60–70% of the power generated by the lower limbs.

Cross-sectional data investigating sex differences in anaerobic fitness are equivocal and generally focused within the very narrow age range of 10–13 years. Studies have reported a higher MP in boys, no sex differences in MP or PP, and higher MP and PP in girls. The conflicting findings are related to lack of control of body size and perhaps also to girls' earlier maturation. To account for body mass, power outputs are usually reported in $W \cdot kg^{-1}$ but ratio-standardized PP and MP data are not reported here, in view of the failure of this statistical technique to fully account for body size (see Chapter 2). Allometric modelling of power data is recommended but the use of the method to analyse young people's anaerobic fitness data is rare. Armstrong et al (1997) used the WAnT to determine the PP and MP of 100 boys and 100 girls aged 12 years. In accord with several other studies, the girls had significantly higher PP and MP (expressed in W) than the boys. However, when the data were adjusted for body mass using a log-linear (allometric) model, the boys' PP and MP were significantly higher than the girls'. The children were categorized into maturity stages using the indices of pubic hair described by Tanner (1962) and analysis of variance revealed significant main effects for maturity for PP, MP, and PP and MP adjusted for body mass in both boys and girls. These data clearly show the importance of accounting for body mass and maturation in the interpretation of anaerobic fitness.

In a study that controlled for body mass using allometric modelling of data from a FVT, Santos et al (2002) compared the PPopt of preteens (9–10 years), teenagers (14–15 years) and adults (21–22 years). Increases in PPopt from preteen to adulthood were 91.0% and 55.6% for males and females, respectively (i.e. the effect of growth and maturation on PPopt in males was more marked than for females). No sex differences were detected in PPopt for preteen subjects, but males had significantly higher PPopt than females in both the teen and adult groups.

Longitudinal studies

Early longitudinal approaches to examining the growth of anaerobic fitness employed either inappropriate statistical techniques to analyse the data or were merely descriptive as the small samples of subjects involved did not allow for any meaningful statistical analysis. A series of recent longitudinal studies of the anaerobic fitness of paediatric subjects have, however, provided valuable insights into the development of anaerobic fitness between 10 and 17 years. These studies, two of which used the WAnT and the other the FVT, are unique in that multilevel modelling was used to analyse the data. In essence, multilevel modelling is more versatile and powerful than traditional methods of analysis such as repeated measures analysis of variance. Multilevel modelling allows for the sensitive interpretation of longitudinal data where age, body size, body fatness and sex effects can be concurrently accounted for within an allometric framework (see Chapter 2).

Armstrong et al (2001) investigated changes in anaerobic fitness in relation to age, sex and maturity by measuring PP and MP on three occasions at 12, 13 and 17 years, respectively. Between 12 and 17 years, PP and MP, expressed in W, in males increased by 121% and 113%, whereas in females PP and MP increased by 66% and 60%, respectively. Across the same age range, blood lactate concentration following the WAnT increased by 23% in females and 31% in males, albeit without any significant sex difference. The negative sex exponents in Table 5.3 show that males generate higher PP and MP than females, even with body mass and body fatness concurrently controlled for. Age exerts a positive but non-linear effect on PP and MP. The negative age by sex interaction term, which is significant for MP only, shows a smaller increase in MP with age for girls over the period studied. However, sexual maturity, assessed using the indices of pubic hair described by Tanner (1962), did not exert an independent effect on PP and MP once body size and body composition had been controlled for.

In a separate study from the same laboratory, De Ste Croix et al (2001) examined the changes in PP and MP in 10-year-olds over a period of 21.6 months using multilevel

Table 5.3 Multilevel regression models for peak power and mean power in 12- to 17-year-olds

Parameter	Peak power estimate (SE)	Mean power estimate (SE)
Fixed:		
Constant	1.884 (0.165)	2.268 (0.165)
Log_e mass	1.232 (0.050)	1.118 (0.051)
Log_e skinfolds	−0.159 (0.024)	−0.228 (0.024)
Age	0.134 (0.010)	0.097 (0.015)
Age^2	−0.034 (0.002)	−(0.012 (0.002)
Sex	−0.054 (0.015)	−(0.066 (0.015)
Age · sex	ns	−(0.017 (0.008)
Random:		
Level 2		
Constant	0.006 (0.001)	0.008 (0.001)
Level 1		
Constant	0.011 (0.001)	0.008 (0.001)

$N = 417$; ns, not significant.
Adapted from Armstrong et al (2001).

modelling. In this narrow age group no sex or maturity effects were evident for PP or MP but an age effect was reported for MP. However, TMV, which was determined using magnetic resonance imaging, exerted a positive and independent effect on both PP and MP.

In another short-term longitudinal study with 6-monthly measurements made over four occasions, the same group used multilevel modelling to examine the FVT-determined PPopt in boys and girls aged 12–14 years. The results showed that PPopt increased with age but PPopt was not significantly different between the sexes. TMV was also shown to be a significant explanatory variable for PPopt even with body size controlled for (Santos et al 2003).

In summary, there is a compelling need for more longitudinal studies that include both boys and girls, throughout childhood and adolescence, to be conducted. Between the ages of 8 and 18 years both PP and MP, determined using different cycle ergometer tests, continue to improve in boys and girls. Though it is likely that PPopt will follow similar trends of improvement from childhood into young adulthood, this has not yet been verified over the whole age range. The tempo and magnitude of the improvements in short-term power output during growth and maturation vary. Improvements in anaerobic fitness are more marked in boys and sex differences in PP, PPopt and MP increase in middle and late adolescence. During adolescence girls' anaerobic performance varies from about 50% to 70% that of boys. Empirical evidence indicates that sexual maturity does not exert an independent effect on PP, MP or PPopt once age, body size and body composition are concurrently accounted for.

DETERMINANTS OF ANAEROBIC FITNESS

The patterns of muscle mass development account for a significant portion but not the entire variance in age- and sex-related differences in anaerobic power during growth and maturation. In males aged 5–18 years, muscle mass increases from 42% to 54% of body mass. This represents almost a fivefold increase in muscle mass from 7.5 to 37 kg. The corresponding increase in females' muscle mass over the same age range is 3.4 times from 7 to 24 kg or from 40% to 45% of body mass. Men attain peak muscle mass at about 30 years of age while women attain peak muscle mass before 20 years. Beyond 7 years of age, males have greater absolute and relative (kg muscle mass/kg body mass) muscle mass than females.

Children and adolescents have smaller muscle cross-sectional areas (CSA) than adults but sex differences in muscle size are small until the middle of puberty. After adolescence, females have about 50% of the muscle size of the upper limb and 70% of the muscle size of the lower limb of males. In female subjects, muscle fibre diameter peaks in adolescence while peak values for muscle fibre diameter in male subjects occur in early adulthood. Boys show a greater size increase in type IIX fibres than girls.

Changes in muscle size alter muscle pennation, which in turn influences force and power output. Data using ultrasonic measurement of muscle fascicles show that fascicle angles (an indicator of changes in muscle pennation) continue to increase in males until the middle of adulthood but the increase in females tapers off in late adolescence. Hence changes in muscle pennation can also help explain some of the age and sex differences in maximal intensity exercise performance during growth and maturation.

Data are sparse but current evidence suggests that genetics account for about 50% of the variance in maximal intensity exercise. Calvo et al (2002) demonstrated that the genetic effect, as estimated using a heritability index (HI), is specific to the anaerobic test used. They reported significant HI values for 5 s PP (HI = 0.74) and MP over 30 s (HI = 0.84) and for maximal post-exercise blood lactate concentration (HI = 0.82). However, the HI for the fatigue index was not significant (HI = 0.43). The HI for AOD was also not significant (HI = 0.22). Importantly, the genetic effects determined using different maximal intensity exercise tests with the same subjects were different. These findings must therefore be extrapolated with caution.

The nature–nurture debate on muscle fibre type distribution remains contentious because it is extremely difficult to apportion the genotype and phenotype effect on muscle fibre distribution. This difficulty is exacerbated by the sparseness of relevant data on children and adolescents and the very small numbers that contribute to the data pool generated using the needle biopsy technique. Data described in Chapter 4 suggest that the percentage distribution of type II fibres is lower in early childhood than in adulthood and that adult proportions are attained in late adolescence. There appears to be a greater prevalence of type IIa than type IIX fibres during childhood and adolescence but the evidence of a sex difference in fibre type distribution in childhood and adolescence is equivocal.

The maximum shortening velocity of type IIa and type IIX muscle fibres is 3 and 10 times faster than that of type I muscle fibres in adults. Therefore, if the relative fibre characteristics are similar in childhood and adolescence and if the evidence of a negative relationship between the percentage of type I muscle fibres and age is accepted (at least in the vastus lateralis), then this partly explains the trend of an age-dependent increase in the anaerobic fitness of the lower limbs.

Magnetic resonance spectroscopy (^{31}P MRS) studies involving single-limb exercise suggest that young people do not attain adult values for end-exercise pH with plantar flexion exercise. Boys develop a smaller oxygen deficit compared to men during strenuous exercise. These observations are supported by several sources of evidence that show an age-dependent capability to use anaerobic metabolism in response to intense exercise (see Chapter 4).

There is speculation that hormonal factors, especially around the period of puberty, may account for some of the characteristic observations in maximal intensity exercise performance. Hormones have both primary and secondary effects. For example, concentrations of circulating growth hormone and testosterone in males and oestradiol in females are markedly increased during puberty. Also, circulating levels of testosterone begin to rise about 12 months before peak height velocity (PHV) and remain elevated, reaching adult levels about 3 years after PHV. While it is tempting to speculate that levels of androgens help to explain sex differences in anaerobic fitness, the evidence is equivocal, partly because of the wide intra-individual variability in levels of circulating hormones. Moreover, the associations between circulating levels of androgens and changes in anaerobic fitness might be coincidental rather than causal.

It is plausible that changes in neural factors during growth and maturation can influence the anaerobic fitness of young people. Research into this area is sparse because of ethical restrictions in the use of invasive procedures with healthy young people. It is not known if children are capable of full muscle activation during maximal intensity exercise but there are data which suggest that adolescents have a higher degree of muscle activation than children. Other neural factors that can help to explain age- and maturation-related differences in anaerobic fitness include increased myelination of nerve fibres (myelination increases the velocity of nerve transmission), improved coordination of muscle synergists and antagonists, and the increased ability to fully activate muscles during maximal intensity exercise. It is also possible that improved coordination with practice and exposure, especially in multi-joint exercise tasks like sprint cycling and sprint running, can also account for some age- and/or maturation-related improvements in maximal intensity exercise performance.

RECOVERY FROM MAXIMAL INTENSITY EXERCISE

The recovery of power is faster in children than in adults during repeated brief maximal intensity exercises that are separated by short rest intervals. For instance, Hebestreit et al (1993) reported that prepubertal boys recovered faster than adult men despite having similar body-mass-related peak $\dot{V}O_2$. Over a series of three separate test sessions, the boys and men completed two 30 s WAnTs (WAnT 1 and WAnT 2) separated by 1, 2 and 10 min recovery intervals, i.e. exercise-to-recovery ratios of 1:2, 1:4 and 1:20. PP and total mechanical work (TMW) in boys was 61.5% and 67. 8% that of the men in WAnT 1, and percent fatigue in WAnT 1 was significantly greater in men than in boys (52.4% vs. 43.8%). Recovery in PPs in WAnT 2 following recovery periods of 1, 2 and 10 minutes were 90.6%, 112% and 105.1% of PPs in WAnT 1 in boys and 58.8%, 70.9% and 95.2% of PPs in WAnT 1 in men. Percentage recovery in PP was significantly higher than recovery in TMW in WAnT 2 in boys and men. The authors suggested that the faster power recovery in boys compared to men could be partially explained by the lower PP, TMW and percent fatigue in WAnT 1 in boys, the lower post-exercise blood lactate concentration in boys, and faster removal of post-exercise metabolites in boys compared to men.

Ratel et al (2002) reported that 10-year-old boys were better able to maintain cycling peak power (0% decrement) during 10 sprints of 10 s, separated by 30 s recovery intervals (i.e. exercise-to-recovery ratio of 1:3 between sprints) than 15-year-old boys and 20-year-old men, where the decrements in CPP were 18.5% and 28.5%, respectively. In another study, the same group required 11-year-old boys and 22-year-old men to perform 10 consecutive maximal 10 s sprints interspersed with 15 s rest periods on both an NMT and a cycle ergometer. On the NMT and cycle ergometer, the boys' PP decreased by 17.7% and 14.3% from sprint one to sprint 10 whereas the decrement in the men's PP was 43.3% and 40.0%, respectively. The boys' MP decrement over the 10 sprints was 28.9% on the NMT and 18.7% on the cycle ergometer compared to 47.0% and 36.7% decreases in the men's MP, respectively. The men experienced a significantly higher increase in blood lactate accumulation than the boys over both the running and cycling exercises. Perceived exertion rates (see Chapter 12) were also significantly higher in the men than in the boys. The authors concluded that the greater fatigue resistance in boys may be explained by their lower work rate in relation to lean leg volume during the earlier sprints, their lower accumulation of lactate and their faster resynthesis of phosphocreatine (PCr) via higher muscle oxidative activity (Ratel et al. 2004).

In the only study to date on female subjects, Chia (2001) examined the power recovery in 13-year-old girls and 25-year-old women using a series of three 15 s maximal cycle sprints (WAnT 1, WAnT 2 and WAnT 3) separated by an active recovery interval of 45 s between the sprints, i.e. an exercise-to-recovery ratio of 1:3. The girls and women had similar body masses and lower limb muscle masses. Peak power in WAnT 1 in girls was 80.6% that of women but MP was not significantly different between girls and women. Girls were able to replicate 82% and 81% of PP and MP of WAnT 1 in WAnT 3 while women replicated 70% and 63% of PP and MP. Blood lactate concentrations before WAnT 1 and 3 min after WAnT 3 were not significantly different between girls and women. These data suggest that despite similar post-exercise blood lactate values, girls exhibit a faster recovery in WAnT PP and MP than women. Girls' higher peak $\dot{V}O_2$ than women, age-related differences in $\dot{V}O_2$ kinetic response to heavy exercise and faster resynthesis of PCr probably accounted for the quicker power recovery in girls.

Further research using a range of exercise–recovery models and modes of exercise is required to map out the physiological mechanisms underlying power recovery during growth and maturation. However, recent work using ^{31}P MRS has provided evidence of faster PCr resynthesis following exercise in 6- to 12-year-olds than in young adults (see Chapter 4 for further details).

SUMMARY

The assessment of anaerobic fitness during growth and maturation is important as daily activities involve both anaerobic and aerobic function. Researchers have to cope with methodological and ethical constraints when studying young people and, compared with aerobic fitness, this has limited the expansion of knowledge of anaerobic fitness with this age group.

Alterations in muscle mass, muscle fibre type or muscle fibre diameter during growth and maturation help to explain some but not all the age- and sex-related changes in anaerobic fitness. Genetics exert a significant influence on anaerobic fitness, notably on PP and MP determined in the WAnT. A greater preponderance of type II muscle fibres in adolescence and adulthood than in childhood helps to explain the increase in anaerobic fitness with age. However, caution must be exercised when interpreting the results of muscle biopsy studies because of methodological limitations, the limited sample sizes analysed and the plasticity of some fibre types to non-genetic and environmental factors. Differences in muscle metabolism between children and adults in their responses to maximal intensity exercise suggest a reduced reliance on anaerobic metabolism during childhood. Levels of circulating hormones, especially around the period of puberty, help to explain some of the sex differences in anaerobic fitness but the evidence is equivocal and current data suggest that sexual maturity does not exert any independent effect on anaerobic fitness, once age, body mass, body composition (including in the WAnT, TMV) are concurrently controlled for. Improvements in neural adaptations with age, complete myelination of nerve fibres, improved muscle coordination during multi-joint exercise and an improved capability to recruit motor units or more fully activate muscles help to explain age-related improvements in anaerobic fitness. However, a full understanding of the development of anaerobic fitness awaits further research.

Despite the range of research protocols used in different laboratories, the results consistently suggest that boys and girls recover more quickly than men and women, respectively, during a series of repeated maximal intensity sprints of short duration separated by short rest periods. The quicker recovery of power output in young people can, at least in part, be attributed to the faster time constant for PCr resynthesis in children and adolescents compared to adults.

Future research directions in paediatric anaerobic fitness worthy of consideration include:

- examining the relevance of anaerobic fitness for sports, exercise performance or physical health
- initiating longitudinal studies that span the entire paediatric age range and into mid-adulthood
- using non-invasive technologies such as magnetic resonance imaging, magnetic resonance spectroscopy, on their own, or in combination with other emergent technologies to examine mechanisms of the anaerobic fitness of children and adolescents
- studying the development of patterns of recovery during repeated maximal intensity exercise, using different exercise-to-recovery models and modes of exercise.

KEY POINTS

1. The outcomes of maximal intensity exercise have been expressed in a number of ways with peak power (PP) and mean power (MP) the conventional terms.
2. Tests of maximal intensity exercise range between 5 s and 60 s duration and require maximal exertion throughout the test.
3. Laboratory tests used to assess maximal intensity exercise include sprint cycling, treadmill sprint running and isokinetic limb extension and flexion.
4. Tests of short duration are more anaerobic while longer tests have a greater aerobic contribution to energy metabolism and the aerobic contribution to maximal intensity exercise in young people is greater than in adult subjects.
5. Maximal power output increases with age between 8 and 18 years and the increase is greater than the corresponding increase in body size.
6. Sex differences in anaerobic fitness are minimal in childhood but increase during adolescence.
7. Potential determinants of anaerobic fitness include muscle mass, muscle size, muscle fibre type distribution, muscle energetics, hormones and neural factors.
8. Recovery during repeated maximal intensity exercise interspersed with brief recovery periods is faster in young people than in adults.
9. The use of non-invasive technologies such as magnetic resonance imaging and magnetic resonance spectroscopy will help elucidate the mechanisms underlying the growth of anaerobic fitness.

References

Armstrong N, Welsman J R, Kirby B J 1997 Performance on the Wingate anaerobic test and maturation. Pediatric Exercise Science 9:253–261

Armstrong N, Welsman J R, Chia M 2001 Short term power output in relation to growth and maturation. British Journal of Sports Medicine 35:118–124

Bland J M, Altman DG 1995 Comparing two methods of clinical measurement: a personal history. International Journal of Epidemiology 24:S7–S14

Calvo M, Rodas G, Vallejo M et al 2002 Heritability of explosive power and anaerobic capacity in humans. European Journal of Applied Physiology 86:218–225

Carlson J, Naughton G 1998 Assessing accumulated oxygen deficit in children. In: Van Praagh E (ed) Pediatric anaerobic performance. Human Kinetics, Champaign, IL, p 119–136

Chia M 2001 Power recovery in the Wingate anaerobic test in girls and women following prior sprints of a short duration. Biology of Sport 18:45–53

Chia M, Armstrong N, Childs D 1997 The assessment of children's anaerobic performance using modifications of the Wingate anaerobic test. Pediatric Exercise Science 9:80–89

De Ste Croix M B A, Armstrong N, Chia M Y H et al 2001 Changes in short-term power output in 10-to-12-year-olds. Journal of Sports Sciences 19:141–148

Doré E, Bedu M, Franca N M et al 2001 Anaerobic cycling performance characteristics in prepubescent, adolescent and young adult females. European Journal of Applied Physiology 84:476–481

Doré E, Duché P, Rouffet et al 2003 Measurement error in short-term power testing in paediatric subjects. Journal of Sports Sciences 21:135–142

Hebestreit H, Minura K-I, Bar-Or O 1993 Recovery of muscle power after high intensity short-term exercise: comparing boys to men. Journal of Applied Physiology 74:2875–2880

Hopkins W G, Schabort E J, Hawley J A 2001 Reliability of power in physical performance tests. Sports Medicine 31:211–234

Inbar O, Bar-Or O Skinner, J S 1996 The Wingate anaerobic test. Human Kinetics, Champaign, IL, p 1–76

Ratel S, Bedu M, Hennegreave A et al 2002 Effects of age and recovery duration on peak power output during repeated cycling sprints. International Journal of Sports Medicine 23:397–402

Ratel S, Williams CA, Oliver J et al 2004 Effects of age and mode of exercise on power output profiles during repeated sprints. European Journal of Applied Physiology 92:204–210

Santos A M C, Welsman J R, De Ste Croix M B A et al 2002 Age- and sex-related differences in optimal peak power. Pediatric Exercise Science 14:202–212

Santos A M C, Armstrong N, De Ste Croix M B A et al 2003 Optimised peak power in relation to age, body size, gender and thigh muscle volume. Pediatric Exercise Science 15:406–418

Sutton N C, Childs D, Bar-Or et al 2000 A non-motorised treadmill test to assess children's short-term power output. Pediatric Exercise Science 12:91–100

Tanner J M 1962 Growth at adolescence, 2nd edn. Blackwell, Oxford

Welsman J R, Armstrong N, Kirby B J et al 1997 Exercise performance and MRI determined muscle volume in children. European Journal of Applied Physiology 76:92–97

Williams C A, Keen P 2001 Isokinetic measurement of maximal muscle power during leg cycling: a comparison of adolescent boys and adult men. Pediatric Exercise Science 13:154–166

Williams C A, Doré E, Alban J et al 2003 Short term power output in 9-yr-old children: typical error between ergometers and protocols. Pediatric Exercise Science 15:302–312

Further reading

Armstrong N, Welsman J R, 1997 Young people and physical activity. Oxford University Press, Oxford, p 32–45, 79–102

Chia M 2000 Assessing paediatric subjects' exercise using anaerobic performance tests. European Journal of Physical Education 5:231–258

Pfitzinger P, Freedson P 1997 Blood lactate responses to exercise in children: part 1. Peak lactate concentration. Pediatric Exercise Science 9: 210–222

Sargeant A J 2000 Anaerobic performance. In: Armstrong N, Van Mechelen W (eds) Paediatric exercise science and medicine. Oxford University Press, Oxford, p 143–152

Van Praagh E, Doré E 2002 Short-term muscle power during growth and maturation. Sports Medicine 32:701–728

Van Praagh E, Franca N M 1998 Measuring maximal short-term power output during growth. In: Van Praagh E (ed) Pediatric anaerobic performance. Human Kinetics, Champaign Il, p 155–190

Welsman J R, Armstrong N 1998 Assessing postexercise lactates in children and adolescents. In: Van Praagh E (ed) Pediatric anaerobic performance. Human Kinetics, Champaign, IL, p 137–154

Williams C A 1997 Children's and adolescents' anaerobic performance during cycle ergometry. Sports Medicine 24:227–240

Chapter **6**

Pulmonary function

Samantha G. Fawkner

LEARNING OBJECTIVES

After studying this chapter you should be able to:

1. describe the important age-related changes in lung size and structure with reference to somatic growth
2. identify and discuss important age-related changes in the mechanical function of the pulmonary system
3. describe age-related changes in static and dynamic lung function at rest
4. discuss age-related changes in minute ventilation ($\dot{V}_E$), breathing frequency and tidal volume at rest and during submaximal and maximal exercise
5. describe the response of $\dot{V}_E$ to an incremental exercise test in children
6. describe the $\dot{V}_E$ kinetic response to exercise and discuss reasons for adult–child differences in $\dot{V}_E$ kinetics
7. discuss the potential mechanisms responsible for adult–child differences in the control of ventilation
8. discuss the possibility that the pulmonary system is limiting to exercise in adults and children
9. consider adaptations of the pulmonary system with training
10. describe sex differences in pulmonary function.

INTRODUCTION

The pulmonary system provides the means to maintaining blood-gas homeostasis during resting and exercise conditions. Its primary function is that of providing an optimum environment for the efficient gas exchange of oxygen (O_2) and carbon dioxide (CO_2) between the ambient air and pulmonary blood. In doing so, the pulmonary system functions to limit the metabolic cost of respiratory work, and maintain acid–base balance even under the most extreme of exercise conditions.

During growth, the various components of the pulmonary system undergo sufficient change such that at all ages in the healthy growing child the pulmonary system is essentially non-limiting to exercise. This is a considerable challenge in view of the quite dramatic difference in the structural and mechanical properties of the prenatal and adult pulmonary systems, and not least due to the need for the pulmonary system to support a basal metabolic rate that in infants and children is two or three times higher than that of an adult. As stated by Polgar & Weng (1979, pp. 660–661):

> It is amazing, although not unexpected, that partially proportional and in other parts seemingly discrepant growth patterns can produce over-all physiologic functions of this complicated organ system, which at any place of development turn out to be just right for an adequate performance under the given circumstances.

This chapter will therefore first identify some of the important structural and mechanical changes that occur in the lung during growth. Second, it will identify some of the apparent age- and sex-related differences in pulmonary function and ventilatory responses during both rest and exercise.

STRUCTURE AND MECHANICS

The lung

The lung increases in both its length and width with age, following growth velocity curves similar in shape to those of both height and mass. The age of peak velocity of lung width occurs at about 12.2 years and 13.8 years in girls and boys, respectively, and coincides closely with peak height velocity (PHV). Peak velocity of lung length, however, occurs some 6–8 months later (Simon et al 1972) and may coincide with the peak velocity of chest depth. Dimensions of the thorax mirror these, and between the ages of 11 and 18 years, thoracic height increases twice as fast as thoracic width (DeGroodt et al 1988), although there are notable sex differences (these will be discussed later). As the lung and thorax increase in size, so do total lung capacity (TLC) and the various subdivisions of lung volume and function. The TLC is well correlated with height, but, as a volume that has three-dimensional properties, has been confirmed to relate most closely to the cube of height (height³). Despite this, prediction equations for TLC are frequently given as simple linear functions, presumably for ease of use. In relation to height, TLC increases from approximately 2 L at 120 cm to 3 L at 140 cm and to 6 L at 180 cm.

Airways and alveoli

At birth the number and branching pattern of the bronchial system are finalized, but subsequently both the diameter and length of the airways increase with age. Conversely, the number of alveoli in the lung only begin to noticeably increase after birth, multiplying exponentially from approximately 24 million to near maximal numbers by the 8th year (280 million) (Dunnill 1962). Concurrently alveolar surface area increases from 2.8 m^2 at birth to 12.2 m^2 at 13 months, 32 m^2 at 8 years and 75 m^2 in adulthood (Dunnill 1962) and, like the TLC, correlates closely with the cube of height. From around 2 years of age, alveoli enlargement coincident with the increasing size of the airways makes the most substantial contribution to the increasing volume of the lung. However, the rate of increase in lung tissue is not necessarily proportional to the rate of the increase in airway diameter, the latter of which is thought to lag behind and 'catch up' in later years.

Respiratory system resistance, compliance and elasticity

The work required to inflate and deflate the lung is governed by the equation: work = total intrapleural pressure × change in lung volume. For a given lung volume, it is therefore the internal pressures opposing inflation and deflation that dictate the efficiency of the lung. Three main components contribute to intrapleural pressure other than the active contraction of the diaphragm and respiratory muscles: airway resistance, respiratory system compliance and elastic recoil. Each of these components change with growth, and have important implications with regard to ventilatory patterns in children.

Airway resistance describes the ease with which air flows through the conducting airways, i.e. the greater the resistance, the greater the pressure that is required to produce a given airflow. During growth, as the lungs increase in size, so do the diameter and length of the airways. Since resistance is increased by the power of four for any reduction in radius, these changes result in an absolute reduction in airway resistance with age whereby respiratory system resistance is closely related to height by an exponent of 1.7 (Lanteri & Sly 1993).

Compliance infers distensibility (stretchiness) of the respiratory system. Essentially, respiratory compliance is the ability of the alveoli and lung tissue to expand on inspiration, i.e. the stiffer the lung, the less the compliance and the more pressure (work) that is required to inflate the lung. Compliance is a measure of the volume of change per unit pressure change, and therefore absolute compliance is dependent upon the size of the lung. Specific compliance, on the other hand, refers to compliance per unit volume of the lung. During growth, lung volume and number and volume of alveoli increase and there is a reduction in the surface area-to-volume ratio and alveolar surface forces. As a result absolute compliance increases with age and is related to height by the exponent 1.76 (Lanteri & Sly 1993). However, at birth, the lungs are extremely flaccid and until late adolescence become increasingly more rigid with the increase in the density of connective tissue. As a result, specific compliance is thought to either decrease or remain stable with age (Lanteri & Sly 1993, Zapletal et al 1976).

The pathological neighbour to compliance is lung elasticity, which refers to the ability of the lung elastic tissues to recoil during expiration. Coincident with the increased density of connective tissue, lung recoil pressure increases throughout childhood until the age of about 18 years (Mansell et al 1977), after which it declines

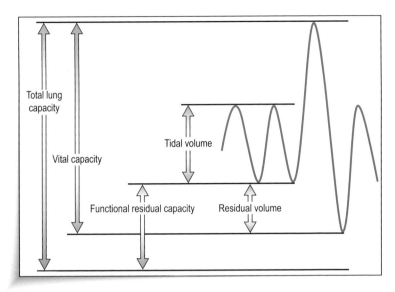

Figure 6.1   Lung volumes. TLC, total lung capacity; VC, vital capacity; FRC, functional residual capacity; TV, tidal volume; RV, residual capacity.

into late adulthood. Counteracting the elastic recoil pressure of the lung is the elastic, opposite recoil of the chest. At functional residual capacity (FRC, the volume of air in the lungs at the end of a normal expiration, Fig. 6.1) the elastic recoil of the lung is balanced by the outward forces of the thoracic cage. This elastic recoil of the thorax is extremely low in the newborn, and increases throughout childhood. It is not known whether the increase in elastic recoil of the lung and thorax are uniform, but there is some evidence that the ratio of FRC to TLC and residual volume (RV) to vital capacity (VC) increases with age (DeGroodt et al 1988, Mansell et al 1977), which may be due to the thoracic elasticity advancing more rapidly than that of the lung.

PULMONARY FUNCTION AT REST

In absolute terms, lung volumes increase with growth. In line with TLC, the increase in the subdivisions of the lung (Fig. 6.1) are well correlated with height and more appropriately with height^3 (Table 6.1). However, due to the various changes in the mechanical properties of the lung the rate at which they increase is not necessarily proportional. As stated above, the ratio of FRC to TLC is thought to be lower in children than in adults and between the ages of 11.5 and 18.5 years the ratio of RV to VC increases by about 1% per year (i.e. RV increases more rapidly than VC (DeGroodt et al 1988)). The ratio of tidal volume (VT) to VC, on the other hand, declines with age. VT has most frequently been reported relative to either body mass or body surface area, but irrespective of the normalization procedure, relative VT declines slightly with age (in a group of 58 children, VT was 11.3 mL · kg^{-1} for children 6–8 years and 10.1 mL · kg^{-1} for children 8–16 years of age (Gaultier et al 1981)). Coincident with a relative reduction in VT, breathing frequency (fR) decreases with age and body size. During early childhood, resting fR will be as high as 25 to 30 breaths · min^{-1}, but falls to around 10 to 15 breaths · min^{-1} in adulthood. The fall in fR is due to proportional

Table 6.1   Prediction equations for lung volumes recommended for use in children and adolescents (data from Cook & Hamann 1961)

	Equation	CC
Males		
TLC (mL)	$0.950 \times 10^{-3} \times H^{3.039}$	0.96
FRC (mL)	$0.125 \times 10^{-3} \times H^{3.298}$	0.92
RV (mL)	$0.162 \times 10^{-3} \times H^{3.099}$	0.79
VC (mL)	$0.767 \times 10^{-3} \times H^{3.028}$	0.95
Females		
TLC (mL)	$1.698 \times 10^{-3} \times H^{2.909}$	0.92
FRC (mL)	$0.286 \times 10^{-3} \times H^{3.136}$	0.86
RV (mL)	$0.320 \times 10^{-3} \times H^{2.972}$	0.77
VC (mL)	$1.213 \times 10^{-3} \times H^{2.920}$	0.94

Volumes in mL BTPS; H, height in cm; TLC, total lung capacity; FRC, functional residual capacity; RV, residual volume; VC, vital capacity, CC; correlation coefficient.

increases in both the inspiratory and expiratory durations and is accompanied by a reduction in mean inspiratory flow relative to body mass. As a result of both a reduced number of breaths and relative volume of air inspired per breath, minute ventilation in relation to body mass ($\dot{V}_E \cdot kg^{-1}$) is quite dramatically lower in children than adults, and mirrors via some as yet unidentified causative mechanism the lower metabolic rate demonstrated by adults at rest.

Measures of dynamic lung function; forced vital capacity (FVC), forced expiratory volume in 1 s (FEV_1), maximal voluntary ventilation (MVV) and peak expiratory flow rate (PEFR) map closely changes in lung size and somatic growth patterns during growth. Before puberty, a linear increase in dynamic lung function with height is evident, with a divergence from linearity during the pubertal growth spurt which is most closely related to thoracic growth (Rosenthal et al 1993). Dynamic lung function is also related to changes with age in muscle strength, since this contributes to forced manoeuvres. Given that peak changes in muscle strength occur some time after PHV, as does peak velocity of thoracic length, it stands to reason that maximum changes in lung function also lag behind PHV from between 6 months to a year.

PULMONARY FUNCTION DURING EXERCISE

Measurement

Fundamental to the study of pulmonary function and the ventilatory response to exercise is the capability to measure ventilation during exercise accurately. This in turn has implications regarding the accurate assessment of exercise response variables that are functions of ventilation such as oxygen uptake ($\dot{V}O_2$) and carbon dioxide production ($\dot{V}CO_2$). Many of the issues concerned with the accuracy of the adopted instrument to measure ventilation are shared when testing either children or adults. Depending on whether a standard pneumotachograph system or turbine system is employed, these issues include problems such as measuring flow temperature, baseline drift, condensation, turbine lag and overspin. Non-linearities of any system can be magnified when measuring ventilation in children, since absolute VT and $\dot{V}E$ may be below the accepted linearity of the device.

In addition, the changing size of the lung with age imposes mechanical problems during the measurement of ventilation and gaseous exchange. The absolute dead space volume of the conducting airways increases from approximately 40 mL at 6 years of age, to 125 mL at ages 12–14 years and 150 mL in adulthood. It is therefore essential that the dead space volume of any valve or measurement ensemble be minimized in order to prevent rebreathing of the expirate.

Minute ventilation response to an increasing metabolic demand

As exercise imposes a greater demand for energy on the working muscles, the demand for O_2 and the need to eliminate CO_2 rises and consequently ventilation has to adapt to maintain normoxia. As a result, fR and VT increase, and $\dot{V}E$ rises with increasing exercise intensity. Up to intensities that equate to the ventilatory threshold (TVENT) (moderate intensities), $\dot{V}E$ increases in parallel to $\dot{V}O_2$, after which $\dot{V}E$ rises proportionately more than $\dot{V}O_2$ in order to eliminate the CO_2 generated as a result of bicarbonate buffering of lactic acid. At very high intensities, an accumulation of H^+ results in a reduction in blood pH and $\dot{V}E$ increases at a disproportionately higher rate than $\dot{V}CO_2$, a situation termed ventilatory compensation. Thus exercise hyperpnoea in most cases maintains arterial gas homeostasis; that is, arterial partial pressure of CO_2 ($PaCO_2$) and O_2 (PaO_2) remain essentially unchanged during exercise near to 40 and 90 mmHg, respectively.

This general pattern of exercise hyperpnoea is similar in children and adults, and with increasing exercise intensity, $\dot{V}E$ increases in a curvilinear fashion (Fig. 6.2). However, there are a number of age-related differences and nuances that are of

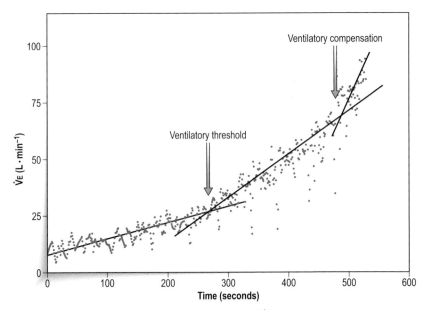

Figure 6.2 Typical breath-by-breath minute ventilation ($\dot{V}E$) response to a ramp incremental exercise test in a 12-year-old child.

significant importance, and reflect some of the most fundamental differences in the response to exercise in children.

Elevated minute ventilation for a given exercise intensity

As with adults, below the TVENT, $\dot{V}E$ increases in parallel to $\dot{V}O_2$. However, $\dot{V}E$ for a given exercise intensity is consistently higher in children than it is in adults, for two fundamental reasons: the higher metabolic cost of exercise in children and the tendency for children to hyperventilate. Firstly, it is considered that children display a greater O_2 cost of work, and demonstrate a higher $\dot{V}O_2$ relative to body mass for a given exercise intensity. As a result, $\dot{V}E$ is higher to accommodate the elevated $\dot{V}O_2$. Much of the data supporting this concept has involved treadmill walking and running and it has been suggested that this poor work efficiency is due to inefficient gait and therefore poor economy of locomotion. The concept certainly seems plausible. However, during cycle ergometry, there is little evidence to suggest that children adopt a less efficient cycling action than adults, and yet the O_2 cost of moderate intensity exercise remains higher in children relative to both body mass and power output. In addition, at moderate intensity, the generation of energy is predominantly aerobic, irrespective of age, and thus age-related changes in the metabolic properties of the working muscles are unlikely to contribute to this greater O_2 cost of work. It is, however, possible that a poorer efficiency of breathing in children results in an elevated cost of ventilation (see later). The reasons for the elevated O_2 cost of work remain unclear, but irrespective of the origins, it will contribute to an elevated $\dot{V}E$ during exercise in children.

Secondly, children display a higher $\dot{V}E$ for a given $\dot{V}O_2$ and lower levels of end-tidal partial pressure of CO_2 ($PETCO_2$) and $PaCO_2$ than adults; in other words, children hyperventilate. This tendency to hyperventilate in childhood is evidenced by a decline in the ventilatory equivalent of oxygen ($\dot{V}E/\dot{V}O_2$) in both cross-sectional and longitudinal studies with age, during both cycle ergometry and treadmill walking and running (Fig. 6.3). Hyperventilation is generally considered to be inefficient, since the work of breathing comes at a metabolic cost, but the reasons for this age-related inefficiency are not entirely understood.

The body of evidence nevertheless points to an age-related adaptation of the neural respiratory drive. The neural respiratory drive of young children (4 years of age), as measured by mouth pressure generated 1 s after airway occlusion ($P_{0.1}$), is two times higher than that of adolescents (16 years of age) and declines with age to the power 0.62 (Gaultier et al 1981). Although this may be a result of the changing mechanics of the lung and the neural afferents arising from the respiratory system, a more plausible explanation lies with age-related changes in the sensitivity to levels of CO_2 in the blood. Put in its most simple terms, it is sufficient to say that for some reason, children will not tolerate high levels of $PaCO_2$, and hence ventilate accordingly. It is therefore not the $\dot{V}E$ for a given $\dot{V}O_2$ that is the physiological paradigm, but $\dot{V}E$ for a given $PaCO_2$. This will be dealt with in more detail later.

Ventilatory threshold (TVENT)

TVENT represents the exercise intensity at which $\dot{V}E$ begins to increase at a faster rate than $\dot{V}O_2$, and is a reflection of both metabolic CO_2 and that resulting from the buffering process. The increase in $\dot{V}E$, which is no longer dependent solely upon metabolic activity, causes a rise in $PETO_2$, and a rise in the $\dot{V}E/\dot{V}O_2$, and respiratory exchange ratio (R), whilst $PETCO_2$ and the ventilatory equivalent for $\dot{V}CO_2$ ($\dot{V}E/\dot{V}CO_2$) remain

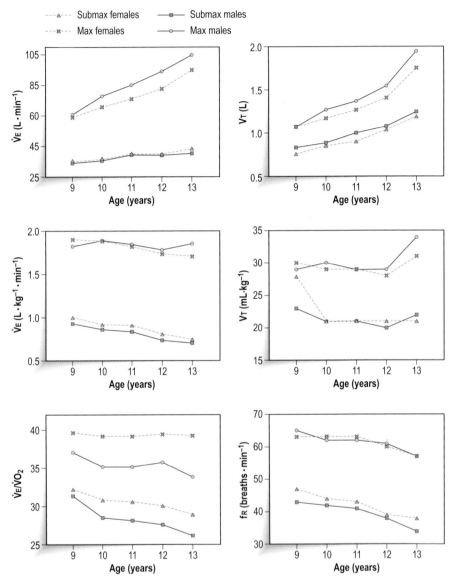

Figure 6.3 Ventilatory response to submaximal and maximal exercise in children 9 to 13 years of age. (Data from Rowland & Cunningham 1997.)

stable. These turning points in ventilatory variables form the basis for the detection of TVENT, which may be subjectively determined from plots of one or more variables against either time or $\dot{V}O_2$. In untrained adults, TVENT occurs at between 45% and 55% of peak $\dot{V}O_2$.

Although there are a number of studies documenting TVENT with children, there is little consensus as to the approximate exercise intensity relative to peak $\dot{V}O_2$ at which it is likely to occur in untrained children. This is possibly due to the number of problems that are associated with the detection of TVENT with both child and adult responses, most notably, that the estimation of TVENT using the above procedures is essentially subjective, and accuracy requires both experience and ideally multiple assessors. However, with children the process is made particularly difficult by the breath-by-breath irregularities (noise) that characterize their ventilatory responses, as well as their tendency to hyperventilate at the beginning of tests, which can impose pseudo thresholds. Generally speaking, though, it is thought that, reflective of age-related changes in metabolic properties of the exercising muscle, TVENT occurs at a higher percentage of peak $\dot{V}O_2$ in children than it does in adults.

Maximal ventilation

Maximal ventilation is a consequence of the by-products of both aerobic and anaerobic metabolism, and with a ramp type protocol and breath-by-breath analysis of the respiratory response the stage of ventilatory compensation is clearly evident in most children (Fig. 6.2). It has traditionally been accepted that MVV at rest far exceeds $\dot{V}E$ at the end of an exercise test to exhaustion ($\dot{V}Emax$) in healthy people. Adults generally use about 70% of their MVV to achieve peak $\dot{V}O_2$, and children near to or slightly less than 70%. It is for this reason that it is generally considered that ventilation does not limit exercise in healthy children and adults (although see later).

In absolute terms, the maximum ventilation that a child achieves during an exercise test increases with age and growth as the lungs increase in size. In one of the few longitudinal studies examining the ventilatory response of children, $\dot{V}Emax$ was found to rise by 8.8 $L \cdot min^{-1}$ a year between the ages of 9 and 13 years (Rowland & Cunningham 1997). However, contrary to changes in the size of the lungs and its subdivisions, the relationships between $\dot{V}Emax$ and body dimensions (height, body surface area and mass) are not well defined. Reports have suggested that $\dot{V}Emax$ increases with mass by the exponent 0.92 (i.e. close to the ratio standard of 1) and height by the exponent 2.5 (Rowland & Cunningham 1997) such that it might appear that absolute $\dot{V}Emax$ increases proportionately with growth of the lung (which increases with height by the exponent of 3). Allometric analysis of $\dot{V}Emax$, on the other hand, has identified exponents quite disparate from these (Armstrong et al 1997, Mercier et al 1991), with allometric exponents of 0.69 and 0.48 for height and mass, respectively. Other authors have suggested that $\dot{V}Emax$ relative to body mass ($L \cdot min^{-1} \cdot kg^{-1}$) is either unchanged, or declines with age, although the limitations of using ratio standards mean that the nature of growth-related changes in $\dot{V}Emax$ remains unresolved. Suggesting normative values for $\dot{V}Emax$ with children should be avoided, or at least treated with caution, not least since $\dot{V}Emax$ is both protocol and ergometer dependent.

More recently, in a study involving 106 children and where height and mass were considered poor predictors of $\dot{V}E$, it was suggested that in order to make comparisons of 'like with like', ventilatory variables should be normalized to absolute power outputs during cycle ergometry, i.e. $\dot{V}E$ per watt (W) at maximum (Rosenthal & Bush, 2000). Using this analysis, relative $\dot{V}Emax$ ($L \cdot min^{-1} \cdot W^{-1}$) decreased with age in males, but not in females. Such a method for normalizing the ventilatory response to exercise may, however, simply reflect children's metabolic efficiency, rather than nuances of the ventilatory response per se.

Breathing frequency and tidal volume

In order to achieve an elevated $\dot{V}E$ during exercise, a child will breathe more rapidly (increase fR) and more deeply (increase VT). However, the ratio of fR to VT appears to be age dependent. The literature is consistently supportive of a fall in fR at both submaximal and maximal intensities with age (Fig. 6.3). Young children may achieve maximum respiratory rates of up to 70 breaths · min^{-1}, whereas the fully mature adult is likely not to exceed 55–60 breaths · min^{-1}. Coincident with the decline in fR at both submaximal and maximal intensities is an increase in absolute VT, but which either declines or remains unchanged when normalized to body mass. Thus the ratio fR/VT declines with age at all exercise intensities. The relationships between fR, V̇E and VT at maximum are nicely illustrated by Godfrey (1974) drawing on some of the earliest work collated in this field (Astrand 1952) (Fig. 6.4). Since then the understanding that the ratio of fR to VT during exercise declines with age has rarely been questioned.

The most likely explanation for this shift in the ratio of fR to VT lies with the mechanical changes that occur from birth through to adulthood, and the interrelationship between the lung size and the elastic and resistive forces of the pulmonary system. Children have a high resistance to flow, which naturally favours a low fR and a large VT. However, a small lung and poor compliance in children favours the opposite. It might be assumed that the high ratio of fR/VT displayed by children is an outcome of the ratio of a high resistance but relatively poorer compliance of the lungs, which in terms of efficiency will favour high respiratory rates and small tidal volumes.

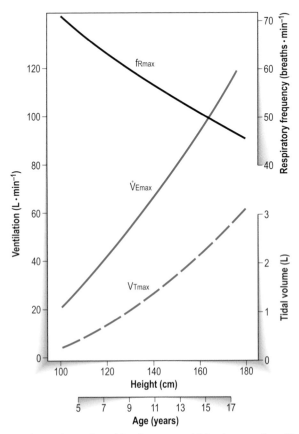

Figure 6.4   Changes in maximum breathing frequency, tidal volume and ventilation with height and age. (Data from Astrand 1952; from Godfrey 1974, with permission of Saunders.)

It should be noted that even if this pattern of response is most economical for the child, compared to the adult lung in which resistance is low and compliance high, the cost of ventilation for any $\dot{V}O_2$ will be comparatively high, and this may contribute to the greater O_2 cost of exercise in children than adults as discussed earlier.

In addition, the ratio of fR to VT in order to achieve $\dot{V}E$ must be adequate in order to maintain optimum alveolar ventilation ($\dot{V}A$). Consider the basic principles which govern the relationships between VT, dead space (VDS) and alveolar volumes (VA):

1. $VA = VT - VDS$ where values are absolute volumes
2. $VA \cdot fR = VT \cdot fR - VDS \cdot fR$
3. $\dot{V}A = \dot{V}E - \dot{V}DS$ where $\dot{V}E$ is minute ventilation, $\dot{V}DS$ is dead space ventilation and $\dot{V}A$ is alveolar ventilation.

It is clear that if the VT falls to extremely low levels, irrespective of the fR, the ratio of VT to $\dot{V}DS$ is compromised at the cost of optimum $\dot{V}A$. Even if it were more economical for a child to achieve a given $\dot{V}E$ by further reducing their VT and increasing their fR, this would severely interfere with $\dot{V}A$. The ratio VT to $\dot{V}DS$ does not appear to change with age, and thus it is also possible that the child's ventilatory response is a compromise between mechanical efficiency and maintaining optimal $\dot{V}A$.

Although the literature is convincing with regard to age-related changes in the ratio of fR to VT during rest and at steady-state exercise, less certain is the pattern of the fR and VT response to a test of increasing exercise intensity in children. For adults, it is generally accepted that VT increases to approximately 60% of VC, at which point it remains stable, and increases in fR bring about the subsequent changes in $\dot{V}E$ (in a similar pattern to changes in cardiac output and stroke volume in response to an increasing exercise intensity). Some data are available that offer support for a similar response in children. During four 3-minute bouts of running at speeds increasing from 7 to 10 $km \cdot h^{-1}$, 11-year-old prepubescent children showed an increase in both fR and VT but also a 19% increase in the ratio fR/VT (Armstrong et al 1997). This implied that fR made a greater contribution to the increasing $\dot{V}E$ at higher exercise intensities than VT. However, contrary to this, other authors have identified the opposite pattern in children, suggesting that fR rises until high intensity, after which it plateaus and VT continues to rise. In terms of pulmonary mechanics, the adult response is indicative of the work required to overcome elastic forces at high tidal volumes, and at 60% of VC, efficiency is minimized by increasing the rate of inflation over and above VT. In children, it is more difficult to suggest why either of the patterns identified earlier might be deemed more efficient at high intensities. However, the former pattern suggests that in line with rest and submaximal exercise, a greater reliance on fR to achieve the required $\dot{V}E$ must be due to poor lung compliance being more costly than airway resistance even at high intensities.

Kinetics of ventilation

Until now, the ventilatory responses to graded exercise intensities have been discussed under the simple pretence that ventilatory parameters are unchanged with time at a set intensity. However, a fundamental component of the respiratory response is the temporal pattern with which $\dot{V}E$ and associated variables respond to exercise, both with the onset of exercise and following prolonged steady-state exercise.

The kinetics of $\dot{V}O_2$ are now reasonably well described in children (see Chapter 9) but studies exploring $\dot{V}E$ kinetics in children are sparse, which is surprising considering the information these data might provide with regard to the control of ventilation.

In adults, $\dot{V}E$ responds to the onset of constant load exercise in three phases. During phase 1, $\dot{V}E$ increases in virtual synchrony with the onset of exercise for approximately 20 s, after which it rises exponentially (with a time constant (τ) of approximately 70 s), and at moderate intensity achieves a steady state by the third minute of exercise. The rapid increase in $\dot{V}E$ at the onset of exercise is accompanied by a rapid increase in cardiac output which causes $\dot{V}O_2$ measured at the mouth to rise, whilst arterial blood gas tensions and R remain constant. The precise control mechanisms responsible for this phase 1 response are not entirely understood. Any form of humoral control is unlikely to be due to the speed of the response and therefore neurogenic mechanisms, originating from the exercising limbs and/or the cerebral cortex, are considered to be likely sources of the rapid hyperpnoea. During phase 2, $\dot{V}O_2$ rises exponentially with a time constant of 30–45 s due to the exponentiality of the oxygen consumption at the muscle, and $\dot{V}CO_2$ and $\dot{V}E$ follow this pattern of response in order to maintain normoxia. However, the kinetics of $\dot{V}CO_2$ lag behind those of $\dot{V}O_2$ due to tissue storage of CO_2, as do the kinetics of $\dot{V}E$, with time constants of some 20 and 25 s slower than those of $\dot{V}O_2$, respectively. The mismatching of $\dot{V}O_2$ to $\dot{V}CO_2$ during this stage explains the fall in R associated with the onset of exercise. Also, as $\dot{V}E$ lags behind $\dot{V}O_2$ quite considerably and $\dot{V}CO_2$ marginally, there is a noticeable fall in $PETO_2$ and short elevation in $PETCO_2$ during this stage.

The general kinetic response pattern of $\dot{V}E$ is thought to be similar in children to that in adults (Fig. 6.5), but data concerning the phase 1 hyperpnoea in children are severely limited by breath-by-breath noise in the response and small amplitudes of $\dot{V}E$ displayed by children. However, there are some data available which are concerned with the phase 2 kinetic response in children. During both square wave exercise transitions and sinusoidal exercise, the $\dot{V}E$ time constant has been demonstrated to be shorter in children than in adults. Most recently, in a comparison of the kinetic

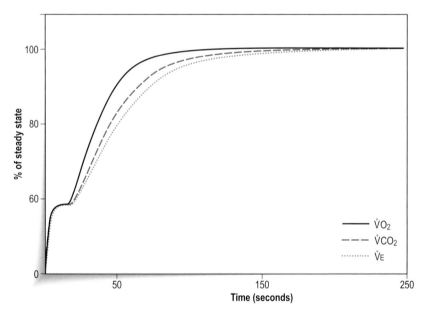

Figure 6.5 Pattern of the kinetic response of $\dot{V}O_2$, $\dot{V}CO_2$ and $\dot{V}E$ following a transition from loadless pedalling to moderate intensity exercise in children.

Table 6.2 Kinetic response to an increase from loadless pedalling to moderate intensity exercise in children and adults (data from Welsman et al 2001)

	Children		Adults	
	Male (n = 12)	Female (n = 10)	Male (n = 12)	Female (n = 9)
τ$\dot{V}O_2$ (s)	19.6 ± 2.5	20.3 ± 4.7	28.3 ± 8.9**	26.1 ± 4.3**
τ$\dot{V}CO_2$ (s)	34.3 ± 3.8	34.7 ± 7.1	55.2 ± 14.0**	48.2 ± 7.1**
τ$\dot{V}E$ (s)	37.9 ± 5.9	41.9 ± 8.4	60.1 ± 16.3**	52.8 ± 9.5*
τ$\dot{V}E$ – τ$\dot{V}CO_2$ (s)	3.7 ± 5.0	7.2 ± 4.8	4.8 ± 5.5	4.5 ± 6.4
τ$\dot{V}CO_2$ – τ$\dot{V}O_2$ (s)	23.8 ± 5.9	22.9 ± 8.4	44.9 ± 14.5**	37.1 ± 7.6**

τ$\dot{V}O_2$, $\dot{V}O_2$ time constant; τ$\dot{V}CO_2$, $\dot{V}CO_2$ time constant; τ$\dot{V}E$, $\dot{V}E$ time constant; τ$\dot{V}E$ – τ$\dot{V}CO_2$, difference between τ$\dot{V}E$ and τ$\dot{V}CO_2$; τ$\dot{V}CO_2$ – τ$\dot{V}O_2$, difference between τ$\dot{V}CO_2$ and τ$\dot{V}O_2$; ** significant within-sex group difference ($P < 0.01$); * ($P < 0.05$).

response between 11- to 12-year-old children and adults, the time constants for $\dot{V}O_2$, $\dot{V}CO_2$ and $\dot{V}E$ in response to a step change to moderate intensity exercise were significantly shorter in the children than in the adults (Table 6.2) (Welsman et al 2001). The shorter $\dot{V}O_2$ time constant suggested a more rapid aerobic response in the children, which would also have resulted in a more rapid $\dot{V}CO_2$ and $\dot{V}E$ response. However, the lag between the $\dot{V}O_2$ and $\dot{V}E$ time constants was significantly smaller in the children. This implies that in fact the $\dot{V}E$ kinetic response undergoes independent change with age.

As had been reported previously, Welsman at al (2001) also identified significantly smaller changes in $PETCO_2$ from baseline to steady-state exercise in the children (mean (standard deviation) children: 2.2 (0.8) and 2.0 (1.0); adults 6.2 (2.7) and 4.7 (2.8) mmHg in males and females, respectively). This is potentially indicative of a lower PCO_2 set point in children than in adults. In line with this, it has been suggested that the shorter $\dot{V}E$ time constant in children may be indicative of a greater sensitivity of the peripheral chemoreceptors, since in adults the carotid bodies are thought to modulate $\dot{V}E$ kinetics. However, it is also likely that the shorter $\dot{V}E$ time constant is simply a function of the shorter $\dot{V}CO_2$ time constant in children. Since children have a smaller capacity for storage of CO_2 in haemoglobin and body fat during exercise, metabolically released CO_2 becomes evident more quickly than it does in adults and therefore invokes a more rapid ventilatory response. Irrespective of the mechanism for a faster $\dot{V}E$ response in children, it results in a closer coupling of $\dot{V}E$ to $\dot{V}O_2$ and less disruption of PaO_2 at the onset of exercise.

The third phase of the kinetic response represents, in theory, a period of steady state. When the exercise is of moderate intensity, oxidative phosphorylation maintains energy turnover, and $\dot{V}O_2$ and $\dot{V}CO_2$ remain stable. Contrary to this, $\dot{V}E$ rises steadily during sustained steady-state exercise by about 10% over a 60-minute period, due to an increase in fR and a small fall in VT. The precise mechanisms responsible for this ventilatory drift are not known, but are most likely related to increases in core temperature. When exercise is above the TVENT, i.e. heavy or very heavy intensity, the ventilatory drift is exaggerated further due to increasing lactic acidosis and the release of CO_2. During sustained heavy intensity exercise in adults, $\dot{V}E$ may increase 50%

defined as a 4% drop in PaO_2 saturation, and a significant reduction in PaO_2 saturation from rest to 75% and 100% of $\dot{V}O_2$max. These children had maximum $\dot{V}O_2$max values ranging from 42 to 62 mL · kg^{-1} · min^{-1}, which were considerably lower than the values reported for the highly trained males usually associated with EIAH, but comparable to some women who had demonstrated EIAH. The seven children who demonstrated EIAH had lower values of $\Delta\dot{V}E/\Delta\dot{V}CO_2$ but showed no difference in end-tidal CO_2 which led the authors to propose that mechanisms other than inadequate compensatory hyperventilation were implicated. There is little evidence to suggest the existence of age-related maturation of $\dot{V}A/\dot{Q}$ inequality or diffusion limitation, and so whether anatomical changes in lung size and mechanics influence children's ability to maintain normoxia during exercise is not known. Clearly, a great deal more work is required to identify whether EIAH, and indeed pulmonary function, is in fact limiting to exercise in children.

Adaptations with training

Understanding the potential for training to induce improvements in pulmonary function in children is fundamentally difficult. There is a shortage of well-controlled longitudinal training studies but conversely a number of cross-sectional studies that are frequently cited as evidence for training adaptations of pulmonary function in children. Cross-sectional studies compare trained children with age-matched controls and have often, although not always, reported superior lung function in those having participated in sports training. Trained children have been shown to demonstrate a larger FVC, greater FEV_1 and MVV and a higher $\dot{V}E$ and lower ratio of fR to VT that suggest a more developed lung. However, such cross-sectional studies cannot discount the problem that trained children may simply be genetically predisposed to better lung function than their untrained counterparts, and have opted into training regimes due to being naturally adept at physical exercise.

Some well-controlled longitudinal data do exist which suggest that training may enhance pulmonary function, at least in swimmers. In five prepubertal girls, a year of swim training invoked improvements in VC, FRC, TLC and airflow per unit lung volume over and above changes in age-matched controls (Courteix et al 1997). Longitudinal studies have also suggested that endurance training that enhances $\dot{V}O_2$max appears to result in an increase in $\dot{V}E$max, which is mostly due to increases in VT rather than fR. Changes in $\dot{V}E$ and respiratory responses during submaximal exercise, however, are less likely.

SEX DIFFERENCES

The sex differences in the size of the lungs shadow to a vast extent those of height. The adolescent growth spurt in length and width of the lung in girls precedes that of boys by approximately 1.6–2.0 years. As we have seen, the ratio of thoracic width to height decreases with age in both males and females, although in girls the increase in thoracic width is minimal, and between the ages of 11.5 and 18.5 years, the increase in thoracic height in males is twice that of females. When matched by height, prepubertal boys tend to have higher TLC than girls, and thereafter the volumes of the lung exceed those in girls and for a given age and height, boys have a greater number of alveoli and a larger alveolar surface area than girls (Thurlbeck 1982). Measures of lung function (FEV_1, FVC and FEV_1/FVC) are greater in height matched boys during pre-puberty, but during the pubertal growth spurt, all measures of lung function apart from FVC are higher in girls than boys. Following the growth spurt, discontinuity in lung function is evident, and males outperform females in all parameters of lung function due to both greater lung and thoracic size as well as muscle strength.

Prepubertal boys have smaller airways in relation to lung size compared with girls, and as a result, girls demonstrate superior airflow per unit lung volume (Rosenthal et al 1993). Subsequently, the growth rate of airways relative to volume is greater in males such that by late adolescence, airways are equal to or relatively larger than in girls (Merkus et al 1993). This prepubertal sex difference in anatomy of the airways has been related to the greater prevalence of respiratory disease in young boys than girls. Equally, sex differences in the mechanical properties of the lung relating to tone of the airways have been reported (Taussig et al 1981) as have consistently lower specific airway resistance in girls than boys (Doershuk et al 1974), although more recent work has failed to support these findings (Lanteri & Sly 1993).

The fundamental pulmonary response to exercise does not appear to differ between prepubertal girls and boys. Armstrong et al (1997) demonstrated that at maximum, and at equal absolute or relative exercise intensity, prepubertal boys demonstrated a higher absolute and body size corrected $\dot{V}E$ and VT than girls. This, however, was attributable to the significantly higher absolute and relative $\dot{V}O_2$ at each exercise intensity. These authors found no significant sex difference in fR, VT/FVC, $\dot{V}E/\dot{V}O_2$ or $\dot{V}E/\dot{V}CO_2$ at all exercise intensities. There are some conflicting data that suggest that in older children, the ventilatory equivalent for girls ($\dot{V}E/\dot{V}O_2$) is higher than for boys at maximal and submaximal exercise intensities, which is more consistent with the adult literature. These data suggest that there might be a divergence in the $\dot{V}E$ response to exercise between males and females which follows the sex differences in changes in lung size and function that occur during puberty. This remains to be proven.

As has already been identified, sex differences in susceptibility to EIAH exist, and women with a relatively low $\dot{V}O_2$max will be more likely to demonstrate excessive widening of the $A - aDO_2$ and hypoventilation than 'fitness'-matched males. However, when male and female subjects are matched for age, height, aerobic power and lung size, women do not experience greater EIAH than men; in fact, they may have better $\dot{V}A/\dot{Q}$ matching than men (Olfert et al 2004) and therefore it is more likely that lung size and aerobic power are the determining factors in EIAH, rather than sex per se. Sex differences have not specifically been explored with regard to EIAH in children, although of the seven prepubertal children that demonstrated EIAH in the study of Nourry et al (2004), five were in fact male. This might suggest that arterial hypoxaemia is independent of sex at this age, although whether this remains so during puberty and adolescence is not known.

SUMMARY

The pulmonary systems of the newly born baby and the fully grown adult are not the same. The lungs and thorax of the newborn are equipped to support prenatal life and easy passage during birth, whereas an adult requires a system that is able to exchange O_2 and CO_2 between the surrounding air and the alveoli efficiently and in the most extreme of environments. The structural and mechanical requirements of the pulmonary system during these life stages are quite different. During the growing years, the pulmonary system adapts, and as the lungs grow and develop, changes in the way in which ventilation is achieved are apparent. Nevertheless, the basic ventilatory response to exercise is similar in children and adults, and during these transitional years, the pulmonary system is more than capable of supporting exercise even at the highest of exercise intensities.

KEY POINTS

1. The lung and thorax increase in size during growth, closely related to increases in height. As the lungs and thorax increase in size relative to height, so do static and dynamic lung volumes.
2. Growth of components of the lung and thorax, and their mechanical properties that contribute to the ventilatory cost of breathing, is not entirely uniform. This invokes age-related changes in the way in which ventilation to sustain normoxia during rest and exercise is achieved.
3. Children have a higher $\dot{V}E$ for a given $\dot{V}O_2$. The evidence to date suggests that this hyperventilation is due to a greater respiratory drive in children and a lower set point for PCO_2.
4. The pattern of the $\dot{V}E$ response to an incremental exercise test is essentially similar in children and adults, although the ventilatory threshold is likely to occur at a higher percentage of peak $\dot{V}O_2$ than it does in adults.
5. At the onset of constant load exercise $\dot{V}E$ responds in three phases with the same basic profile as adults. The phase 2 time constant of the $\dot{V}E$ response is faster than it is in adults, and during phase 3 at moderate intensity (steady state) end-tidal PCO_2 is lower than in adults.
6. Lower exercising end-tidal PCO_2, a higher ventilatory equivalent for CO_2 and a greater neural respiratory drive in children suggests that the control of ventilation undergoes maturation with age. The reasons for this are not entirely understood.
7. Pulmonary function is not generally considered to be limiting to exercise. However, there is some evidence to suggest that exercise-induced arterial hypoxaemia, which is normally evident in highly trained males, may occur in some children at high exercise intensities.
8. Training adaptations of the pulmonary response to exercise might occur, but the lack of well-controlled longitudinal studies means that it is difficult to identify if the enhanced pulmonary response in trained children is due to training overload or natural predisposition to sporting participation.
9. Girls have smaller lungs and static and dynamic lung volumes than boys at all ages, apart from the short period when girls begin their adolescent growth spurt earlier than boys. Sex differences in the ventilatory response to exercise may exist in older children, but data are not conclusive.

References

Armstrong N, Kirby B J, McManus A M et al 1997 Prepubescents' ventilatory responses to exercise with reference to sex and body size. Chest 112:1554–1560

Astrand P O 1952 Experimental studies of physical working capacity in relation to sex and age. Munksgaard, Copenhagen

Cook C D, Hamann J F 1961 Relation of lung volumes to height in healthy persons between the ages of 5 and 38 years. Journal of Pediatrics 59:710–714

Courteix D, Obert P, Lecoq A M et al 1997 Effect of intensive swimming training on lung volumes, airway resistance and on the maximal expiratory flow–volume relationship in prepubertal girls. European Journal of Applied Physiology 76:264–269

DeGroodt E G, van Pelt W, Borsboom G J et al 1988 Growth of lung and thorax dimensions during the pubertal growth spurt. European Respiratory Journal 1:102–108

Doershuk C F, Fisher B J, Matthews L W 1974 Specific airway resistance from the perinatal period into adulthood. Alterations in childhood pulmonary disease. American Review of Respiratory Disease 109:452–457

Dunnill M S 1962 Postnatal growth of the lung. Thorax 17:329–333

Gaultier C, Perret L, Boule M et al 1981 Occlusion pressure and breathing pattern in healthy children. Respiration Physiology 46:71–80

Godfrey S 1974 Exercise testing in children. Saunders, London

Hammond M D, Gale G E, Kapitan K S et al 1986 Pulmonary gas exchange in humans during exercise at sea level. Journal of Applied Physiology 60:1590–1598

Harms C A, McClaran S R, Nickele G A et al 1998 Exercise-induced arterial hypoxaemia in healthy young women. Journal of Physiology 507 (Pt 2):619–628

Lanteri C J, Sly P D 1993 Changes in respiratory mechanics with age. Journal of Applied Physiology 74:369–378

Mansell A L, Bryan A C, Levison H 1977 Relationship of lung recoil to lung volume and maximum expiratory flow in normal children. Journal of Applied Physiology 42:817–823

Mercier J, Varray A, Ramonatxo M et al 1991 Influence of anthropometric characteristics on changes in maximal exercise ventilation and breathing pattern during growth in boys. European Journal of Applied Physiology and Occupational Physiology 63:235–241

Merkus P J, Borsboom G J, Van Pelt W et al 1993 Growth of airways and air spaces in teenagers is related to sex but not to symptoms. Journal of Applied Physiology 75:2045–2053

Nourry C, Fabre C, Bart F et al 2004 Evidence of exercise-induced arterial hypoxemia in prepubescent trained children. Pediatric Research 55:674–681

Olfert I M, Balouch J, Kleinsasser A et al 2004 Does gender affect human pulmonary gas exchange during exercise? Journal of Physiology 557(Pt 2):529–541

Polgar G, Weng T R 1979 The functional development of the respiratory system from the period of gestation to adulthood. American Review of Respiratory Disease 120:625–695

Potter C R, Childs D J, Houghton W et al 1999 Breath-to-breath 'noise' in children's ventilatory and gas exchange responses to exercise. European Journal of Applied Physiology 80:118–124

Rosenthal M, Bush A 2000 Ventilatory variables in normal children during rest and exercise. European Respiratory Journal 16:1075–1083

Rosenthal M, Bain S H, Cramer D et al 1993 Lung function in white children aged 4 to 19 years: I – spirometry. Thorax 48:794–802

Rowland T W, Cunningham L N 1997 Development of ventilatory responses to exercise in normal white children. A longitudinal study. Chest 111:327–332

Simon G, Reid L, Tanner J M et al 1972 Growth of radiologically determined heart diameter, lung width, and lung length from 5–19 years, with standards for clinical use. Archives of Disease in Childhood 47:373–381

Springer C, Cooper D M, Wasserman K 1988 Evidence that maturation of the peripheral chemoreceptors is not complete in childhood. Respiration Physiology 74:55–64

Taussig L M, Cota K, Kaltenborn W 1981 Different mechanical properties of the lung in boys and girls. American Review of Respiratory Disease 123:640–643

Thurlbeck W M 1982 Postnatal human lung growth. Thorax 37:564–571

Welsman J R, Fawkner S G, Armstrong N 2001 Respiratory response to non-steady state exercise in children and adults (abstract). Pediatric Exercise Science 13:263–264

Zapletal A, Paul T, Samanek M 1976 Pulmonary elasticity in children and adolescents. Journal of Applied Physiology 40:953–961

Further reading

Cooper D M 1995 Rethinking exercise testing in children: A challenge. American Journal of Respiratory and Critical Care Medicine 152:1154–1157
Ohuchi H, Kato Y, Tasato H et al 1999 Ventilatory response and arterial blood gases during exercise in children. Pediatric Research 45:389–396
Nagano Y, Baba R, Kuraishi K et al 1998 Ventilatory control during exercise in normal children. Pediatric Research 43:704–707
Nixon P A 2000 Pulmonary function. In: Armstrong N, Van Mechelen W (eds) Paediatric exercise science and medicine. Oxford University Press, Oxford, p 47–56

Chapter **7**

Cardiovascular function

Richard J. Winsley

CHAPTER CONTENTS

LEARNING OBJECTIVES

After studying this chapter you should be able to:
1. describe the determinants of cardiac output
2. evaluate the different methods of assessing cardiac output in children
3. equate for differences in body size in cardiac function
4. describe resting cardiac function in children
5. discuss cardiac function during exercise in children
6. discuss the changes in cardiac function as a result of endurance training in children.

INTRODUCTION

The cardiovascular system plays an integral role in allowing a person to exercise. Without an efficiently functioning pump and blood distribution network the exercising muscle would not receive the necessary oxygenated blood and nutrients to allow exercise to continue for more than a minute or so. Additionally, the by-products of

oxidative and anaerobic metabolism could not be removed nor would the heat generated by muscular activity be adequately dissipated, all potentially limiting the ability
of an individual to exercise.

Although we have a relatively complete understanding of how an adult's cardiovascular system responds to exercise, the practical, technological and ethical limitations in
assessing cardiovascular function in the exercising child mean that our knowledge
of children's responses is only slowly taking shape. There is also the added challenge
of interpreting these responses in relation to growth and maturation, so that fair
comparison can be made with the responses of adults.

INTEGRATION OF CARDIAC OUTPUT, STROKE VOLUME AND HEART RATE

It is important to understand the factors that interact to regulate cardiac output ($\dot{Q}$).
Although this is well covered in most standard anatomy and physiology texts (see
Silverthorn 2001), its revision is useful so that the terms and interactions of the
variables involved are familiar when discussed later.

As can be seen in Figure 7.1 cardiac output is the product of heart rate (HR) and
stroke volume (SV) and changes in either or both of these variables will affect $\dot{Q}$.
Stroke volume refers to the amount of blood expelled by the heart in each beat and is

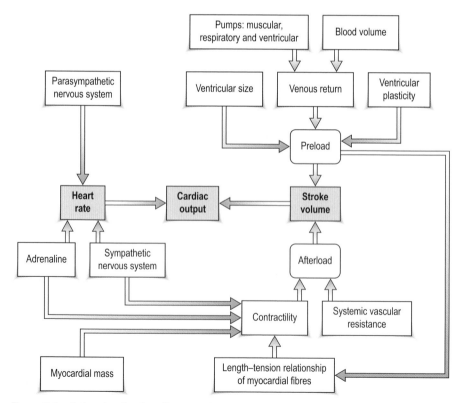

Figure 7.1   Determinants of cardiac output.

measured in millilitres (mL). It represents the difference between the volume of blood in the ventricles before contraction (preload) and that remaining in the ventricles after the heart has contracted (afterload). Preload is influenced by the capacity of the ventricles, how much they distend as they fill with blood – although this is quite small and limited by the pericardium – and most importantly venous return. The heart can only pump out the amount of blood it receives back from the systemic circulation; therefore venous return is critical in determining SV. Muscular, thoracic and ventricular 'pumps' all aid venous return and will be described in more detail later. Although blood volume usually stays fairly constant during exercise of short to moderate duration, if blood volume reduces or increases this can affect SV. For example, in exercise of a longer duration without adequate rehydration, or if an individual starts exercising in a state of dehydration this may result in hypovolaemia potentially reducing venous return. Conversely, training-induced expansion in blood volume leads to an increase in SV. Thus acute or chronic changes in blood volume can be important determinants of SV.

Afterload is determined by the strength with which the heart muscle contracts to eject the blood contained within the ventricles and by the systemic vascular resistance. Systemic vascular resistance refers to the resistance to flow provided by the vascular network. If resistance is high then it will be more difficult to eject the blood from the ventricles into the circulation, more blood will remain in the heart after contraction, increasing afterload and reducing SV. Conversely, if systemic vascular resistance is low, afterload will be reduced and SV will increase. Contractility is influenced firstly by preload – the stretching of the myocardial fibres through the volume of blood filling the ventricles promotes the Frank–Starling mechanism that in turn aids contractility. Secondly, contractility is related to the size and thickness of the myocardial mass – an increased cardiac muscle mass produces more force facilitating ejection of blood from the ventricles. Finally, the inotropic effects of noradrenaline released by the sympathetic nervous system and adrenaline secreted by the adrenal glands both act to increase contractility. Activation of the myocardial beta-receptors by these substrates allows an increased entry of calcium ions into the myocardial cell from the extracellular fluid; this then triggers an increase in the release of stored calcium ions from the sarcoplasmic reticulum, the combined result of which leads to an enhanced delivery of calcium to the actin–troponin complexes, resulting in an enhanced contractile strength.

The sympathetic nervous system and circulating adrenaline also have a chronotropic effect, serving to increase HR. Conversely the parasympathetic nervous system, through the release of its neurotransmitter acetylcholine (ACh), reduces HR. The heart's intrinsic rhythm is set by the sinoatrial node (SA node), which will produce a rate of approximately 100–120 bts $\cdot$ min^{-1} without any neural or hormonal input. These myocardial auto-rhythmic cells have the attribute of being able to generate innate action potentials and thus safeguard a basic HR. However, the net effect of sympathetic and parasympathetic autonomic modulation is to increase and decrease heart rate, respectively. A predominance of sympathetic autonomic modulation increases HR above its intrinsic level and vice versa for parasympathetic modulation.

The sympathetic nervous system innervates the SA node, the atrioventricular (AV) node, the atria and the ventricles of the heart, and its regulation of HR occurs through a combination of both neural and hormonal pathways. Sympathetic efferent impulses travel from the brain towards their target organs and release the catecholamines noradrenaline and adrenaline. As discussed previously, the catecholamines facilitate the influx of calcium ions into the myocardial cells, speeding depolarization of the myocardial cell and initiating contraction. Additionally, there is also a shorter duration of contraction because of an enhanced recycling of the calcium ions back to the sarcoplasmic reticulum combined with their faster removal from the cell to the extracellular fluid. Thus the cell is repolarized more quickly, allowing it to be ready for the next heartbeat.

Parasympathetic nerve impulses reach the heart via the right and left vagus nerves. These innervate the SA and AV nodes and the atrial myocardium. In contrast to the response of the sympathetic nervous system, there is no parasympathetic innervation of the ventricular myocardium. Vagal efferent impulses trigger the release of ACh at their synapses. Acetylcholine combines with the myocardial muscarinic receptors, which results in an increased efflux of potassium ions and a reduced influx of calcium ions. This results in cell hyperpolarization, slowing the rate of depolarization and thus HR.

With $\dot{Q}$ being influenced by a range of modifiable factors, it can be more sensitively up- or downregulated depending on the metabolic demands of the body at any moment in time.

MEASURING CARDIAC OUTPUT AND STROKE VOLUME

Although the assessment of HR at rest and during exercise in children can be performed easily, cheaply and non-invasively, unfortunately the same is not true for $\dot{Q}$ and SV.

Our understanding of children's cardiac function during exercise has been limited by the lack of safe, accurate and non-invasive means of assessing $\dot{Q}$. Most techniques require a period of steady-state exercise, making measurements during high intensity exercise virtually impossible. Additionally, there is no 'gold standard' by which such techniques can be measured and validated. Even using the same methodology, variability as high as 10–20% is observed, and it is uncertain whether such variability can be attributed to biological or technical factors. With these caveats stated at the outset, a brief overview of the different methods available to assess $\dot{Q}$ and SV follows. Interested readers should refer to the reviews by Barber (2000) and Driscoll et al (1989) for further details.

Invasive methods

Direct Fick

This method calculates $\dot{Q}$ directly according to the Fick principle:

$$\text{Cardiac output} = \frac{O_2 \text{ uptake}}{\text{arterial } O_2 \text{ concentration} - \text{mixed venous } O_2 \text{ concentration}}$$

$$\text{i.e. } \dot{Q} = \frac{\dot{V}O_2}{CaO_2 - CvO_2}$$

Arterial oxygen content and mixed venous oxygen content are measured directly from the blood within the systemic and pulmonary arteries concurrently with a measure of oxygen uptake ($\dot{V}O_2$). Invasive cardiac catheterization is necessary to collect this measure and its accuracy is only verified during steady-state conditions, restricting its use during exercise at higher exercise intensities. However, with a reproducibility error of approximately 5%, it represents the closest thing to a gold standard for such measurements.

Dye dilution and thermodilution

The dye dilution method involves injecting a known quantity of dye into the circulation using either a pulmonary artery catheter or a central venous line. The concentration of the dye in blood is then determined over time giving an estimate of $\dot{Q}$. It has been successfully validated against the direct Fick method, but a measurement variation of between 5% and 30% has been described for the dye dilution technique, resulting from errors of incomplete mixing of the dye with blood, especially during rapid flow rates (e.g. during exercise). This method has, however, been used with children despite its inherent limitations.

The thermodilution technique requires injection of a cold fluid into the circulation with subsequent assessment of its temperature change to measure $\dot{Q}$ and SV. However, loss of coolant from the circulation to the interstitial fluid can affect the accuracy of the measurement.

The use of direct methods to determine $\dot{Q}$ in healthy children is normally agreed to be unethical and although these methods have been used with children, studies are few in number and generally limited to clinical populations. Consequently, non-invasive measures for the assessment of $\dot{Q}$ and SV are essential.

Non–invasive methods

The rebreathing techniques have conventionally been the methods of choice for the non-invasive assessment of $\dot{Q}$. They are indirect and remove the need for invasive arterial and mixed venous blood sampling by catheterization, so are well suited for use with children. The techniques measure the change in concentration of a reference gas as it diffuses from the lungs and into the blood. They rely on the assumption that the rate of disappearance of the gas is proportional to pulmonary blood flow and that pulmonary blood flow and $\dot{Q}$ are essentially equal.

Carbon dioxide rebreathing

This method uses carbon dioxide (CO_2) to represent the inert gas and employs the Fick principle written for CO_2 as follows:

$$\text{Cardiac output} = \frac{CO_2 \text{ production}}{\text{mixed venous } CO_2 \text{ concentration} - \text{arterial } CO_2 \text{ concentration}}$$

$$\text{i.e. } \dot{Q} = \frac{\dot{V}CO_2}{CvCO_2 - CaCO_2}$$

$\dot{V}CO_2$ can be measured directly using a flow meter and CO_2 gas analyser. However, it is more difficult to estimate CO_2 content within arterial and mixed venous blood. $CaCO_2$ estimates can be established from end-tidal CO_2 concentration, whilst $CvCO_2$ is estimated by the subject rebreathing a gas mixture containing CO_2 at a concentration predicted to be close to that of the mixed venous concentration. The subject continually rebreathes this CO_2 mixture and eventually the concentration in the bag plateaus at a concentration equal to that of the mixed venous circulation. These estimates of arterial and mixed venous CO_2 concentrations are then converted into further estimates of CO_2 content to predict $\dot{Q}$.

Herein lies the problem with this method: several formulae and conversion equations exist to calculate $\dot{Q}$. As Marks et al (1985) observed, the variety of possible equations to measure $CvCO_2$ and $CaCO_2$ created the potential for 36 different estimates of $\dot{Q}$ ranging from 2 to 11.1 L · min^{-1} from a single data set. Errors with young subjects can also arise through poor choice of rebreathing bag size: if the bag is too small it may collapse during rebreathing, but if it is too large it can delay or even preclude the attainment of a plateau. Similarly, if the chosen CO_2 concentration is too low or high equilibrium, may not be reached during the rebreathing manoeuvre. These disadvantages are further confounded by the fact that if rebreathing continues for too long, the possibility of recirculation increases, which will overestimate $\dot{Q}$ values. Therefore technical experience is required to appropriately select subject-specific bag volumes and CO_2 concentrations. Finally, the rebreathing of CO_2 is unpleasant, particularly at the high flow rates experienced during exercise, making the compliance of young subjects difficult.

In adults, the CO_2 rebreathing method has been reported to under- and overestimate $\dot{Q}$ by as much as 31% and 11%, respectively. A similarly wide variation has been reported in children, $\dot{Q}$ values differing by as much as 9–21% depending on the equations used. However, the reliability of this method has been shown to be high. During submaximal exercise, test–retest correlation coefficients have been reported to be >0.80 in both adults and children. Because of the necessity to be in a steady state for the technique's assumptions to be met, estimates of validity and reliability at maximal exercise, although reported, should be treated with caution.

Acetylene rebreathing

The acetylene (C_2H_2) rebreathing technique is similar to CO_2 rebreathing, except C_2H_2 is used as the inert gas. The rebreathing bag contains a soluble gas (C_2H_2) and an insoluble gas (helium). The soluble gas readily diffuses into the passing pulmonary blood, whilst the insoluble gas concentration stays constant. By measuring the rate of decline in C_2H_2 concentration in the expired air, $\dot{Q}$ can be estimated.

The C_2H_2 rebreathing technique in adults has been validated against direct techniques. Correlation coefficients of >0.80 are reported against both the direct Fick and dye dilution methods during submaximal exercise. However, under/overestimations of $\dot{Q}$ ranging from −12% to +8% have been observed during submaximal exercise in adults. Few investigators have validated the technique during maximal exercise due to the technical and theoretical difficulties involved. As regards reproducibility, coefficients of variation of 3–5% have been reported for adults, but with children substantially larger coefficients of variation (in the region of 25%) have been observed.

Doppler echocardiography

Doppler echocardiography has markedly progressed the assessment of cardiovascular function in children. It is non-obtrusive, less constraining and significantly, it is one of the few methods that does not require steady-state exercise conditions for validity. Consequently, it has been used successfully to evaluate children's $\dot{Q}$ and SV in conditions ranging from rest to maximal exercise.

SV is estimated as the product of aortic blood flow velocity and aortic cross-sectional diameter:

Stroke volume = aortic blood velocity × cross-sectional area of the aorta

The cross-sectional diameter of the aorta is determined at rest, allowing subsequent calculation of area. The Doppler transducer is placed in the suprasternal notch of the subject, allowing the ultrasound signal to be parallel with aortic blood flow. The Doppler shift of the blood can then be measured and its velocity determined. The signal pattern used can be either a continuous-wave or pulse-wave depending on equipment employed.

This technique is not without its drawbacks. The optimal site for cross-sectional aortic measurement is undecided. Its precise measurement is important, as small errors can have a profound effect on SV calculations. Moreover, the assumption that the resting cross-sectional area of the aorta is circular and that it remains constant during exercise is debatable. The technique is dependent on the ultrasound beam being parallel with the direction of aortic blood flow, which is presumed to be uniform, and it must match the position of the aortic cross-sectional area that was measured. Failure to satisfy these conditions will lead to errors in measurement. During intensive exercise the increased movement resulting from ventilation, muscular effort and heart motion all make obtaining reliable measurements difficult.

With adults, Doppler echocardiography has been successfully validated against the direct techniques with correlations of 0.60 for resting and submaximal exercise SV. However, underestimations of $\dot{Q}$ by Doppler echocardiography may be as much as 15–30%. The reliability of this technique in children at rest and during exercise has been reported to be in the region of 5–9%.

Thoracic electrical bioimpedance

Thoracic electrical bioimpedance (TEB) works on the principle that transthoracic electrical impedance changes in proportion to changes in thoracic blood volume and in turn that the change in thoracic blood volume is equal to SV.

This concept, albeit elegant in its simplicity, has some potential problems. The relationship between electrical impedance and blood volume is dependent on the geometry of the thorax. The original equations relied on an oversimplified assumption that the thorax was a homogeneous cylinder of blood with a specific resistivity. For this reason newer equations based on modelling the thorax as a truncated cone were developed and blood resistivity has been eliminated as an independent variable. However, the equations used in the TEB method have proved problematic. Electrical impedance depends upon multiple factors such as thorax morphology, homogeneity of thorax perfusion, thoracic gas and fluid content and subcutaneous adiposity. Additionally, poor electrical contact, movement artefacts from respiration and muscular contraction all affect the impedance signal. Notwithstanding these problems, TEB is cost-effective, safe, does not require steady-state conditions and combines simplicity of use with non-invasive measurements of $\dot{Q}$ and SV in conditions ranging from rest to maximal exercise. For these reasons TEB has been successfully used to characterize children's $\dot{Q}$ and SV responses to exercise.

Correlation coefficients to validate TEB against direct techniques of >0.70 have been described for resting and submaximal exercise in adults, with mean differences reported to be approximately 15–20%. Therefore the validity of TEB to measure $\dot{Q}$ during rest and exercise conditions is at least as good as the more established non-invasive methodologies. The reliability of TEB measurement of $\dot{Q}$ in children has been reported as 9% (Welsman et al 2005).

To summarize, in the absence of being able to assess $\dot{Q}$ directly in healthy children, employing any of the indirect methods comes with a reduced level of accuracy of measurement. Therefore the following description of our knowledge about cardiovascular function in children, especially during exercise, must be interpreted in this context.

BODY SIZE AND CARDIAC FUNCTION

Body size has a strong influence on heart size and dimensions and in order to compare fairly individuals of different body sizes we need to be able to equate for these body size differences. The different methods available to remove the effects of body size from physiological data are discussed in detail in Chapter 2, and the generic issues raised are equally pertinent to cardiac data.

Relationship between cardiovascular variables and body size

Stroke volume is often expressed in absolute terms (mL), but SV increases with increasing body size. Correlation coefficients of 0.8 to 0.9 are reported between resting SV and body mass or body surface area (BSA) in children. This indicates that SV is a size-dependent variable, thus the removal of body size is necessary to facilitate meaningful inter-individual comparisons. Normalization of SV is most commonly performed by the ratio standard approach using BSA as the size denominator, with the resultant variable known as the stroke index (SI) (mL · m^{-2}).

As with SV, resting absolute $\dot{Q}$ (L · min^{-1}) is also related to body size. Correlation coefficients between $\dot{Q}$ and stature, BSA and body mass of 0.7 to 0.9 have been reported. Conventionally, the effects of body size on $\dot{Q}$ have been expressed as a ratio standard with BSA – the cardiac index (CI) (L · min^{-1} · m^{-2}).

With regard to heart dimensions, research has demonstrated that body size relates closely to left ventricular size. Typically correlations of >0.85 have been found between left ventricular end-diastolic diameter (LVEDD) and body mass, stature or BSA in children. An autopsy study with children indicated that heart weight and ventricular wall thickness also increased relative to body mass, stature and BSA (Scholz et al 1988). Finally, the ratio of heart volume to body mass stays constant through 8–18 years; hence it is clear that heart size increases in direct proportion with body size. Consequently, body size must be taken into account when comparing individuals of different sizes.

Equating for differences in body size

In order to remove the effects of body size, cardiac variables have been expressed in relation to body mass, stature, lean body mass and BSA. However, using the ratio standard is only applicable when the two variables under scrutiny are related in a particular manner; failure to meet these assumptions can mean that body size is not appropriately removed and the data become distorted. But which is the appropriate denominator to use?

These dilemmas were explored by Batterham et al (1999) who addressed the allometric relationships between cardiac and body size variables. They argued that volumes are 3-dimensional parameters and include variables such as SV, left ventricular end-diastolic volume (LVEDV), left ventricular end-systolic volume (LVESV), heart mass and left ventricular mass. Lengths are one-dimensional and thus variables such as myocardial wall thickness, LVEDD and left ventricular end-systolic diameter (LVESD) should be so considered. Areas such as aortic cross-sectional area are two-dimensional. Because $\dot{Q}$ ($L \cdot min^{-1}$) is a product of a volume (three-dimensional) over time (one-dimensional), it should also be considered as a two-dimensional parameter. Consequently, to remove the effects of body size using either body mass, stature or BSA the following dimensional exponents should apply:

- SV, LVEDV, LVESV, heart mass, LV mass
    Body mass$^{1.0}$ (volume/volume)
    BSA$^{1.5}$ (volume/area)
    Stature^{3} (volume/length)
- Wall thicknesses, LVEDD, LVESD
    Body mass$^{0.33}$ (length/volume)
    BSA$^{0.5}$ (length/area)
    Stature$^{1.0}$ (length/length)
- $\dot{Q}$
    Body mass$^{0.66}$ (area/volume)
    BSA$^{1.0}$ (area/area)
    Stature$^{2.0}$ (area/length)

Bearing in mind that the ratio standard approach is only valid when the scaling exponent between the two variables is equal to 1.0, what exponents have been reported in children? Cardiac index is theoretically sound because $\dot{Q}$ and BSA are allometrically related to the power of 1.0, and indeed several authors have reported scaling coefficients of 1.0 between BSA and resting $\dot{Q}$. However, others have indicated that it is <1.0 and have therefore questioned the appropriateness of the CI.

Although SI is traditionally reported, it is clear that the theoretical rationale is somewhat debatable; indeed body mass may be a better divisor to use. However, exponents close to 1.0 for BSA and resting and exercise SV have been observed in children, supporting the idea that the use of the SI is appropriate. There also exists a debate about which scaling coefficients to use; one school of thought recommends that theoretically derived exponents be used, whilst others suggest that the unique exponents for the population under investigation be calculated and applied, as regardless of the actual exponent itself these are most appropriate for the group under scrutiny (see Chapter 2).

Recent work by Sluysmans & Colan (2005) concluded that BSA alone was the most important determinant of cardiac size, volumes, areas and diameters. With allometric exponents close to 1.0 reported for $\dot{Q}$ and SV in relation to BSA, it appears that calculating the CI and the SI to equate for differences in body size may be the most pragmatic approach.

CARDIOVASCULAR FUNCTION AT REST

Stroke volume at rest

When interpreting SV data, it is important to recognize that resting SV is affected by body position in both adults and children – SV is approximately 25% greater in the supine than the seated position. This is as a consequence of a reduced venous return in the seated position because of blood pooling in the lower extremities due to the effects of gravity. Direct comparison should only therefore be made between data collected in similar body positions.

Adults and children

Resting SV in absolute terms is greater in adults than children. Absolute values have been reported of 5 mL at birth, 25 mL aged 5 years and 85 mL aged 15 years; hence the strong positive correlation between age and resting SV is unsurprising.

However, why do adults have a greater absolute SV than children? De Simone et al (1998) found that left ventricular mass correlated strongly with SV ($r = 0.85$) from birth, through childhood and into adulthood. As the heart grows in size in parallel with the age-related increase in body size, so does absolute SV. These findings suggest that increases in resting absolute SV during childhood can be accounted for entirely by increases in left ventricular size; there are no data to suggest alterations in myocardial function (i.e. contractility). Resting left ventricular ejection fraction has been demonstrated to be stable with advancing age at approximately 65–70%; measurements of left ventricular shortening fraction (34–36%) and ejection periods by systolic time intervals also show no significant differences in children of different ages or between children and adults. Thus as contractile function appears to be age independent, any age-related differences in absolute SV arise due to body-size-dependent differences in left ventricular size.

When comparing resting SV in relation to body size, as the stroke index, SI stays constant with age, so that adults' resting SI is similar to that of children. Most studies describe resting supine SI of 40–45 mL $\cdot$ m^{-2} in children, reducing to 35 mL $\cdot$ m^{-2} in the upright body position.

Sex differences

Although the data suggest that the SI of boys and girls at rest is similar, with values of 35–53 mL $\cdot$ m^{-2} being reported, this issue remains unclear. Anxiety, body position and whether the measurement taken was at rest or simply pre-exercise all affect the resultant data. In addition, there is the indication that boys' resting SI is higher than that of girls, although statistical significance is not always achieved due to the wide standard deviation of this measure. Whether sex differences in resting SI do exist requires further clarification.

Heart rate at rest

Similar to SV, body position and emotional state can all affect resting HR. Seated resting values are typically 15 bts $\cdot$ min^{-1} higher than those obtained in basal conditions (post-absorptive, lying quietly for at least 30 minutes). Likewise, anxiety or arousal, for example, can also influence HR at rest.

Adults and children

Resting HR declines by 10–20 bts $\cdot$ min^{-1} in children between the ages of 5 and 15 years such that basal HR aged 5 years is typically 80 bts $\cdot$ min^{-1}, declining to about 62 bts $\cdot$ min^{-1} at age 15 years.

But why does a child's resting HR decline with age? Studies that have pharmacologically induced autonomic blockade to the SA node have shown that intrinsic HR declines with age in children. This is thought to arise because of a loss of pacemaker cells in the SA node. In addition to the decline in intrinsic HR, there are data to suggest that there is a maturation of the vagal modulation on HR from birth to young adulthood; however, these data are not conclusive. Rowland (2005) suggested that HR declined at the same rate as basal metabolic rate (BMR). He argued that the decline in resting HR with age parallels that of mass-related BMR. The allometric relationship between HR and body mass has been demonstrated as HR $\propto$ body mass$^{-0.25}$. With a similar allometric relationship between BMR and body mass (BMR $\propto$ body mass$^{-0.25}$) it is plausible that the two are interlinked.

Sex differences

Girls' resting HR is typically 3–5 bts $\cdot$ min^{-1} faster than that of boys. Although some authors argue that this is only evident in children after the age of 10 years, there is evidence that girls' HR is higher than boys' HR from birth onwards. Girls' higher resting HR may be a compensatory mechanism to offset a lower SV in order to maintain $\dot{Q}$.

Cardiac output at rest

Resting $\dot{Q}$ can show considerable intra- and inter-individual variability and is affected by emotional state and body position. Supine resting $\dot{Q}$ is greater than $\dot{Q}$ in the upright body position due to blood pooling in the lower extremities in the latter. Supine CI has been reported as 4 L $\cdot$ min^{-1} $\cdot$ m^{-2} and in the sitting position somewhat lower at 3–4 L $\cdot$ min^{-1} $\cdot$ m^{-2}.

Adults and children

In general, resting absolute $\dot{Q}$ increases with age secondary to increased body size. Resting $\dot{Q}$ of an adult is approximately 5 L $\cdot$ min^{-1}, which is the same as the total adult blood volume of approximately 5 L. Unsurprisingly, children have a lower absolute resting $\dot{Q}$ than adults, ranging from 3 to 4 L $\cdot$ min^{-1} and reflecting their smaller body size.

When $\dot{Q}$ is expressed relative to body size as CI a different picture emerges. Mass-related BMR declines with age and therefore so does $\dot{V}O_2$ in relation to body mass. With a close relationship between $\dot{Q}$ and $\dot{V}O_2$ this means that $\dot{Q}$ relative to body size also declines. From ages 6 to 18 years there is a 20% decline in BMR relative to BSA; thus CI declines to a similar extent; typically resting CI is 6 L $\cdot$ min^{-1} $\cdot$ m^{-2} at 4 years of age, dropping to 4 L $\cdot$ min^{-1} $\cdot$ m^{-2} during adolescence. For this reason the CI of children is often higher than that of adults, with child values of resting CI being approximately 4–5 L $\cdot$ min^{-1} $\cdot$ m^{-2}, whilst in adults values of 3–4 L $\cdot$ min^{-1} $\cdot$ m^{-2} are typical. However, some studies have reported no difference in CI between adults and children.

Sex differences

There appears to be no sex difference in resting CI between boys and girls, although some reports have indicated that boys have a greater resting CI. A similar CI between the sexes could either arise because there is no difference in resting SI and HR between boys and girls, or, as is more plausible, that resting CI is the same in both sexes because females have a lower SI but compensate for this through a higher resting HR.

CARDIOVASCULAR FUNCTION DURING EXERCISE

Stroke volume response to exercise

Stroke volume increases progressively with exercise up to moderate submaximal intensities (approximately 40–50% peak $\dot{V}O_2$) and then plateaus until termination of exercise. This response is, however, dependent on body position. In the supine position there is no significant increase in SV from rest to exercise (Fig. 7.2). Ventricular filling is optimized both at rest and during exercise, as there are no gravitational effects to overcome. Conversely, in the upright body position at the commencement of exercise there is a rapid increase in SV. Stroke volume increases approximately 30–40%, soon attaining its maximal level even during submaximal exercise. This increase in SV reflects the combined effects of venoconstriction and the action of the skeletal muscle pump in redistributing the blood that had been naturally residing in the lower extremities at rest. It has been suggested that there is a small (<5%) increase in SV reflecting an enhanced contractility, in the supine as well as the upright body positions, but this is not always demonstrated. There are, however, no significant differences in maximal SV between supine or upright exercise.

The relative contributions of preload, contractility and afterload to exercise SV have been little researched in children. However, a response similar to that seen in adults is becoming apparent. As displayed in Figure 7.3, there are marked changes with exercise in ventricular end-diastolic diameter (EDD), representing preload, and end-systolic diameter (ESD), representing afterload. Stroke volume corresponds to the difference between EDD and ESD.

Left ventricular EDD initially rises, remains stable and then declines slightly. The initial rise in EDD at the start of exercise has been attributed to mechanisms that augment systemic venous return, which increases preload. As discussed in detail by Rowland (2001), the factors that produce an increase in venous return include:

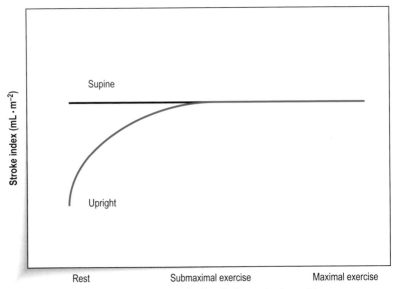

Figure 7.2   Stroke volume response to exercise in relation to body position.

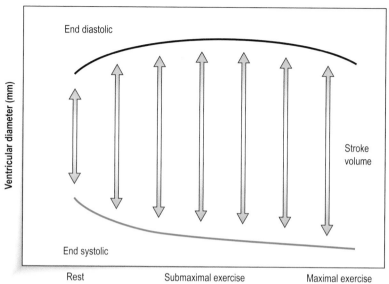

Figure 7.3   Change in end-diastolic and end-systolic ventricular dimensions during upright exercise.

1. Blood flowing back towards the heart due to a pressure difference between systemic venules and the right atrium.
2. Skeletal muscle pump – the dynamic activity of skeletal muscles during exercise enhances venous return. Muscular contractions compress intramuscular venules, imparting kinetic energy to the blood, which aids its return to the heart by overcoming the effects of gravity. This milking action by the skeletal muscles is facilitated by the one-way valve structure of the venous system. Additionally, the ejection of the blood back towards the heart causes a negative pressure during the muscle relaxation period; this creates a 'suction' effect for the blood to be moved through the vascular system.
3. Respiratory pump – the very action of breathing itself promotes blood return to the heart. During inspiration the pressure within the thorax declines, sucking blood into the inferior vena cava and enhancing venous return.
4. Ventricular pump – after ejecting its blood content the ventricle becomes temporarily a low pressure environment. As a result, blood is actively sucked into it during ventricular diastole.
5. Constriction of the veins by sympathetic nervous activity, which reduces venous capitance so that blood is shunted out of the venous system towards the heart.

With increasing exercise intensities venous return continues to rise but due to a reduced filling time caused by the increasing HR, EDD stays stable. However, towards maximal exercise the rapidity of the HR can outpace venous return, such that ventricular filling is reduced slightly, reflected in a slight decline in EDD.

Left ventricular ESD reduces with increasing exercise intensity, representing an enhancement in myocardial contractility with exercise. This is evidenced by the improvement in shortening fraction (SF) during exercise. SF increases from approximately 35% at rest to 50% at maximal exercise and is a result of a stable EDD but a declining ESD $(SF = (EDD - ESD)/EDD))$. The increase in contractility is brought about through:

1. Increased preload – a greater preload increases left ventricular EDD, thus SV rises in response to the Frank–Starling mechanism. According to this concept, enhanced preload stretches myocardial muscle fibres and stimulates stretch receptors, which creates a more powerful force of contraction during ventricular systole. The enhanced contractility of stretched muscle is due to an improved arrangement of myofilaments in the myocardium, as increasing the length of muscle fibres (within limits) improves their force-generating potential. The greater the preload, the more forceful the ensuing contraction, expelling the greater volume of blood in the ventricle.
2. Reduced systemic vascular resistance during exercise due to peripheral vasodilation.
3. Catecholamines – as discussed previously, the release of adrenaline and noradrenaline enhances contractile strength.

Contractile indices such as SF, ejection fraction (EF) and peak aortic velocity all steadily increase with exercise to exhaustion. Ejection fraction increases from approximately 60% at rest to 80% at peak exercise. Additionally, the time period that systole represents increases during exercise – at rest about 40% of cardiac cycle time is taken up by systole, but at maximal exercise this increases to 65%; therefore relatively more time is spent ejecting the blood from the heart. This ultimately means that the quantity of blood left in the heart after contraction is reduced; hence ESD declines during exercise.

Yet why does SV plateau? Although filling time is reduced with increasing HRs, as both filling speed and contractility also increase, the same amount of blood can be ejected during each heartbeat. Indeed it has been suggested that the body tries to defend an optimal SV. If venous return was to increase without a parallel increase in HR, the ventricles could become overfilled. An increase in ventricular size would not only overstretch the myocardial fibres beyond their elastic limits and compromise any benefits from the Frank–Starling mechanism, but also, according to the law of Laplace, an increase in ventricular size (thus ventricular radius) with a constant wall thickness increases wall tension, making the myocardial fibres less mechanically efficient and increases myocardial work. Thus the defence of the optimal SV is brought about through regulation of HR. The increase in HR is triggered by the activation of mechanoreceptors, chemoreceptors and baroreceptors but also through deformation of stretch receptors located in vena cava and right atria. The stretching of these receptors in the right hand side of the heart directly reflects the enhanced venous return from the systemic circulation. Known as the Bainbridge reflex, it means that HR increases in parallel with increased venous return. In addition, to ensure that HR does not outpace venous return, potentially reducing SV, stretch receptors in the ventricle wall, if activated by a declining EDV, give rise to a reciprocal increase in vagal cardiac modulation, slowing the rise in HR so that venous return and HR keep pace with each other.

Adults and children

During submaximal exercise, children typically have a lower absolute SV than adults at all levels of submaximal exercise or when working at a given $\dot{V}O_2$. This is characterized by a smaller SV and a higher HR to deliver the same $\dot{Q}$. This evidence has been used to suggest that children have a blunted SV response to exercise in relation to adults. Indeed, adults nearly double SV from rest to maximal exercise, with ratios between resting and peak SV being 1.28–1.94, whilst children demonstrate ratios of 1.10–1.40. But why might children show a blunted SV? It has been suggested that children show both a reduced production of and sensitivity to catecholamines. Lower noradrenaline concentrations are seen in children compared to adults during exercise and there is also a positive correlation between age and beta-adrenergic receptor density on the myocardium, potentially reducing contractility. In addition, blood volume in relation to BSA increases as children grow, augmenting venous return in adults.

However, the suggestion that children have a blunted SV has been challenged. There is no suggestion that SF, EF or aortic velocity during exercise are different between adults and children; thus contractile function appears to be similar. Although blood volume in relation to BSA may be reduced, when expressed relative to body mass no difference is seen between children and adults. Rowland (2005) argued that comparing children and adults at fixed exercise intensities or fixed absolute $\dot{V}O_2$ levels is unfair, as children are working at a higher relative percentage, and this situation rarely occurs. As heart size increases, so does absolute SV as a consequence of a greater left ventricular size, so it is unsurprising that adults have a larger absolute SV compared to children. When SV is expressed in relation to body size, no significant differences in submaximal exercise SI are noted between adults and children. Rowland et al (1997) compared adults and children at similar relative exercise intensities (approximately 50% and 70% peak $\dot{V}O_2$); by so doing they saw no difference in SI or peak:rest SV ratio between adults and children, suggesting that although absolute SV may be lower, relative SV is similar between children and adults.

Maximal SV shows a similar pattern to that described above, with maximal absolute SV increasing with age. In children aged 6–8, 9–10 and 11–13 years, observed SVs were 59.2, 61.4 and 67.9 mL, respectively. Unsurprisingly, children's maximal SV (mL) is less than adults. Maximal SI, however, is similar between adults and children and also stable across childhood at 50–65 mL · m^{-2}.

Sex differences

Stroke volume is greater in boys than girls at given submaximal exercise intensities as well as at equivalent work rates. SI has been shown to be approximately 10% lower in girls compared to boys during submaximal exercise. However, the sex differences are small and in some cases statistically insignificant.

Sex differences in maximal SV are also evident. Absolute SV is greater in boys than in girls. Vinet et al (2003) illustrated that boys have a significantly higher SV than girls, 64.1 mL versus 53.9 mL, respectively, with similar findings reported by Rowland et al. (2000): boys (82 mL) versus girls (78 mL). The sex difference persists even when expressed relative to body size; maximal SI in boys is reported in the range 50–65 mL · m^{-2}, whilst for girls 45–55 mL · m^{-2} is normal with a typical sex difference of about 10–20%.

There is a pattern of data to indicate that boys have a greater SV at rest, during submaximal exercise and maximal SV, but why is this so? By the time that children are old enough to be involved in exercise-related studies (approximately 5 years of age), boys have bigger hearts than girls. Left ventricular mass and EDV have been frequently shown to be greater in prepubertal, pubertal and postpubertal boys than in girls of a similar level of maturity. The autopsy study of Scholz et al (1988) indicated that even from the age of 3 years boys have thicker right ventricular, left ventricular and septal walls and that from a body mass of 32 kg upwards, boys' heart mass is greater than that of girls. Some studies do suggest, however, that boys' heart size is greater even from birth, although the difference is slight and of little practical benefit. The work of Vinet et al (2003) suggested that the larger left ventricle seen in boys might be a reflection of their larger lean body mass because when the left ventricular mass was allometrically normalized for lean body mass, the difference was no longer apparent. Although boys might have a quantitative advantage, SV is also dependent on the contractility of the myocardium. Consistently SF, EF and peak aortic velocity have been shown to be similar between boys and girls, suggesting contractility is comparable. In addition, no difference in systemic vascular resistance is apparent, leading to the conclusion that differences in SV between boys and girls are simply due to boys having bigger and more muscled hearts.

Heart rate response to exercise

Heart rate increases in parallel with increasing exercise intensity. Heart rate is stimulated to increase through the activation of mechano-, chemo- and baroreceptors sending afferent signals to the cardiovascular control centre in the brain. This in turn adjusts sympathovagal balance to the SA node bringing about a change in HR. At the onset of exercise, there is a rapid increase in HR. Due to its speed of response, this is suggested to arise through a withdrawal of parasympathetic modulation which enables the HR to increase up to the intrinsic rate of approximately 100 bts · min^{-1}. Thereafter, any increase in HR is stimulated through an increased sympathetic modulation. Increased sympathetic cardiac modulation is evident from approximately 25% peak $\dot{V}O_2$ onwards and by the time exercise reaches an intensity of 50–60% of peak $\dot{V}O_2$, data suggest that vagal modulation disappears all together. Very few studies have reported the dynamics of autonomic control of HR during exercise in children. Those studies that have been performed report similar findings to those observed in adults.

Heart rate deflection point

Although it is generally reported that HR rises linearly with increasing exercise intensity until maximal HR is reached, it is frequently observed that HR deviates from linearity, such that HR continues to rise but at a slower rate after approximately 60–70% peak $\dot{V}O_2$. This phenomenon is known as the HR deflection point (HRDP) and has been noted in children and adults alike (Bodner & Rhodes 2000). It is variable in its expression, but typically 40–90% of individuals will demonstrate an HRDP on a single exercise test to exhaustion. What causes the HRDP is still unclear. Possible reasons include a rising blood lactate accumulation and hyperkalaemia, but recently it has been suggested that it might result from the heart trying to defend an optimal SV. In adults, the HRDP occurs at the same exercise intensity at which SV reaches its peak, but this is yet to be confirmed in children. Studies that have induced parasympathetic blockade noted a reduced magnitude of deflection. This suggests that the HRDP might result from a rebound increase in vagal modulation towards higher exercise intensities such that the rise in HR is slowed so that it keeps pace with venous return, optimizing SV through to exhaustion. With no conclusive answer available, further research into this intriguing phenomenon is clearly warranted.

Cardiovascular drift

During light and moderate submaximal exercise at a fixed exercise intensity, children like adults also demonstrate a steady state in HR. However, during heavy exercise HR does not show such a plateau but drifts upwards towards maximum HR.

Prolonged steady-state exercise will also result in cardiovascular drift in children. Cardiovascular drift is defined as the progressive rise in HR and decline in SV observed during prolonged (>40 minutes) submaximal exercise.

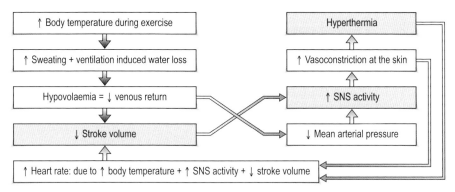

Figure 7.4 Contemporary view of mechanisms responsible for cardiovascular drift. SNS, sympathetic nervous system.

The traditional explanation for this phenomenon is that the decline in SV with the compensatory rise in HR arose to maintain $\dot{Q}$, because of a shifting of blood from the central circulation to the cutaneous vessels to facilitate heat loss and maintain a stable body temperature. However, the contemporary explanation suggests that the decline in SV and increase in HR may arise through a combination of factors (Coyle & Gonzalez-Alonso 2001). As displayed in Figure 7.4, the rise in body temperature with exercise increases fluid loss through sweating and ventilation. If this fluid loss is not replaced, it results in hypovolaemia. The hypovolaemia reduces venous return, lowering SV and triggering the sympathetic nervous system to increase HR to maintain $\dot{Q}$. The hypovolaemia also initiates a cascade of events to further exacerbate the situation. Mean arterial pressure declines as a result of the hypovolaemia, triggering a response by the sympathetic nervous system. The increased sympathetic autonomic tone leads to vasoconstriction at the skin, which compromises heat loss, further exacerbating the hyperthermic situation. Increased body temperature acts to speed HR independently. A rapidly beating heart in an environment of reduced venous return further reduces SV, which in turn stimulates the sympathetic nervous system to increase HR further. It is clear that multiple mechanisms seem to be responsible for cardiovascular drift and whether similar mechanisms are at work in children is unknown. Research that has been performed with children has shown that the magnitude of change in both HR and SV does appear to be less, such that the rise of HR and decline in SV is greater in adult subjects in both absolute and percentage terms. The explanation for such observations is unclear.

Adults and children

During submaximal exercise, when compared at a given $\dot{V}O_2$ or absolute exercise intensity, children have higher HRs than adults. Similar findings are seen regardless of mode of exercise. This is expected, as the oxygen cost required to exercise at a specific workload is fixed regardless of age; thus a critical $\dot{Q}$ is necessary to complete this exercise. With absolute SV being greater in adults the same fixed $\dot{Q}$ can be delivered with a lower HR. For instance, Rowland (1996) reported that submaximal HR declines from about 140 to 100 bts · min^{-1} in males between the ages 8 and 18 years while pedalling at 30 watts.

Maximal exercise HR is dependent upon exercise protocol, ergometer and crucially, subject motivation. Peak HRs obtained during cycle testing are typically about

5 bts $\cdot$ min^{-1} less than those obtained during treadmill exercise, and values during treadmill running are usually higher than with walking protocols. Notwithstanding this it is consistently documented that maximal HR is stable throughout the growing years in both sexes, with typical values of 195–210 bts $\cdot$ min^{-1}. It is important to recognize that formulae used for estimating maximal HR (such as 220 minus age) are inappropriate for use with children. Maximal HR has a large inter-individual variation as reflected by standard deviations of approximately 5–12 bts $\cdot$ min^{-1}. Such variation may be due to a genetic component.

Rowland (1996) highlighted the advantage that a stable maximal HR confers as the child ages. As resting HR falls while maximal values are stable, the difference (HR reserve) increases. For instance, in a typical boy between the ages of 6 and 12 years, HR reserve increases from 120 to 133 bts $\cdot$ min^{-1} and may contribute to the maturity-associated improvement in aerobic fitness.

Sex differences

The sex difference in HR is readily apparent during exercise, with females having a higher HR during submaximal exercise than males. This is frequently demonstrated whether HRs are compared at fixed or relative exercise intensities. But why is this so? As discussed previously, boys have a greater SV than girls as a result of their bigger left ventricles, so to deliver a fixed $\dot{Q}$, this can be achieved by boys with a lower HR. Additionally, it has been reported that females may have a higher intrinsic HR than boys, but this remains contentious.

However, there is no difference in maximal HRs between boys and girls. This finding is evident regardless of exercise protocol, ergometer or training status of the subjects.

Cardiac output response to exercise

Cardiac output increases linearly with $\dot{V}O_2$ such that for every 1 L $\cdot$ min^{-1} increase in $\dot{V}O_2$, $\dot{Q}$ increases by about 5 L $\cdot$ min^{-1}. This is the same for adults and children, males and females. During light to moderate exercise, both the increase in SV and HR contribute to the increase in $\dot{Q}$, but as exercise intensity increases further, SV plateaus and the increase in HR is the prime mechanism by which $\dot{Q}$ rises towards its maximum.

Adults and children

Studies have consistently demonstrated absolute $\dot{Q}$ to be significantly lower in children than adults at a given submaximal exercise level or at fixed levels of $\dot{V}O_2$. Children's response is characterized by a smaller SV than adults, with a compensatory higher HR, combined with a greater arteriovenous oxygen difference. This response is unsurprising as children have smaller hearts than adults and are working at a relatively greater percentage of maximum. Such comparisons are therefore fundamentally unfair. When adults and children are compared expressing $\dot{Q}$ as CI and at similar relative workloads (Rowland et al 1997, Vinet et al 2002), there are no significant differences in CI between adults and children.

Since maximal HR during childhood is stable, the rise in maximal $\dot{Q}$ in children as they grow is entirely due to an increase in SV. Maximal $\dot{Q}$ (L $\cdot$ min^{-1}) of adults is greater than that of children. Vinet et al (2002) reported Doppler echocardiography determined $\dot{Q}$ to be less in children compared to adults (mean (standard deviation)):

16.5 (3.6) L $\cdot$ min^{-1} versus 24.3 (4.6) L $\cdot$ min^{-1}, respectively. However, once again this is simply a reflection of body size differences between adults and children. The growth-related changes in $\dot{Q}$ are exemplified by the earlier cross-sectional study of Miyamura & Honda (1973). They indicated that absolute maximal $\dot{Q}$ increased from 12.5 to 21.1 L $\cdot$ min^{-1} in males between 10 and 20 years of age and from 10.5 to 15.5 L $\cdot$ min^{-1} in girls of the same ages.

Adults' maximal $\dot{Q}$ is approximately four times bigger than resting $\dot{Q}$. In comparison, children's maximal $\dot{Q}$ typically rises just threefold from resting values. Although this implies some inadequacy in cardiac performance in children, other methods of examining myocardial function with exercise do not reveal any such insufficiency in children. The ratio of change of $\dot{Q}$ to change in $\dot{V}O_2$ during exercise (the exercise factor) has been interpreted as an indicator of myocardial performance, and values of 5.0 to 7.0 are typical in adult subjects. Among seven investigations of children, the average exercise factor was 5.8, suggesting a similar magnitude of response for increased myocardial functionality (Rowland 1996).

When maximal $\dot{Q}$ is expressed independent of body size as CI, children and adults have similar maximal values. Vinet et al (2002) noted no significant difference in maximum CI (L $\cdot$ min^{-1} $\cdot$ m^{-2}) for adults (13.6 (2.6)) and children (12.9 (2.9)). It appears that values for maximal CI are reasonably consistent throughout childhood at approximately 10–12 L $\cdot$ min^{-1} $\cdot$ m^{-2}.

Sex differences

Although not consistently reported, it appears that there is no sex difference in absolute $\dot{Q}$ between boys and girls when both are exercising submaximally at the same relative percentage of peak $\dot{V}O_2$. Maximal absolute $\dot{Q}$ and CI are, however, lower in girls. This is not unexpected as maximum HR is similar between the sexes but maximum SV and SI are greater in boys. Girls' maximal CI is on average 10–20% less than that of boys. Rowland et al (2000) reported maximal CI to be significantly larger at 12 years of age in boys compared to girls, 12.34 (2.16) L $\cdot$ min^{-1} $\cdot$ m^{-2} versus 10.90 (1.75) L $\cdot$ min^{-1} $\cdot$ m^{-2} for the boys and girls, respectively. In general, maximal CI for boys is approximately 10–12 L $\cdot$ min^{-1} $\cdot$ m^{-2}, whilst for girls it is 8–10 L $\cdot$ min^{-1} $\cdot$ m^{-2}.

TRAINABILITY OF CARDIOVASCULAR FUNCTION

It is commonly noted that the trainability of aerobic fitness, particularly of prepubertal children, is less than that of adults; typically an adult would expect a 15–30% increase in peak $\dot{V}O_2$ after participating in an endurance training programme, whilst changes of 10% or less are seen in children (see Chapter 10 for further details). Why children should show a blunted training effect is unclear, but clearly both central and peripheral factors are implicated. The effect of training on peripheral factors is discussed by Rowland (2005), but there is evidence to suggest that central adaptations to exercise training might be reduced in children compared with adults.

SV is greater in trained compared to sedentary children and it increases after participation in an endurance exercise-training programme. With maximum HR unaffected by training, the increased SV leads directly to an enhanced $\dot{Q}$, thus positively affecting peak $\dot{V}O_2$ in children. This increase in SV occurs primarily through an increase in left ventricular dimensions and myocardial mass, as contractility appears to be little affected by training. Favourable changes with training in SVR, haemoglobin and plasma volume will promote an increase in SV and the oxygen-carrying capacity of the blood, but evidence to support training-induced changes in children is limited. Although in general, the data suggest a similar direction of training responses in children to those observed in adults, the magnitude of the changes is slightly lower than in adults. Possible causes include differences in anabolic hormone concentrations reducing the magnitude of expansion in plasma volume and cardiac hypertrophy, a reduced density of testosterone receptors on the myocardium in children and differences in the magnitude of response in cardiac autonomic balance. However, all these mechanisms have been challenged and as yet many questions remain unanswered.

SUMMARY

Understanding of cardiovascular function in children, particularly during exercise, is slowly taking shape. The ability to measure $\dot{Q}$ and SV during exercise is limited and the accuracy of the measurements uncertain, but improvements in technology should allow further clarification of the pattern of response in the future.

It had been proposed that myocardial function was inferior in children, but once interpreted appropriately in relation to body size, the data suggest that children's cardiac function is equal to that of adults. Both $\dot{Q}$ and SV change in parallel with growth in body size, but proportionally stay similar in adults and children. There is little evidence to suggest that myocardial contractility differs between adults and children. Differences between the sexes are more apparent. Boys' larger hearts bestow a greater SV, which results in a lower HR at rest and during submaximal exercise, but ultimately allows them to deliver a greater maximum $\dot{Q}$. On balance, it seems that cardiac changes after participation in an endurance exercise-training programme are similar to those seen in adults. However, the magnitude of adaptations may be reduced. Why this is so remains unclear.

Many questions remain, but with technological developments allowing a more detailed assessment of both the quantitative and qualitative aspects of children's cardiovascular function, it is hoped that the answers may be found.

KEY POINTS

1. Measurement of $\dot{Q}$ and SV in children is challenging and therefore our knowledge of cardiovascular function during exercise must be interpreted in this context.
2. Heart size increases in proportion with increasing body size – most closely with body surface area.
3. SI remains constant at rest from childhood into adulthood. However, resting CI and HR both decline.
4. Children's SV response to exercise appears similar in nature to adults, increasing initially from resting values but then levelling off at its maximum from approximately 40% of peak $\dot{V}O_2$.
5. Submaximal exercise SI is similar between adults and children when exercising at comparable relative exercise intensities. Maximal SI is also similar between adults and children and stable across childhood at 50–65 mL · m^{-2}.
6. Children have higher HR than adults during submaximal exercise due to their smaller SV. Maximal HR is higher than that of adults and remains stable through adolescence at approximately 195–205 bts · min^{-1}.
7. CI is comparable when adults and children are exercising at similar relative exercise intensities. There is no significant difference in maximal CI between adults and children (approximately 10–12 L · min^{-1} · m^{-2}).

8. Boys have a higher SI than girls; this allows them to have a lower HR during rest and submaximal exercise. With no sex difference in maximal HR, boys' larger maximal SI results in a 10–20% greater maximal CI.

References

Barber G 2000 Cardiovascular function. In: Armstrong N, van Mechelen W (eds) Paediatric exercise science and medicine. Oxford University Press, Oxford, p 57–64

Batterham A M, George K P, Whyte G et al 1999 Scaling cardiac structural data by body dimensions: a review of theory, practice, and problems. International Journal of Sports Medicine 20:495–502

Bodner M E, Rhodes E C 2000 A review of the concept of the heart rate deflection point. Sports Medicine 30:31–46

Coyle E F, Gonzalez-Alonso J 2001 Cardiovascular drift during prolonged exercise: new perspectives. Exercise and Sport Sciences Reviews 29:88–92

De Simone G, Devereux R B, Kimball T R et al 1998 Interaction between body size and cardiac workload: influence on left ventricular mass during body growth and adulthood. Hypertension 31:1077–1082

Driscoll D J, Staats B A, Beck K C 1989 Measurement of cardiac output in children during exercise: a review. Pediatric Exercise Science 1:102–115

Marks C, Katch V, Rocchini A et al 1985 Validity and reliability of cardiac output by CO_2 rebreathing. Sports Medicine 2:432–446

Miyamura M, Honda Y 1973 Maximum cardiac output related to sex and age. Japanese Journal of Physiology 23:645–656

Rowland T W 1996 Developmental exercise physiology. Human Kinetics, Champaign, IL

Rowland T W 2001 The circulatory response to exercise: role of the peripheral pump. International Journal of Sports Medicine 22:558–565

Rowland T W 2005 Children's exercise physiology. Human Kinetics, Champaign, IL

Rowland T W, Popowski B, Ferrone L 1997 Cardiac responses to maximal upright cycle exercise in healthy boys and men. Medicine and Science in Sports and Exercise 29:1146–1151

Rowland T, Goff D, Martel L et al 2000 Influence of cardiac functional capacity on gender differences in maximal oxygen uptake in children. Chest 117:629–635

Scholz D G, Kitzman D W, Hagen P T et al 1988 Age-related changes in normal human hearts during the first 10 decades of life. Part I (Growth): A quantitative anatomic study of 200 specimens from subjects from birth to 19 years old. Mayo Clinic Proceedings 63:126–136

Silverthorn D G 2001 Human physiology: an integrated approach. Prentice-Hall, Upper Saddle River

Sluysmans T, Colan S D 2005 Theoretical and empirical derivation of cardiovascular allometric relationships in children. Journal of Applied Physiology 99:445–447

Vinet A, Nottin S, Lecoq A M et al 2002 Cardiovascular responses to progressive cycle exercise in healthy children and adults. International Journal of Sports Medicine 23:242–246

Vinet A, Mandigout S, Nottin S et al 2003 Influence of body composition, hemoglobin concentration, and cardiac size and function of gender differences in maximal oxygen uptake in prepubertal children. Chest 124:1494–1499

Welsman J R, Bywater K, Farr C et al 2005 Reliability of peak $\dot{V}O_2$ and thoracic bioimpedance maximal cardiac output in children. European Journal of Applied Physiology 94:228–234

Further reading

Rowell L 1993 Human cardiovascular control. Oxford University Press, Oxford

Rowland T W 2000 Cardiovascular function. In: Armstrong N, van Mechelen W (eds) Paediatric exercise science and medicine. Oxford University Press, Oxford, p 163–171

Chapter **8**

Aerobic fitness

Neil Armstrong and Samantha G. Fawkner

LEARNING OBJECTIVES

After studying this chapter you should be able to:
1. address whether peak oxygen uptake can be accepted as the criterion measure of young people's aerobic fitness
2. evaluate the methodological factors involved in the determination of peak oxygen uptake
3. design an exercise test to determine the aerobic fitness of children and adolescents
4. analyse methods of interpreting peak oxygen uptake in relation to age, growth and maturation
5. discuss peak oxygen uptake in relation to age, growth and maturation
6. compare and contrast the aerobic fitness of boys and girls during growth and maturation
7. discuss peak oxygen uptake in relation to habitual physical activity
8. evaluate secular trends in aerobic fitness
9. evaluate the theoretical and methodological factors involved in the assessment and interpretation of blood lactate accumulation
10. discuss blood lactate responses to exercise in relation to age and maturation.

INTRODUCTION

Aerobic fitness may be defined as the ability to deliver oxygen to the exercising muscles and to utilize it to generate energy during exercise. Aerobic fitness therefore depends upon the pulmonary, cardiovascular and haematological components of oxygen delivery and the oxidative mechanisms of the exercising muscle.

Maximal oxygen uptake ($\dot{V}O_2$max), the highest rate at which an individual can consume oxygen during exercise, is widely recognized as the best single measure of adults' aerobic fitness. Maximal oxygen uptake conventionally implies the existence of a $\dot{V}O_2$ plateau (see later) but this response is not typical of children and adolescents and it has gradually become more common to use the term peak $\dot{V}O_2$, the highest $\dot{V}O_2$ elicited during an exercise test to exhaustion, to describe young people's aerobic fitness. Peak $\dot{V}O_2$ limits the capacity to perform aerobic exercise but it does not describe fully all aspects of aerobic fitness and a more comprehensive analysis requires consideration of the transient kinetics of $\dot{V}O_2$, the non-steady-state response to changes in metabolic demand with exercise. Furthermore, peak $\dot{V}O_2$ is not the most sensitive measure of the ability to sustain aerobic exercise at submaximal intensities and despite its origins in anaerobic metabolism, blood lactate accumulation provides a valuable indicator of submaximal aerobic fitness. As $\dot{V}O_2$ kinetics is addressed in Chapter 9, here we will focus on aerobic fitness as described by peak $\dot{V}O_2$ and blood lactate accumulation.

Robinson (1938) published the first laboratory study of boys' aerobic fitness almost 70 years ago and Åstrand (1952) conducted his studies of the aerobic fitness of both boys and girls over 50 years ago. Since these pioneering studies aerobic fitness has become the most researched variable in paediatric exercise physiology, with over 20% of papers published in the journal *Pediatric Exercise Science* involving the determination of peak $\dot{V}O_2$. Yet, the understanding of aerobic fitness during childhood and adolescence is still shrouded in controversy.

Evaluation of young people's peak $\dot{V}O_2$ and blood lactate responses to exercise is clouded by methodological issues. The interpretation of aerobic fitness in relation to age and sex is confounded by inappropriate means of controlling for growth and maturation. In this chapter we examine the methodological problems involved in determining peak $\dot{V}O_2$ and appropriate submaximal blood lactate indices in young people and clarify the development of aerobic fitness during childhood and adolescence.

MAXIMAL OR PEAK OXYGEN UPTAKE?

In a progressive exercise test to exhaustion $\dot{V}O_2$ rises with increasing exercise intensity up to a point beyond which no further increase in $\dot{V}O_2$ takes place, despite well-motivated participants being able to increase further the intensity of their exercise. Exercise above the intensity where $\dot{V}O_2$ levels off or plateaus is assumed to be supported by anaerobic resynthesis of adenosine triphosphate (ATP) resulting in an intracellular accumulation of lactate, acidosis, and inevitably termination of exercise. Maximal oxygen uptake is conventionally regarded as the point where $\dot{V}O_2$ reaches a plateau. However, an absolute plateau of $\dot{V}O_2$ with increasing exercise intensity seldom occurs and a number of age-related criteria to define a plateau have been proposed. The most commonly applied plateau criterion with young people is a body mass-related requirement for an increase in $\dot{V}O_2$ of not more than 2.0 mL $\cdot$ kg^{-1} $\cdot$ min^{-1} for a 5–10% increase in exercise intensity.

Table 8.1 Peak physiological data of children and adolescents who showed a plateau and no plateau in oxygen uptake

	Status	Group	N	$\dot{V}O_2$ (L · min⁻¹)	HR bts · min⁻¹	Blood lactate (mmol · L⁻¹)
Girls	Children	No plateau	34	1.49 (0.26)	202 (7)	5.0 (2.0)
		Plateau	19	1.41 (0.14)	201 (7)	5.3 (1.9)
	Adolescents	No plateau	65	1.93 (0.40)	201 (8)	6.1 (1.8)
		Plateau	39	1.86 (0.30)	203 (8)	5.9 (1.7)
Boys	Children	No plateau	84	1.81 (0.24)	200 (7)	4.7 (1.4)
		Plateau	27	1.72 (0.27)	199 (7)	4.4 (1.4)
	Adolescents	No plateau	80	2.34 (0.62)	200 (8)	5.2 (1.7)
		Plateau	33	2.24 (0.57)	202 (9)	5.5 (2.2)

Values are mean (standard deviation).
Data are from Armstrong & Welsman (1997).

Åstrand (1952) was the first to document that many children and adolescents complete an incremental exercise test to exhaustion without meeting the plateau criterion for $\dot{V}O_2$max and subsequent studies have confirmed that only a minority of young people exhibit a conventional $\dot{V}O_2$ plateau. It could be argued that failure to demonstrate a $\dot{V}O_2$ plateau following an exercise test to exhaustion is related to poor motivation and that peak $\dot{V}O_2$ is not a maximal value. However, data from Armstrong & Welsman (1997) (Table 8.1) have shown, with large samples of both prepubertal children and adolescents, that those who plateau (i.e. show $\dot{V}O_2$max) do not have higher $\dot{V}O_2$, heart rate or post-exercise blood lactate values than those who do not plateau (i.e. show peak $\dot{V}O_2$).

To address whether peak $\dot{V}O_2$ can be accepted as a maximal index of children's aerobic fitness Armstrong et al (1996a) determined the peak $\dot{V}O_2$ of 18 girls and 17 boys aged 9 years on three occasions 1 week apart (Table 8.2). The first test comprised a discontinuous, incremental protocol with the treadmill belt speed held at 1.94 m · s⁻¹ and the slope increasing every 3 min. The children exercised until voluntary exhaustion. Seven girls and 6 boys demonstrated a $\dot{V}O_2$ plateau but no significant differences in either anthropometrical or peak physiological data were revealed between those who exhibited a plateau and those who did not. The second and third tests were performed at treadmill slopes that were 2.5% and 5.0% greater, respectively, than the highest slope achieved on the first occasion. Although the children were exercising more intensely, mean peak $\dot{V}O_2$ was not significantly different in tests two and three than in the first test. This study indicates that $\dot{V}O_2$ does not increase with higher exercise intensities above the peak $\dot{V}O_2$ values observed in a progressive exercise test to voluntary exhaustion. Peak $\dot{V}O_2$ therefore reflects the limits of aerobic fitness in young people and, because $\dot{V}O_2$max conventionally implies the existence of a plateau, peak $\dot{V}O_2$ is widely recognized as the appropriate term to use with children and adolescents.

DETERMINATION OF PEAK OXYGEN UPTAKE

The laboratory assessment of peak $\dot{V}O_2$ requires technical expertise and sophisticated apparatus and as a result a number of performance tests have been developed to

Table 8.3   Guidelines for the determination of peak oxygen uptake

1. The time of day is not critical but the test should be conducted at least 2 h after the consumption of food
2. The participant should not have exercised vigorously on the day of testing
3. The participant should be wearing appropriate physical education kit and suitable footwear
4. The participant should be habituated to the laboratory environment and familiar with either treadmill running or cycle ergometry
5. The young person's safety and well-being are paramount and contraindications to exercise must be ruled out before the test begins
6. A low intensity exercise warm-up is advisable
7. The child's age, maturity and therefore attention span should be considered when designing the protocol
8. The optimal test duration involves about 9–12 min of exercise following warm-up and the exercise periods may be interspersed with standard rest periods (e.g. 1 min)
9. Ancillary measures such as blood sampling are facilitated by discontinuous tests although the length of exercise stage should be at least 3 min for blood lactate to reflect the exercise intensity
10. Changes in belt speed or slope or cycling resistance should not be excessive and gradients, speeds and resistances should be appropriate to the size, age and maturity of the participant
11. Subjective and objective end-points should be decided prior to the test (e.g. facial flushing, sweating, hyperpnoea, unsteady gait; HR levelling off at about 195 or 200 bts · min^{-1}; R $\geq$1.00)
12. The participant should be allowed to gradually warm down following the test

untenable. For example, Table 8.2 illustrates the range of a group of 9-year-olds' blood lactates at peak $\dot{V}O_2$ determined using different protocols.

There is no easy solution to the problem of whether in the absence of a $\dot{V}O_2$ plateau the child or adolescent has delivered a maximal effort. However, if in a progressive treadmill (or cycle ergometer) exercise test to voluntary exhaustion, the participant exhibits clear subjective symptoms of fatigue, supported by a HR which is levelling off at about 200 (or 195 for a cycle ergometer) bts · min^{-1} and an R $\geq$1.00, a maximal effort can be assumed. Using these criteria across three tests a week apart, the typical error expressed as a coefficient of variation is about 4.0% for children's peak $\dot{V}O_2$, which compares very favourably with the repeatability of adults' $\dot{V}O_2$max. Guidelines for determining the peak $\dot{V}O_2$ of young people are outlined in Table 8.3.

PEAK OXYGEN UPTAKE AND AGE

The heritability of aerobic fitness has been estimated from twin studies as about 50% but no studies have considered fluctuations with age during growth and maturation. Few studies have considered the stability (or tracking) of aerobic fitness in healthy, untrained children but limited evidence suggests that it tracks at moderate levels from childhood into adolescence and through adolescence into young adulthood.

Peak $\dot{V}O_2$ data are available for children as young as 3 years of age but studies are difficult to interpret and often confounded by small sample sizes, data pooled from boys and girls, an absence of objective exercise termination criteria, and a tendency to report only mass-related data. Young children typically have short attention spans and poor motivation to participate in an exercise test lasting several minutes. They have small tidal volumes and their $\dot{V}O_2$ scores are influenced by the size of respiratory valves, mouthpieces and tubing. Dead space in the analysis system can be reduced but this must be balanced against the resulting increase in resistance to flow. This chapter therefore focuses on the more secure database of boys and girls aged 8–18 years.

Young people's peak $\dot{V}O_2$ in relation to age has been extensively documented and Figure 8.1 represents almost 5000 treadmill-determined peak $\dot{V}O_2$ scores of untrained 8- to 16-year-olds. The figure must be interpreted cautiously as the data points represent reported means from studies with varying sample sizes. No information is available on randomly selected youngsters, and since participants are volunteers, selection bias cannot be ruled out. Nevertheless, the figure clearly illustrates an almost linear increase in boys' peak $\dot{V}O_2$ in relation to age. Girls' data demonstrate a similar but less consistent trend, with a tendency to plateau at about 14 years of age. The regression equations indicate that peak $\dot{V}O_2$ increases by 150% in boys over the age range 8–16 years and by 80% in girls over the same time period.

Longitudinal studies of peak $\dot{V}O_2$ determined on a treadmill provide a safer analysis in relation to age than cross-sectional studies (see Chapter 1) but few studies of untrained children and adolescents have coupled rigorous determination of peak $\dot{V}O_2$ with substantial sample sizes. The only studies to have satisfied these criteria are investigations of Canadian and Dutch boys and girls, and Czech boys which were initiated in the 1970s and, more recently, of British children and adolescents (Table 8.4).

The boys' data reflect the cross-sectional findings in Figure 8.1 and show a clear picture of a gradual increase in peak $\dot{V}O_2$ from 8 to 18 years. Canadian boys' peak $\dot{V}O_2$

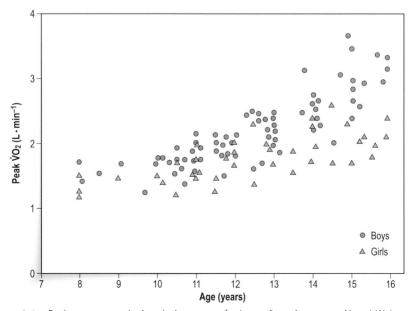

Figure 8.1   Peak oxygen uptake in relation to age (redrawn from Armstrong N and Welsman J Assessment and interpretation of aerobic fitness in children and adolescents. Exercise and Sports Sciences Reviews 22:435–476, 1994. Reprinted with permission of Lippincott, Williams and Wilkins).

Table 8.4 Longitudinal studies of treadmill-determined peak oxygen uptake

Citation	Country	Age (years)	N	Peak $\dot{V}O_2$ (L · min^{-1})
Boys				
Mirwald & Bailey (1986)	Canada	8	75	1.42 (0.21)
		9	75	1.60 (0.20)
		10	75	1.77 (0.22)
		11	75	1.93 (0.25)
		12	75	2.12 (0.29)
		13	75	2.35 (0.38)
		14	75	2.66 (0.46)
		15	75	2.98 (0.48)
		16	75	3.22 (0.45)
Sprynarova et al (1987)	Czechoslovakia	11	90	1.74 (0.23)
		12	90	2.02 (0.31)
		13	90	2.20 (0.35)
		14	90	2.76 (0.45)
		15	90	3.24 (0.47)
		16	39	3.38 (0.47)
		17	39	3.38 (0.48)
		18	39	3.53 (0.48)
Armstrong & Van Mechelen (1998)	Netherlands	13	83	2.66 (0.39)
		14	80	3.07 (0.48)
		15	84	3.37 (0.43)
		16	79	3.68 (0.52)
Armstrong et al (1999) Armstrong & Welsman (2001)	United Kingdom	11.2	71	1.80 (0.25)
		12.1	71	2.15 (0.34)
		13.1	71	2.45 (0.47)
		17.0	37	3.55 (0.55)
Girls				
Mirwald & Bailey (1986)	Canada	8	22	1.27 (0.14)
		9	22	1.39 (0.15)
		10	22	1.53 (0.20)
		11	22	1.72 (0.28)
		12	22	1.97 (0.36)
		13	22	2.20 (0.39)
Armstrong & Van Mechelen (1998)	Netherlands	13	97	2.45 (0.31)
		14	97	2.60 (0.35)
		15	96	2.58 (0.34)
		16	96	2.65 (0.33)
Armstrong et al (1999) Armstrong & Welsman (2001)	United Kingdom	11.2	61	1.63 (0.28)
		12.2	61	1.93 (0.28)
		13.1	61	2.14 (0.28)
		17.0	26	2.39 (0.40)

Values are mean (standard deviation).

increased by 164% from 8 to 16 years, with annual increases averaging 11%. The peak $\dot{V}O_2$ of the Czech and British boys doubled from 11 to 17/18 years. The largest annual increases occurred between 13 and 15 years in the three studies that monitored this age range. Dutch boys showed a 38% increase in peak $\dot{V}O_2$ between 13 and 16 years. Girls' data are less consistent and peak $\dot{V}O_2$ appears to progressively rise to 13 years and then level off from about 14 years of age. The Canadian girls' peak $\dot{V}O_2$ increased by 73% from 8 to 13 years, with annual increases of 12%. The British girls showed an increase of only 12% from 13 to 17 years. The Dutch girls' peak $\dot{V}O_2$ exhibited a more marked levelling off, with only a 2% increase from 14 to 16 years of age. These findings are similar to those of several cross-sectional studies which have observed an apparent plateauing of girls' peak $\dot{V}O_2$ in the mid to late teens.

The increase in aerobic fitness with age during childhood and adolescence can be explained by examining the components of peak $\dot{V}O_2$.

Minute ventilation at peak $\dot{V}O_2$ seldom exceeds values greater than 70% of maximal voluntary ventilation although there are age, growth, maturation and sex differences in minute ventilation and its constituents, tidal volume and respiratory rate. Ventilation does not appear to limit the peak $\dot{V}O_2$ of healthy children and adolescents, but see Chapter 6 for a discussion of recent evidence concerning the effects of exercise-induced arterial hypoxaemia on children's maximal minute ventilation.

Peak $\dot{V}O_2$ is a function of $\dot{Q}$ and arteriovenous oxygen difference but understanding of $\dot{Q}$ is clouded by the methodological limitations of measuring it during maximal exercise. Nevertheless, the few data that are available consistently indicate that $\dot{Q}$ at peak $\dot{V}O_2$ increases with age in both boys and girls. The components of $\dot{Q}$ are HR and stroke volume (SV) and as HRmax is independent of age during adolescence, the increase in $\dot{Q}$ with age is wholly due to SVmax, which increases in parallel with growth of the left ventricle (see Chapter 7 for further details).

Arteriovenous oxygen difference at peak $\dot{V}O_2$ is calculated from measurements of peak $\dot{V}O_2$ and estimates of the related $\dot{Q}$ via the Fick equation (oxygen uptake = cardiac output × arteriovenous oxygen difference) and therefore few reliable data from young people are available. Evidence is equivocal, with some investigators observing age-related increases in arteriovenous oxygen difference and others reporting no relationship with age. Children's lower blood haemoglobin concentration than adults supports the premise that adults have higher arterial oxygen content and therefore potentially a greater arteriovenous oxygen difference. However, children appear to at least partially compensate for their lower blood haemoglobin concentration by having a greater facility than adults for unloading oxygen at the tissues. This might be due to the age-related decline in 2,3-diphosphoglycerate.

The rise in peak $\dot{V}O_2$ with age during childhood and adolescence appears to be primarily due to an increase in SVmax and therefore $\dot{Q}$max. Arteriovenous oxygen difference might increase with age, but additional insights into oxygen delivery to the muscle and subsequent oxidative metabolism at peak $\dot{V}O_2$ are dependent on technological advances in non-invasive methodology.

PEAK OXYGEN UPTAKE AND GROWTH

Peak $\dot{V}O_2$ is strongly related to body size, with correlation coefficients describing its relationship with body mass or stature typically exceeding $r = 0.70$. Thus, much of the age-related increase in peak $\dot{V}O_2$ reflects the overall increase in body size during the transition from childhood through adolescence and into young adulthood. As most physical activities involve moving body mass from one place to another, to compare the aerobic fitness of young people who differ in body mass, peak $\dot{V}O_2$ is conventionally expressed in ratio with body mass as millilitres of oxygen per kilogram body mass per minute ($mL \cdot kg^{-1} \cdot min^{-1}$). When expressed in this manner, a different picture emerges from that apparent when absolute values of peak $\dot{V}O_2$ (in $L \cdot min^{-1}$) are used. Boys' mass-related peak $\dot{V}O_2$ remains remarkably stable over the age range 8–18 years, with values approximating 48–50 $mL \cdot kg^{-1} \cdot min^{-1}$. Girls' peak $\dot{V}O_2$ generally falls with increasing age, from about 45 to 35 $mL \cdot kg^{-1} \cdot min^{-1}$. Boys show higher mass-related peak $\dot{V}O_2$ than girls throughout childhood and adolescence, with the sex difference being reinforced by girls' greater accumulation of body fat during puberty.

The expression of peak $\dot{V}O_2$ in ratio with body mass is the conventional method of controlling for body mass during growth but in Chapter 2 compelling arguments are presented to question the validity of using ratio scaling to remove the influence of body size from size-related measures such as peak $\dot{V}O_2$. Several studies have produced findings that show how ratio scaling has led to misinterpretation of physiological variables whereas studies in which appropriate scaling techniques have been used have provided new insights into the development of peak $\dot{V}O_2$ during growth.

To specifically address this issue, Williams et al (1992a) used a linear regression model to investigate changes in peak $\dot{V}O_2$ with age in samples of boys aged 10 and 15 years. The mean values for mass-related peak $\dot{V}O_2$ were, as expected, not significantly different (i.e. 49 vs. 48 $mL \cdot kg^{-1} \cdot min^{-1}$). However, the regression lines for the relationship between peak $\dot{V}O_2$ and body mass described two clearly different populations and led to the conclusion that for a given body mass, older boys have a significantly higher peak $\dot{V}O_2$ than younger ones (Fig. 8.2). This is, of course, in accord with adolescents' performance in events dependent on aerobic fitness but involving the transport of body mass (see Fig. 4.3).

The same research group used both ratio and allometric (log-linear analysis of covariance) scaling to remove effects of body size from peak $\dot{V}O_2$ in samples of

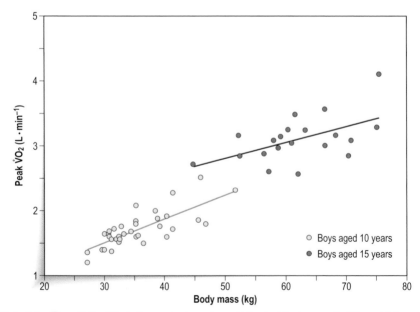

Figure 8.2   The relationship between peak oxygen uptake and body mass in 10- and 15-year-old boys (redrawn from Williams et al 1992a).

Table 8.5 Scaling peak oxygen uptake for differences in body size

Males	1M (n = 29)	2M (n = 26)	3M (n = 18)
Age (years)	10.7 (0.2)	14.1 (0.3)	22.8 (2.9)
Peak $\dot{V}O_2$ in ratio with body mass (mL · kg^{-1} · min^{-1})	50 (4)	53 (4)	53 (3)
Allometry adjusted peak $\dot{V}O_2$ (L · min^{-1})	2.25*	2.50**	2.80

Females	1F (n = 33)	2F (n = 34)	3F (n = 16)
Age (years)	10.7 (0.2)	13.0 (0.2)	21.7 (2.8)
Peak $\dot{V}O_2$ in ratio with body mass (mL · kg^{-1} · min^{-1})	45 (3)[†]	47 (4)[††]	43 (3)
Allometry adjusted peak $\dot{V}O_2$ (L · min^{-1})	1.99[†]	2.19	2.13

Values are mean (standard deviation).
* Significantly different ($P < 0.05$) from 2M and 3M; ** significantly different ($P < 0.05$) from 3M.
† Significantly different ($P < 0.05$) from 2F and 3F; †† significantly different ($P < 0.05$) from 3F.
Data are from Welsman et al (1996).

prepubertal boys and girls, circumpubertal boys and girls, and adult men and women (Table 8.5). In males, the conventional ratio analyses were consistent with the extant literature and showed no significant differences between the groups. In contrast, the allometric analyses revealed significant, progressive increases in peak $\dot{V}O_2$ across groups, indicating that relative to body mass peak $\dot{V}O_2$ increases with age rather than remaining static. Analysis of the females' data also challenged conventional findings. Mass-related peak $\dot{V}O_2$ followed the expected pattern, with no change from pre-puberty to circumpuberty but a significant decrease from circumpuberty to adulthood. The allometrically scaled data demonstrated that with body mass controlled females' peak $\dot{V}O_2$ increases into puberty and is then maintained into young adulthood.

The application of allometry to longitudinal data is complex but multilevel modelling techniques provide a sensitive and flexible approach which enables body size, age and sex effects to be partitioned concurrently within an allometric framework (see Chapter 2 for details). Armstrong et al (1999) applied multilevel modelling to the interpretation of peak $\dot{V}O_2$ in 11- to 13-year-old boys and girls, and founded the analysis on 590 peak $\dot{V}O_2$ determinations over three annual occasions. The initial model incorporated body mass, stature, age and sex (Table 8.6). Body mass and stature were significant covariates but there was an additional significant positive effect for age, which was larger for boys than girls as indicated by the significant negative age by sex interaction term, which is deducted from the age term for girls. Girls' peak $\dot{V}O_2$ was shown to be significantly lower than boys' as reflected by the negative term for sex. These data confirm the earlier cross-sectional findings and challenge the traditional view of peak $\dot{V}O_2$ during growth. They demonstrate that there is a progressive increase in peak $\dot{V}O_2$ in both sexes independent of body size, at least in the age range 11–13 years. Sixty-three of the children were retested at age 17 years and the results indicate that with body size controlled for, peak $\dot{V}O_2$ increases with age through to 17 years. The girls' data from this study are particularly noteworthy as previous studies suggest little change in females' peak $\dot{V}O_2$ from about 14 years of age even with body mass controlled for.

Table 8.6   Multilevel regression analysis for peak oxygen uptake in 11- to 13-year-olds

Parameter	Estimate (SE)
Fixed:	
Constant	−1.3903 (0.0970)
Log_e mass	0.5011 (0.0322)
Log_e stature	0.9479 (0.1162)
Age	0.0585 (0.0111)
Sex	−0.1378 (0.0093)
Age · sex	−0.0134 (0.0068)
Random:	
Level 2	
Constant	0.0042 (0.0005)
Age	0.0007 (0.0003)
Covariance	
Level 1	
Constant	0.0030 (0.0004)

$N = 590$.
Adapted from Armstrong et al (1999).

PEAK OXYGEN UPTAKE AND MATURATION

As children grow they also mature and the physiological responses of adolescents must be considered in relation to biological as well as chronological age. Few studies have investigated the relationship between peak $\dot{V}O_2$ and maturation, perhaps because of the difficulty in assessing maturation (see Chapter 1).

Cross-sectional studies have reported skeletal age and serum testosterone concentration to make no significant contribution to the explained variance in peak $\dot{V}O_2$ beyond that accounted for by chronological age and body size. Mass-related peak $\dot{V}O_2$ ($mL \cdot kg^{-1} \cdot min^{-1}$) has been shown to be unrelated to the stages of maturation described by Tanner (1962). However, Armstrong et al (1998a) hypothesized that as previous investigations had used ratio scaling to account for body size this might have obscured any relationship between maturation and peak $\dot{V}O_2$. To examine this premise the maturation of 176 12-year-olds was classified according to indices of pubic hair and their peak $\dot{V}O_2$ was determined using a discontinuous, incremental treadmill test to voluntary exhaustion (Table 8.7). In accord with previous studies, peak $\dot{V}O_2$ in ratio with body mass remained unchanged with stage of maturation. An allometric analysis, however, yielded a mass exponent common to both boys and girls of 0.65 which was not significantly different from the theoretical exponent of 0.67 (see Chapter 2). In contrast to previous studies using the ratio standard, with body mass appropriately accounted for using allometry a significant effect of maturation on peak $\dot{V}O_2$ independent of body mass was observed.

Longitudinal studies indicate that there is a spurt in peak $\dot{V}O_2$ in boys which reaches a maximum gain at about the time of peak height velocity but there is insufficient evidence to support a similar spurt in girls (see Table 8.4). The data from the longitudinal study of British children and adolescents described in Table 8.4 were analysed using multilevel modelling. The initial model showed a significant, additional and

Table 8.7   Peak oxygen uptake in relation to stage of maturation in 12-year-olds

	Stage of maturation according to pubic hair development			
Boys	1 ($n = 32$)	2 ($n = 34$)	3 ($n = 18$)	4 ($n = 9$)
Peak $\dot{V}O_2$ in ratio with body mass (mL · kg^{-1} · min^{-1})	50 (6)	54 (5)	52 (6)	52 (5)
Allometrically adjusted peak $\dot{V}O_2$ (L · min^{-1})	2.01	2.17	2.20	2.30
Girls	1 ($n = 19$)	2 ($n = 25$)	3 ($n = 25$)	4 ($n = 14$)
Peak $\dot{V}O_2$ in ratio with body mass (mL · kg^{-1} · min^{-1})	45 (7)	44 (5)	44 (3)	46 (5)
Allometrically adjusted peak $\dot{V}O_2$ (L · min^{-1})	1.78	1.84	1.85	1.99

Values are mean (standard deviation).
Significant ($P < 0.01$) main effects for maturity were demonstrated for allometrically adjusted peak $\dot{V}O_2$; no significant ($P > 0.05$) main effects for maturity were demonstrated for peak $\dot{V}O_2$ in ratio with body mass.
Data are from Armstrong et al (1998a).

incremental effect of stage of maturation on peak $\dot{V}O_2$ with both age and body size controlled for (Table 8.8, model 1). The positive effect of maturation on aerobic fitness was consistent for both girls and boys. When triceps and subscapular skinfolds were introduced into the analysis there was a significant improvement in fit but maturation stages two to four remained significant, additional and incremental explanatory variables of peak $\dot{V}O_2$ in both sexes (Table 8.8, model 2 and see Chapter 2 for explanation of log-likelihood in determining statistical significance). The magnitude of the maturation effect was, however, reduced with the introduction of the sum of two skinfolds. This indicates the importance of maturity-related changes in fat-free mass on the differential growth of boys' and girls' peak $\dot{V}O_2$.

PEAK OXYGEN UPTAKE AND SEX

Boys' peak $\dot{V}O_2$ values are consistently higher than those of girls by late childhood and the sex difference becomes more pronounced as young people progress through adolescence. The British boys described in Table 8.4 showed a 10.4% higher peak $\dot{V}O_2$ (in L · min^{-1}) than the girls at age 11 years and the difference increased to 48.5% by age 17 years. Over the age range 11–17 years the boys almost doubled their peak $\dot{V}O_2$ whereas the increase in girls' scores was less than 50%, with the boys having significantly higher scores at each age examined. The negative sex exponent in Table 8.8 shows that even with body size controlled for, boys have higher peak $\dot{V}O_2$ than girls and the negative age by sex interaction indicates that the sex difference progressively increases with age.

Sex differences during adolescence have been attributed to a combination of factors including habitual physical activity, body size and composition, and blood haemoglobin concentration.

Boys are generally more physically active than girls but the evidence relating habitual physical activity to young people's peak $\dot{V}O_2$ is weak and the issue is further

Table 8.8   Multilevel regression model for peak oxygen uptake in 11- to 17-year-olds

Parameter	Model 1 Estimate (SE)	Model 2 Estimate (SE)
Fixed:		
Constant	−1.20203 (0.1474)	−1.9005 (0.1400)
Log_e mass	0.4454 (0.0460)	0.8752 (0.0432)
Log_e stature	1.0082 (0.1607)	ns
Log_e skinfolds	Not entered	−0.1656 (0.0174)
Age	0.0452 (0.0101)	0.0470 (0.0094)
Sex	−0.1608 (0.0135)	−0.1372 (0.0121)
Age · sex	−0.0258 (0.0051)	−0.0214 (0.0053)
Maturity 2	0.0511 (0.0116)	0.0341 (0.0094)
Maturity 3	0.0655 (0.0135)	0.0361 (0.0102)
Maturity 4	0.0988 (0.0169)	0.0537 (0.0116)
Maturity 5	0.0770 (0.0301)	ns
Random:		
Level 2		
Constant	0.0042 (0.0007)	0.0030 (0.0005)
Age	0.0002 (0.0001)	0.0004 (0.0001)
Level 1		
Constant	0.0033 (0.0004)	0.0032 (0.0004)
−2* log (like)	−844.2189	−870.6431

$N = 388$.
ns, not significant.
Adapted from Armstrong & Welsman (2001).

confounded by problems with accurately assessing physical activity patterns during youth. Regular bouts of sustained high intensity exercise are required to increase aerobic fitness (see Chapter 10) and the sporadic nature of children's daily physical activity is not conducive to the promotion of peak $\dot{V}O_2$ and unlikely to contribute to sex differences (see later in this chapter).

Muscle mass increases through childhood and although girls have less muscle mass than boys from an early age, marked sex differences do not become apparent until the adolescent growth spurt. Between 5 and 16 years, boys' relative muscle mass increases from 42 to 54% of body mass. Girls do experience an adolescent spurt in muscle mass but it is less dramatic than that of boys with increases from 40 to 45% of body mass between 5 and 13 years and then, in relative terms, a decline due to an increase in fat accumulation during adolescence. Boys have slightly less body fat than girls during childhood but during the adolescent growth spurt, boys' body fat declines to about 12–14% of body mass while girls' body fat increases to about 25% of body mass. These dramatic changes in body composition during puberty contribute significantly to the progressive increase in sex differences in peak $\dot{V}O_2$ over this period. This is illustrated in Table 8.8 where the introduction of skinfold thicknesses into the model reduces the sex exponent. Boys' greater muscle mass not only facilitates the use of oxygen during exercise but also enhances the peripheral muscle pump, supplements the venous return to the heart and therefore augments SV.

There is no sex difference in blood haemoglobin concentration in childhood, with typical values of about 134 g · L⁻¹. During puberty the effect of testosterone on red blood cell production stimulates a noticeable increase in boys' haemoglobin concentration which is not reflected in girls. By the mid teens boys' values are about 10% higher than those of girls and boys' enhanced oxygen-carrying capacity is likely to augment muscle mass-related differences in peak $\dot{V}O_2$. Peak $\dot{V}O_2$ is significantly correlated with blood haemoglobin during the teen years but it should be noted that when Armstrong & Welsman (2001) introduced it into their multilevel analysis of 11–17-year-olds' peak $\dot{V}O_2$ it proved to be a non-significant explanatory variable once body size, body composition and maturation had been controlled for (Table 8.8). In addition, there is no strong experimental evidence to support sex-related differences in maximal arteriovenous oxygen difference.

Prior to puberty there are small sex differences in muscle mass and haemoglobin concentration, yet even with body size appropriately controlled for prepubertal boys have peak $\dot{V}O_2$ values that are about 10% higher than those of prepubertal girls. The Fick equation suggests that the explanation lies in either HRmax, SVmax or maximal arteriovenous oxygen difference.

Two studies have addressed the issue but although sex differences in SVmax, stroke index and SVmax in relation to lean body mass (LBM) were common findings in both studies the authors' interpretation of their data is conflicting. Rowland et al (2000) used Doppler echocardiography to determine the cardiac function of 49 12-year-olds (25 prepubertal boys and 24 premenarcheal girls) during maximal exercise. The girls were taller and fatter than the boys but there was no significant difference in LBM. No significant sex differences in HRmax or maximal arteriovenous oxygen difference were observed but the boys displayed significantly higher SVmax (by 4.9%) and stroke index (by 12.7%). When SV was expressed in ratio with LBM, the sex difference diminished to 5.2% and when allometrically normalized to LBM it remained fundamentally the same with a 5.1% difference. These authors therefore suggested that factors influencing SV during exercise such as skeletal muscle pump function, systemic vascular resistance, and adrenergic responses rather than intrinsic left ventricular size might be responsible for the sex differences in SVmax during childhood.

Vinet et al (2003) also used Doppler echocardiography to measure maximal cardiac function. The participants in this investigation were 17 girls and 18 boys with a mean (standard deviation) age of 10.5 (0.4) years. There were no significant sex differences in body mass, stature or haemoglobin concentration but LBM was higher in the boys. The findings confirmed boys' significantly greater SVmax (by 18.9%) and stroke index (by 10.9%) with no significant sex differences in HRmax or maximal arteriovenous oxygen difference. However, when SVmax was normalized for LBM using allometry the sex difference (4.8%) was no longer significant. In contrast to Rowland et al (2000), Vinet et al (2003) therefore concluded that cardiac size rather than function explains boys' greater SVmax (see Chapter 7 for further details).

HABITUAL PHYSICAL ACTIVITY AND PEAK OXYGEN UPTAKE

The measurement of habitual physical activity is one of the most difficult tasks in epidemiological research. Self-report is the most frequently used method of assessment but data need to be interpreted cautiously. Children are less time conscious than adults and tend to engage in physical activities at sporadic times and intensities rather than consistent bouts. The self-recall of the intensity, frequency and duration of bouts of activity by children is therefore even more problematic than with adults. The problem is further confounded by leisure time activity, which is more difficult to quantify than occupational activity, making up a greater proportion of total physical activity time in children. Of the more objective estimates of physical activity heart rate monitoring and accelerometry have provided valuable insights into young people's activity patterns, although sample sizes tend to be small and non-representative of populations (see Armstrong & Van Mechelen, 1998 for a review of methods of assessing physical activity).

Regardless of methodology, data are remarkably consistent. Boys of all ages participate in more physical activity than girls and the sex difference is more marked when moderate to vigorous physical activity is considered. The physical activity levels of both boys and girls are higher during childhood and decline as young people move through their teen years. Periods of physical activity are brief and sustained periods of vigorous activity are seldom experienced by many children and adolescents (Armstrong & Van Mechelen 1998).

Few studies have analysed the directly determined peak $\dot{V}O_2$ of children and adolescents in relation to their habitual physical activity. Investigations involving European children have been collated in Table 8.9. The results of each of these studies suggest that there is little or no relationship between physical activity and peak $\dot{V}O_2$. In the more recent studies, Armstrong and his associates (1990, 1996b, 1998b) assessed the physical activity of 231 boys and 217 girls, aged 10–16 years, using 3-day heart rate monitoring and reported no significant relationships with peak $\dot{V}O_2$. Ekelund et al (2001) used the same measurement techniques and noted no significant correlations between moderate to vigorous activity ($min \cdot day^{-1}$) and peak $\dot{V}O_2$ in either girls or boys but observed significant correlations between 'activity-related energy expenditure' and peak $\dot{V}O_2$ in both girls ($r = 0.45$) and boys ($r = 0.30$). However, after controlling for body fat and maturation none of the physical activity variables were significantly correlated to peak $\dot{V}O_2$ in boys. When the highly active boys were compared to the rest of the boys, no significant differences were noted in peak $\dot{V}O_2$.

In a study of 101 girls and 127 boys, aged 8–11 years, Dencker et al (2006) estimated habitual physical activity from accelerometry over 3 to 4 days and determined peak $\dot{V}O_2$ using cycle ergometry. They observed no relationship between peak $\dot{V}O_2$ and moderate physical activity but found a weak but significant correlation ($r = 0.27$ to 0.30) between vigorous physical activity and peak $\dot{V}O_2$. A major limitation of this study, however, is that the peak $\dot{V}O_2$ of some children included in the analysis is likely to have been underestimated as only 71% reached even 85% of predicted maximal HR (range 132–220 $bts \cdot min^{-1}$) before terminating the exercise test. With such a wide range of observed 'peak $\dot{V}O_2$' the reported correlations need to be interpreted cautiously.

Armstrong et al (2000) used multilevel modelling to examine moderate and vigorous activity in a longitudinal study of 104 boys and 98 girls, from the ages of 11–13 years. They introduced peak $\dot{V}O_2$ into the model once age, sex, and maturation had been controlled for and reported that a non-significant parameter was obtained.

Empirical evidence therefore supports the view that habitual physical activity is not related to peak $\dot{V}O_2$. This is not an unexpected finding as the typical physical activity patterns of children and adolescents lack the intensity and duration necessary to improve peak $\dot{V}O_2$.

SECULAR TRENDS IN PEAK OXYGEN UPTAKE

Analysis of laboratory-based studies over the last 50 years suggests a consistency over time in aerobic fitness but no study involving the direct determination of peak $\dot{V}O_2$ has appropriately controlled for body mass and addressed the issue of secular trends.

Table 8.9   Habitual physical activity and peak oxygen uptake in European youth

Citation	Participants	PA measures	Mode of exercise	Outcomes
Seliger et al (1974)	11 boys; aged 12 years Czechoslovakia	1 day heart rate monitoring; questionnaire interview	Cycle ergometer	No significant relationships
Saris (1982)	Approx 400 girls, 400 boys; aged 6–10 years The Netherlands	1 day heart rate monitoring; questionnaire	Treadmill	No significant relationship between peak $\dot{V}O_2$ in any of the age groups when TDEE was used as an index for daily physical activity
Andersen et al (1984)	21 girls, 27 boys; aged 13–18 years The Netherlands	1 day accelerometry; questionnaire	Cycle ergometer	No significant relationships
Sunnegardh & Bratteby (1987)	49 girls, 52 boys; aged 8–13 years Sweden	1 day accelerometry; questionnaire	Cycle ergometer	No significant relationships between accelerometry and peak $\dot{V}O_2$. Significant relationship between questionnaire data and peak $\dot{V}O_2$ in 8-year-old boys and 13-year-old boys and girls
Armstrong et al (1990)	111 girls, 85 boys; aged 11–16 years England	3 day heart rate monitoring	Cycle ergometer or treadmill	No significant relationships. Non-significant correlation coefficients ranged from $r = 0.01$ to -0.26
Armstrong et al (1996b)	43 girls, 86 boys; aged 10–11 years England	3 day heart rate monitoring	Treadmill	No significant relationships. Non-significant correlation coefficients ranged from $r = -0.15$ to 0.09
Armstrong et al (1998b)	63 girls, 60 boys; aged 12.2 years England	3 day heart rate monitoring	Treadmill	No significant relationships. Non-significant correlation coefficients ranged from $r = 0.13$ to 0.16 in boys and from $r = -0.02$ to 0.04 in girls

(continued)

Table 8.9   Continued

Citation	Participants	PA measures	Mode of exercise	Outcomes
Ekelund et al (2001)	40 girls, 42 boys; aged 14–15 years Sweden	3 day heart rate monitoring	Treadmill	No significant relationships between MVPA and peak $\dot{V}O_2$ AEE significantly correlated with peak $\dot{V}O_2$ in both girls and boys but after controlling for body fat and maturity level the relationship in boys was non-significant
Dencker et al (2006)	101 girls, 127 boys; aged 8–11 years Sweden	3–4 day accelerometry	Cycle ergometer (note that only 71% of children reached 85% of HRmax before terminating the exercise test)	Moderate physical activity was not significantly correlated with peak $\dot{V}O_2$. VPA and MDPA were significantly but weakly ($r = 0.23$ to 0.32) related to peak $\dot{V}O_2$. In a multiple forward regression analysis VPA and MDPA explained 10% of the variability in peak $\dot{V}O_2$ (VPA 9% and MDPA 1%)

PA, physical activity; TDEE, total daily energy expenditure; MVPA, moderate to vigorous physical activity; AEE, activity-related energy expenditure; VPA, vigorous physical activity; MDPA, mean daily physical activity.

As participants are required to give informed consent to take part in an exercise test, published values of peak $\dot{V}O_2$ are not population-representative. The data could therefore be interpreted as indicating that the aerobic fitness (i.e. peak $\dot{V}O_2$ in L · min^{-1}) of children and adolescents volunteering for exercise studies has not changed much over five decades.

In contrast, data from performance tests consistently indicate a decrease in aerobic fitness over the last 20 years. For example, Tomkinson et al (2003) reviewed 55 studies of aerobic fitness determined using the 20mSRT, from 11 countries, over the period 1980–2000 and reported a reduction of 0.5% per year in the performance of European children and 1% per year in adolescents. The authors noted, however, that performance fitness measured by running can be reduced by increased body mass or fatness and that children and adolescents were fatter in 2000 than in 1980.

A recent study by Wedderkopp and his associates (2004) provides valuable insights into changes in aerobic fitness over time. They analysed secular trends through two cross-sectional surveys performed 12 years apart on representative samples of 9-year-old children from Odense in Denmark. In 1985–1986, 670 girls and 699 boys participated in the study and in 1997–1998 310 girls and 279 boys participated. On both occasions fitness was determined by a maximal work test (watt-max test) which involved the children exercising to exhaustion on a cycle ergometer. Unfortunately respiratory gases were not measured but the watt-max test was validated against directly determined peak $\dot{V}O_2$ in a subsample of the children and the regression equations were used to predict peak $\dot{V}O_2$ in mL · kg⁻¹ · min⁻¹ from the watt-max data. The boys in 1997–1998 had a lower fitness level and a higher fatness percentage than those in 1985–1986, whereas no overall differences in fitness or fatness were found between girls in 1997–1998 or 1985–1986.

Wedderkopp et al (2004) split their sample into deciles and noted that in 1997–1998 the fittest boys had the same level of fitness as in 1985–1986, and the fittest girls had a significantly higher level of fitness in 1997–1998 than in 1985–1986. Both the boys and girls with the poorest fitness level in 1997–1998 had a significantly lower level of fitness than the poorest fitness levels of boys and girls in 1985–1986, respectively. The authors noted that the difference between the least fit and the most fit increased over time in both sexes. In girls, the difference between the top 10% and the lowest 10% in peak $\dot{V}O_2$ expressed in ratio with body mass was 37% in 1985–1986 and 44% in 1997–1998. The same polarization was found in boys, with a difference between the top 10% and the lowest 10% of 38% in 1985–1986 and 45% in 1997–1998. However, the decrease in predicted peak $\dot{V}O_2$ (mL · kg⁻¹ · min⁻¹) from 1985–1986 to 1997–1998 in the least fit was partly explained by a higher body mass.

Data examining secular trends in aerobic fitness are sparse and although predictions of peak $\dot{V}O_2$ indicate a decrease in aerobic fitness the methodology used suggests that it might be a reflection of the rise in body fatness over the last two decades rather than a true reduction in peak $\dot{V}O_2$. Nevertheless, Wedderkopp et al's (2004) observations indicate an emerging polarization with the difference between fit and unfit young people increasing over time. It appears that the secular increase in body mass is not being accompanied by a proportional increase in aerobic fitness with the inevitable result that in activities which involve moving body mass young people's aerobic performance is declining.

BLOOD LACTATE

As described in Chapter 4, lactate is continuously produced in skeletal muscle, even at rest, but with the onset of exercise, increases in the glycolytic resynthesis of ATP result in a correspondingly greater production of lactate in active fibres. Lactate metabolism is a dynamic process and while some fibres produce lactate, adjacent fibres simultaneously consume it as an energy source. Nevertheless, during exercise lactate accumulates within the muscle and, although output does not match production, some lactate will diffuse into the blood where, during submaximal exercise, it can be sampled, assayed and analysed to provide an estimate of the anaerobic contribution to exercise and therefore a measure of aerobic fitness.

Lactate is continuously eliminated from the blood by oxidation in the heart or skeletal muscles or through conversion to glucose in the liver and kidneys. The lactate concentration of sampled blood is therefore a function of several dynamic processes including muscle production, muscle consumption, rate of diffusion into the blood and rate of removal from the blood. Consequently, measures of blood lactate accumulation must be interpreted cautiously as lactate measured in the blood cannot be assumed to reflect a consistent or direct relationship with either muscle lactate production or muscle lactate accumulation.

Assessment of blood lactate concentration

Blood lactate sampling is a routine procedure in many paediatric exercise physiology laboratories but interpretation of the extant literature is confounded by methodological issues. Children's blood lactate responses to exercise are influenced by variations in mode of exercise, exercise protocol, time of sampling, site of sampling, blood treatment and assay procedures and these factors are often overlooked in comparative analyses.

Children's blood lactate responses to submaximal cycle ergometry cannot be directly compared to those from treadmill running as, for reasons described earlier, the restriction of blood flow during part of the pedal revolution will promote anaerobic metabolism and therefore lactate production during cycling. Blood lactate accumulation is influenced not only by exercise intensity but also by the timing of sampling. In an incremental test each exercise stage must be of sufficient duration to allow adequate diffusion of lactate from muscle to blood. If sampled too soon, the lactate will not reflect the intensity of exercise and with children and adolescents an incremental stage of at least 3 min is required. Similarly, in a peak $\dot{V}O_2$ test, blood lactate reaches its maximum 2–3 min following the termination of the exercise. The post-exercise blood lactate concentration is highly dependent on the test protocol and specifically the interplay between exercise intensity, size of incremental exercise increase and duration of exercise. Table 8.2 clearly shows how post-exercise blood lactate varies according to exercise test protocol although the peak $\dot{V}O_2$ remains relatively constant.

Blood for lactate sampling may be drawn from arteries, veins or capillaries. Lactate produced in skeletal muscles during leg exercise diffuses into the femoral veins, then rapidly appears in the arterial circulation. Arterial arm blood is therefore the preferred indicator of muscle lactate production as lactate concentrations here closely approximate those in the femoral venous blood draining the muscle groups active during leg exercise. The ethical, technical and potential medical complications associated with arterial sampling preclude its use with children but during treadmill running arterial lactate concentration is closely reflected by capillary blood lactate if a good flow is maintained at the sampling site. Most paediatric exercise studies therefore measure lactate in capillary blood drawn from either the fingertip or ear lobe. To ensure a free flow of blood the site should be warmed and the application of an anaesthetic cream or spray to the sampling site reduces children's anxiety. The sampling site must remain clean to prevent contamination by sweat and squeezing the site to obtain a larger blood sample must be avoided to prevent dilution of the sample by tissue fluid.

Once sampled, blood may be analysed immediately or undergo some preparation or chemical treatment prior to assay. The nature of treatment is dictated by the specific analytical technique which might require either serum, plasma, lysed blood, whole blood or a protein-free preparation (Table 8.10). Early studies of blood lactate used an assay that required a protein-free preparation but referred to their results as 'blood lactate'. Modern semi-automatic analysers analyse whole blood immediately following sampling and results are also reported as 'blood lactate'. The two values must not be directly compared.

The variation in the data obtained from different assays is considerable and depends on two main factors. First, whether the solids (cells, proteins, etc.) have been removed (as in serum, plasma and protein-free preparations) or not, and second, whether the sample has been haemolysed to release red blood cell lactate (as in lysed

Table 8.10   Blood preparations for lactate assay

Lysed blood	Blood is treated with chemicals which break open (lyse) the red blood cells releasing the intracellular lactate
Plasma	Blood is centrifuged to separate the liquid (plasma) and solid constituents. The plasma is assayed
Protein-free preparation	Blood is treated with chemicals which break down proteins and then centrifuged to separate the solids and liquids. The liquid portion is assayed
Serum	Blood is allowed to clot and then centrifuged to separate the clear, straw-coloured serum, which is then assayed
Whole blood	Blood is collected into a capillary tube or cuvette coated with heparin to prevent clotting and is assayed without further treatment

blood and protein-free preparations). The volume difference accounts for much of the observed variation in lactate concentration. In whole blood assays, only the lactate in the plasma fraction is assayed but the blood still contains the solid fraction. Lactate concentrations measured in whole blood are therefore lower than in preparations from which solids have been removed. For example, lactate concentrations in plasma are about 30% higher than in whole blood. The addition of a chemical lysing agent releases lactate from the red blood cells. Lysed blood assays measure plasma plus red blood cell lactate and report higher concentrations than those in whole blood, with the difference becoming more marked at higher lactate concentrations. Haematocrit is therefore a confounding factor in the assessment of blood lactate concentration during growth and maturation.

The effect of different assays upon children's blood lactate concentrations can be estimated from the regression equations determined by Williams et al (1992b). If a sample taken during exercise gives a lactate value in whole blood of 4 mmol $\cdot$ L^{-1}, simply lysing the blood increases it to 4.4 mmol $\cdot$ L^{-1} and a value of 5.5 mmol $\cdot$ L^{-1} is obtained from a plasma assay of the same sample.

Blood lactate thresholds and reference values

During an incremental exercise test blood lactate concentration typically increases as illustrated in Figure 8.3. The early stages of the test are associated with minimal change in blood lactate, with values not increasing much above resting concentrations of about 1–2 mmol $\cdot$ L^{-1}. As discussed in Chapter 4, it is not unusual for blood lactate concentrations to initially increase and then fall back to near resting values, due to the interplay between type 1 and type 2 muscle fibre recruitment at the onset of submaximal exercise. As exercise progresses, an inflection point is reached where blood lactate accumulation begins to increase rapidly with a subsequent steep rise until exhaustion.

The point at which blood lactate accumulation increases non-linearly in response to progressive exercise is defined as the lactate threshold (T$_{LAC}$) and serves as a measure of submaximal aerobic fitness. The T$_{LAC}$ represents the upper border of moderate exercise (see Chapter 9) and has been determined using visual inspection, mathematical interpolation or by defining it as a 1 mmol $\cdot$ L^{-1} increase over the resting value. To avoid blood sampling, some authors have preferred to use the T$_{VENT}$ to estimate the T$_{LAC}$ (see Chapter 6). With a discontinuous, incremental exercise

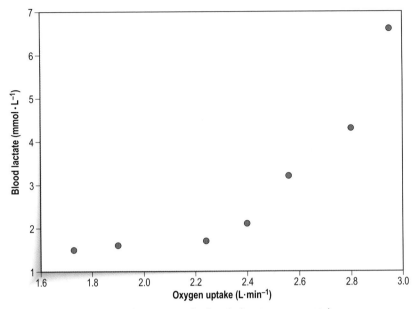

Figure 8.3   Blood lactate response to exercise in relation to oxygen uptake.

protocol, where peak $\dot{V}O_2$ is attained within relatively few stages, a clear inflection point may not be discernible. To circumvent this, fixed blood lactate reference values have been used to estimate aerobic fitness but these are not recommended for use with young people as they are not physiologically equivalent to T_{LAC}. Both the fixed reference value and T_{LAC} vary both within an individual and independently with age. At any time during growth and maturation, a lactate reference point (e.g. 4 mmol · L^{-1}) might be above or below the T_{LAC} and therefore not comparable with the relative performance of another child or adolescent.

Maximal lactate steady state (MLSS) defines the highest exercise intensity which can be maintained without incurring a progressive increase in blood lactate. It reflects the highest point at which the diffusion of lactate into the blood and removal from the blood are in equilibrium. Maximal lactate steady state therefore corresponds to a different and subsequent physiological incident to T_{LAC} and it acts as the criterion of the onset of very heavy exercise (see Chapter 4). Maximal lactate steady state represents the highest individual rate of anaerobic glycolysis at which the amount of pyruvate produced can be catabolized by aerobic oxidation. The MLSS is therefore a sensitive indicator of submaximal aerobic fitness but few studies have investigated it with children as the determination of the MLSS requires multiple blood samples during extended periods (about 20 min) of exercise at the border of heavy and very heavy exercise and it is difficult to motivate children to participate in this type of test.

Blood lactate responses to exercise in relation to sex, age and maturation

The measurement and definition issues discussed earlier make it very difficult to interpret blood lactate responses to exercise during growth and maturation. Lactate

Table 8.11 Potential mechanisms for children's lower blood lactate accumulation during progressive exercise

Factor	Potential mechanism
Muscle metabolic characteristics	Higher proportion of type 1 fibres
	Higher ratio of aerobic to anaerobic enzymes
	Greater use of fat as an energy substrate
Hormonal differences	Subdued catecholamine response to exercise
	Lower levels of testosterone
Cardiorespiratory factors	Faster oxygen uptake kinetics
	Faster circulation time due to smaller body size

threshold has been reported to lie in the range 65–70% of peak $\dot{V}O_2$ in most studies of young people and, although relatively few investigations have included girls, data indicate that there is no sex difference when T_{LAC} is expressed in relation to peak $\dot{V}O_2$. Consistent findings show that T_{LAC} occurs at a higher percentage of peak $\dot{V}O_2$ in children than in adults. Few studies, mostly of boys, have examined MLSS during childhood and adolescence and a plethora of different methodologies confound interpretation of the results. For example, MLSS has been reported to occur at blood lactate concentrations ranging from 2.1 to 5.0 mmol $\cdot$ L^{-1} in similarly aged boys. There is no secure evidence to suggest a relationship between lactate concentration at MLSS and age, or between MLSS as a percentage of peak $\dot{V}O_2$ and age. Post-exercise blood lactate concentration following a peak $\dot{V}O_2$ test is positively related to age and, despite a tendency for girls to exhibit higher values in some studies, a significant sex difference is not supported.

Potential causal mechanisms underlying a relationship between maturation and blood lactate markers of aerobic fitness are discussed in detail in Chapter 4 and summarized in Table 8.11. However, very few studies have directly addressed this topic and empirical evidence relating maturation to blood lactate responses to exercise during adolescence is equivocal.

SUMMARY

Aerobic fitness depends upon the pulmonary, cardiovascular and haematological components of oxygen delivery and the oxidative mechanisms of the exercising muscles. Maximal oxygen uptake is widely recognized as the criterion measure of adults' aerobic fitness but only a minority of children and adolescents demonstrate the $\dot{V}O_2$ plateau conventionally associated with $\dot{V}O_2$max. Peak $\dot{V}O_2$ is therefore the appropriate term to use with young people and it can be accepted as a maximal measure of aerobic fitness provided subjective indices of exhaustion are demonstrated and supported by the achievement of appropriate HR and R values. Ergometric protocols and analytical equipment used with adults are often unsuitable for use with children and the precise methodology, apparatus, and criteria of a maximal effort used in the determination of peak $\dot{V}O_2$ should be carefully reported.

There is an almost linear increase in peak $\dot{V}O_2$ with age, although some studies indicate that from about 14 years of age girls' peak $\dot{V}O_2$ begins to plateau. The rise in peak $\dot{V}O_2$ with age is strongly correlated with body size and inappropriate analyses have clouded our understanding of the independent contributions of age and maturation to the increase of peak $\dot{V}O_2$. Studies using the conventional ratio standard have reported mass-related peak $\dot{V}O_2$ to be unchanged in boys over the age range 8–16 years, whereas girls' values steadily decline. The removal of the influence of body size using allometric techniques has provided further insights and showed that boys' peak $\dot{V}O_2$ improves during growth independently of body size whereas girls' values increase through adolescence and then level off in adulthood. In contrast to findings using ratio standards, data analysed using allometry have indicated that maturation induces increases in peak $\dot{V}O_2$ independent of age and body size.

Boys' peak $\dot{V}O_2$ is higher than that of girls at least from late childhood and there is a divergence in boys' and girls' values during the teen years. The prepubertal sex difference in peak $\dot{V}O_2$ is probably a function of girls' lower SVmax. During puberty boys' progressively greater increase in muscle mass enhances the sex difference in peak $\dot{V}O_2$ and from about 14 years of age this might be augmented by the marked increase in boys' blood haemoglobin concentration and the subsequent boost in blood oxygen-carrying capacity.

The heritability of peak $\dot{V}O_2$ is about 50% and it appears to moderately track from childhood through adolescence and into adult life. It is not related to habitual physical activity during youth. Data examining secular trends in peak $\dot{V}O_2$ are sparse and laboratory data can be interpreted as indicating that the aerobic fitness of young people who volunteer for fitness tests has not changed over the last 50 years. Predictions of peak $\dot{V}O_2$ from performance tests suggest a decrease in aerobic fitness over time but it is plausible that these data are more a reflection of the secular rise in body mass than a change in aerobic fitness. Nevertheless, this indicates that the rise in body mass and fatness is not being accompanied by a similar increase in aerobic fitness, with the result that in activities which involve moving body mass aerobic performance is declining.

The determination of blood lactate accumulation during exercise is highly dependent on measurement issues and this has limited our understanding of the development of blood lactate responses to exercise in relation to age, maturation and sex. Blood lactate thresholds or reference values are not directly comparable between studies unless identical protocols and assay procedures have been followed. Much remains to be elucidated but current evidence shows that TLAC is negatively correlated with age and when it is expressed in relation to percent peak $\dot{V}O_2$ there are no sex differences. Age effects on MLSS during adolescence are unproven. Adult blood lactate concentrations following peak $\dot{V}O_2$ tests are higher than those of children, with no sex difference apparent during youth. Any relationship between maturation and blood lactate markers of aerobic fitness remains obscure.

KEY POINTS

1. The majority of children and adolescents complete an incremental exercise test to exhaustion without demonstrating a plateau in oxygen uptake.
2. Peak oxygen uptake reflects the limits of aerobic fitness in young people and its reliability compares favourably with the reliability of maximal oxygen uptake in adults.
3. In determining peak oxygen uptake, paediatric exercise physiologists must consider carefully the use of respiratory equipment designed for adults, mode of exercise (cycle ergometer vs. treadmill), exercise protocol and test termination criteria in relation to the age, size and maturity of participants.

4. Boys' peak oxygen uptake $(L \cdot min^{-1})$ rises in an almost linear manner with age. Girls' data demonstrate a similar but less consistent trend, with some studies showing a tendency for peak oxygen uptake to level off at about 14 years of age.

5. The use of the ratio standard has clouded understanding of peak oxygen uptake during growth. Allometrically scaled data demonstrate that there is a progressive increase in peak oxygen uptake with age in both sexes independent of body size.

6. Maturation has a significant additional effect on peak oxygen uptake with both age and body size controlled for.

7. Boys have a higher peak oxygen uptake than girls and this is due to their larger stroke volume and greater muscle mass which might be augmented in the mid to late teens by boys' higher blood haemoglobin concentration.

8. There is little or no relationship between habitual physical activity and peak oxygen uptake.

9. Evidence supporting a secular trend in peak oxygen uptake is equivocal but the secular increase in body mass and body fatness is not being accompanied by an increase in peak oxygen uptake. Performance in activities involving moving body mass appears to have declined.

10. Blood lactate accumulation must be interpreted cautiously as lactate measured in the blood cannot be assumed to reflect a consistent or direct relationship with either muscle lactate production or accumulation.

11. Blood lactate responses to exercise are influenced by a number of methodological issues which must be carefully considered in comparative analyses.

12. Adults demonstrate higher post-exercise blood lactate concentrations following incremental exercise tests to determine peak oxygen uptake.

13. The lactate threshold is negatively related to age but age effects on maximal lactate steady state remain to be proven. Neither lactate threshold nor maximal lactate steady state have been shown to be related to either sex or maturation.

References

Andersen K L, Ilmarinen J, Ruttenfranz J 1984 Leisure time sport activities and maximal aerobic power during late adolescence. European Journal of Applied Physiology 52:431–436

Armstrong N, Van Mechelen W 1998 Are young people fit and active: In: Biddle S, Sallis J, Cavill N (eds) Young and active. Health Education Authority, London, p 69–97

Armstrong N, Welsman J R 1994 Assessment and interpretation of aerobic fitness in children and adolescents. Exercise and Sports Sciences Reviews 22:435–476

Armstrong N, Welsman J R 1997 The assessment and interpretation of aerobic fitness in children and adolescents: An update. In: Froberg K, Lammert O, St Hansen H, Blimkie C J R (eds) Exercise and fitness – benefits and limitations. University Press, Odense, p 173–180

Armstrong N, Welsman J R 2001 Peak oxygen uptake in relation to growth and maturation. European Journal of Applied Physiology 28:259–265

Armstrong N, Balding J, Gentle P et al 1990 Peak oxygen uptake and habitual physical activity in 11- to 16-year-olds. Pediatric Exercise Science 2:349–358

Armstrong N, Welsman J R, Winsley R J 1996a Is peak $\dot{V}O_2$ a maximal index of children's aerobic fitness? International Journal of Sports Medicine 27:356–359

Armstrong N, McManus A M, Welsman J R et al 1996b Physical activity patterns and aerobic fitness among prepubescents. European Physical Education Review 2:7–18

Armstrong N, Welsman J R, Kirby B J 1998a Peak oxygen uptake and maturation in 12-year-olds. Medicine and Science in Sport and Exercise 30:165–169

Armstrong N, Welsman J R, Kirby B J 1998b Physical activity, peak oxygen uptake and performance on the Wingate anaerobic test in 12-year-olds. Acta Kinesiologiae Universitatis Tartuesis 3:7–21

Armstrong N, Welsman J R, Nevill A M et al (1999) Modeling growth and maturation changes in peak oxygen uptake in 11–13-year-olds. Journal of Applied Physiology 87:2230–2236

Armstrong N, Welsman J R, Kirby B J 2000 Longitudinal changes in '11–13-year-olds' physical activity. Acta Paediatrica 89:775–780

Åstrand P O 1952 Experimental studies of physical working capacity in relation to sex and age. Munksgaard, Copenhagen

Dencker M, Thorsson O, Karlsson M K et al 2006 Daily physical activity and its relation to aerobic fitness in children aged 8–11 years. European Journal of Applied Physiology 96:587–592

Ekelund U, Poortvleit E, Nilsson A et al 2001 Physical activity in relation to aerobic fitness and body fat in 14-to-15 year-old boys and girls. European Journal of Applied Physiology 85:195–201

Kemper H C G, Vershuur R 1981 Maximal aerobic power in 13 and 14 year old teenagers in relation to biological age. International Journal of Sports Medicine 2:97–100

Mirwald R L, Bailey D A 1986 Maximal aerobic power. Sports Dynamics, London, Ontario

Robinson S 1938 Experimental studies of physical fitness in relation to age. Arbeitsphysiologie 10:251–323

Rowland T W, Goff D, Martel L et al 2000 Influence of cardiac functional capacity on gender differences in maximal oxygen uptake in children. Chest 117:629–635

Saris W H M 1982 Aerobic power and daily physical activity in children. Kripps Repro, Meppel, Netherlands

Seliger V, Trefny S, Bartenkova S et al 1974 The habitual physical activity and fitness of 12 year old boys. Acta Paediatrica Belgica 28:54–59

Sprynarova S, Parizkova J, Bunc V 1987 Relationships between body dimensions and resting and working oxygen consumption in boys aged 11 to 18 years. European Journal of Applied Physiology 56:725–736

Sunnegardh J, Bratteby L E 1987 Maximal oxygen uptake, anthropometry and physical activity in a randomly selected sample of 8 and 13 year old children in Sweden. European Journal of Applied Physiology 56:266–272

Tanner J M 1962 Growth and adolescence, 2nd edn. Blackwell Scientific, Oxford

Tomkinson G R, Léger L A, Olds T et al 2003 Secular trends in the performance of children and adolescents (1980–2000). Sports Medicine 33:285–300

Vinet A S, Mandigout S, Nottin S et al 2003 Influence of body composition, haemoglobin concentration, cardiac size and function on gender differences in maximal oxygen uptake in prepubertal children. Chest 124:1494–1499

Wedderkopp N, Frobert K, Hansen H S et al 2004 Secular trends in physical fitness and obesity in Danish 9-year-old girls and boys: Odense school child study and Danish substudy of the European youth heart study. Scandinavian Journal of Medicine and Science in Sports 14:1–6

Welsman J R, Armstrong N, Kirby B J et al 1996 Scaling peak $\dot{V}O_2$ for differences in body size. Medicine and Science in Sports and Exercise 28:259–265

Williams J, Armstrong N, Winter E et al 1992a Changes in peak oxygen uptake with age and sexual maturation in boys: physiological fact or statistical anomaly? In: Coudert J, Van Praagh E (eds) Children and exercise XVI. Masson, Paris, p 35–37

Williams J R, Armstrong N, Kirby B J 1992b The influence of the site of sampling and assay medium upon the measurement and interpretation of blood lactate responses to exercise. Journal of Sports Sciences 10:95–107

Further reading

Armstrong N, Welsman J R 1997 Young people and physical activity. Oxford University Press, Oxford, p 25–45, 56–102

Armstrong N, Welsman J R 2000 Development of aerobic fitness during childhood and adolescence. Pediatric Exercise Science 12:128–149

Bar-Or O, Rowland T W 2004 Pediatric exercise medicine. Human Kinetics, Champaign, IL, p 3–59

Pfitzinger P, Freedson P 1997 Blood lactate responses to exercise in children: Part 2, lactate threshold. Pediatric Exercise Science 9:299–307

Rowland T W 1993 Aerobic testing protocols. In Rowland T W (ed) Pediatric laboratory exercise testing. Human Kinetics, Champaign, IL, p 19–42

Rowland T W 2005 Children's exercise physiology. Human Kinetics, Champaign, IL, 89–112

Chapter 9

Oxygen uptake kinetics

Samantha G. Fawkner and Neil Armstrong

LEARNING OBJECTIVES

After studying this chapter you should be able to:

1. describe the basic pattern of the $\dot{V}O_2$ kinetic response to exercise
2. describe how the $\dot{V}O_2$ kinetic response differs between exercise intensity domains
3. understand the basic principles underpinning control of the $\dot{V}O_2$ kinetic response
4. appreciate the problems involved with measuring and quantifying the $\dot{V}O_2$ kinetic response, especially with regard to children's responses
5. understand the basic principles of the mathematical models used in quantifying the response at various exercise intensities
6. identify the main age differences in the three phases of the kinetic response relative to the exercise intensity domains
7. identify sex differences in the $\dot{V}O_2$ kinetic response
8. consider the potential explanations for age- and sex-related differences in the $\dot{V}O_2$ kinetic response
9. consider the application of the $\dot{V}O_2$ kinetic response to athletic and everyday situations.

INTRODUCTION

Throughout the process of growth and maturation and irrespective of the size of the human body, human movement is supported by a complex interaction of physiological responses. Through these the body is able to maintain a homeostatic balance despite the additional metabolic demands under which it is placed. The way in which this balance between demand and response is achieved depends upon the function of the combined cardiovascular, respiratory and muscular systems, and laboratory-based exercise tests have allowed us to explore age and maturational changes in these systems. However, to date the literature concerned with the paediatric response to exercise has been somewhat preoccupied with the use of peak oxygen uptake (peak $\dot{V}O_2$) and the cardiorespiratory response to the demands of near-steady-state exercise, which have been deemed as representative of the functioning efficiency and capacity of the exercising child. Such testing protocols have provided invaluable insights into the changing characteristics of the exercising body during growth and have allowed investigations to proceed non-invasively where ethical constraints have prevented more thorough investigation. However, to what extent do such testing modalities really represent the body's ability to support the demands of everyday activity? Children in particular display patterns of activity that are sporadic and rarely, if ever, steady state and they may never actually require the maximum potential of their cardiorespiratory system. More appropriate therefore might be to explore how the cardiorespiratory system is able to cope with transient changes in metabolic demand.

The oxygen uptake ($\dot{V}O_2$) kinetic response to exercise provides such information pertaining to the transient cardiorespiratory response following a shift from one metabolic state to another. When a sudden change in exercise intensity is imposed during an exercise test, $\dot{V}O_2$ does not increase in direct synchrony with the changing metabolic demand, but lags behind, increasing gradually until achieving an optimum level for the given intensity (Fig. 9.1). It is the nature and speed of this response that is of fundamental interest when studying $\dot{V}O_2$ kinetics, although as will become clear in the following paragraphs, the $\dot{V}O_2$ kinetic response is by no means this simple. Nevertheless, when the exercise protocols are carefully selected and the $\dot{V}O_2$ response suitably quantified, this form of exercise testing provides insights into the ability to cope with everyday activity, essential information regarding athletic performance, and also provides a useful non-invasive window into metabolic activity at the muscular level.

Although the delayed $\dot{V}O_2$ response at the onset of exercise has been recognized since the beginning of the twentieth century, it is only in the last 20–30 years that exercise physiologists have become aware of the true nature of $\dot{V}O_2$ kinetics. This has evolved due to the advent of online metabolic systems capable of measuring $\dot{V}O_2$ with the high temporal resolution necessary to identify the dynamics of the $\dot{V}O_2$ response. Even so, much of our understanding of the $\dot{V}O_2$ kinetic response stems from data collected with adults, and literature concerned with children is scarce. The general pattern of the kinetic response is considered to be similar in children and adults, but both age- and sex-related differences in the detail of the dynamics have been demonstrated.

This chapter will therefore first overview the main principles governing the $\dot{V}O_2$ kinetic response to exercise before looking at age- and sex-related differences.

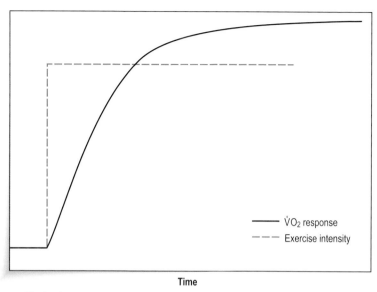

Figure 9.1   The basic oxygen uptake kinetic response to a step change in exercise intensity. Oxygen uptake does not rise to match the increase in intensity, but lags behind, finally achieving a steady state.

PRINCIPLES OF OXYGEN UPTAKE KINETICS

Exercise intensity domains

The characteristics of the $\dot{V}O_2$ kinetic response are governed by the exercise intensity to which the body is having to adjust. These exercise intensities are termed moderate, heavy, very heavy and severe, and exercise intensities within these domains may be set in relation to specific demarcation thresholds. Exercise intensities within the moderate domain do not involve a sustained anaerobic contribution to adenosine triphosphate (ATP) synthesis, and therefore the upper threshold of moderate intensity has been expressed as the anaerobic threshold (T_{AN}), or a suitable derivative such as the ventilatory threshold (T_{VENT}) or lactate threshold (T_{LAC}). Exercise within the heavy domain results in an increase in $\dot{V}O_2$ and blood lactate concentration and a decrease in pH that eventually may be stabilized. The upper boundary of heavy exercise coincides with the fatigue threshold or critical power (CP). Exercise intensities that involve the eventual achievement of peak $\dot{V}O_2$ are classed as very heavy, and exercise intensities that require a theoretical $\dot{V}O_2$ above peak $\dot{V}O_2$ as severe. In order to assess the kinetic response, especially when comparing highly heterogeneous groups (such as children and adults), it is critical that individuals exercise at the same exercise intensity relative to these demarcators.

Oxygen uptake kinetic response model

At the onset of a step change transition in exercise intensity, a cardiodynamic phase (phase 1) which is independent of oxygen uptake at the muscle ($\dot{Q}O_2$) is followed

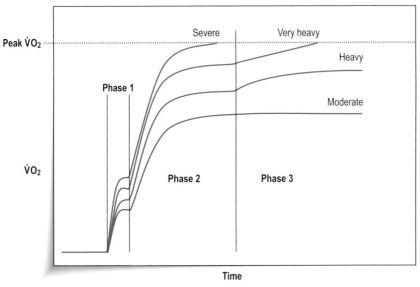

Figure 9.2 The three phases of the kinetic rise in oxygen uptake in response to a step change in exercise in four different exercise intensity domains.

by an observable exponential rise in $\dot{V}O_2$ (phase 2) towards a steady state (phase 3) (Fig. 9.2). When the exercise is of moderate intensity, this steady state is achieved within approximately 2–3 min. However, when the exercise is in the heavy intensity domain (i.e. above TAN) the steady state in $\dot{V}O_2$ is delayed, and an additional slow component of $\dot{V}O_2$ causes an eventual but elevated $\dot{V}O_2$ steady state. Above CP in the very heavy intensity domain, $\dot{V}O_2$ rises rapidly during phase 3 and the slow component results in the eventual attainment of peak $\dot{V}O_2$. When exercise is of severe intensity, peak $\dot{V}O_2$ is attained during the phase 2 response, the exponentiality of which is maintained, but truncated (Fig. 9.2).

The three phases

At the onset of exercise, there is a rapid cardiodynamic and respiratory response. Heart rate (HR), stroke volume (SV) and consequently cardiac output ($\dot{Q}$) increase almost in synchrony with exercise, as does minute ventilation ($\dot{V}E$). This results in an increased flow of pulmonary blood and pulmonary ventilation, and hence $\dot{V}O_2$ measured at the mouth rises. However, this rise in $\dot{V}O_2$ is independent from $\dot{Q}O_2$ due to the muscle–lung transit delay, and phase 1 is characterized by stable end-tidal partial pressures of oxygen ($P_{ET}O_2$) and carbon dioxide ($P_{ET}CO_2$), and respiratory exchange ratio (R). The explanation for this rapid cardiodynamic and hyperpnoeic response independent from changes in mixed venous partial pressures arising from the working muscles is a topic of some debate. Due to the rapidity of the response it seems most likely that some neural mechanism affecting the control centres, such as affectors originating in the joints and muscles, are responsible for the phase 1 response, but other factors may also contribute (see also Chapters 6 and 7).

Following the muscle–lung transit delay (which is approximately 10–20 s), hypoxic and hypercapnic blood arising from the working muscles arrives at the lung, and $\dot{V}O_2$

is closely representative of $\dot{Q}O_2$ (despite some disassociation due to muscle utilization of O_2 stores and differences in blood flow at the muscle and lung). $\dot{Q}O_2$, representative of oxidative phosphorylation in the mitochondria of the working muscle, rises in an exponential fashion towards a steady state that is proportional to the exercise intensity. During this stage, the ATP required for muscular contraction that is not provided by oxidative phosphorylation of inspired O_2 is predominantly provided by the breakdown of phosphocreatine (PCr), with some contribution from anaerobic glycolysis and usable O_2 stores. The O_2 equivalent of these sources of energy is termed the O_2 deficit. Thus, the quicker that aerobic metabolism is able to 'switch on', the smaller is the O_2 deficit and the less is the drain on exhaustible sources of energy.

The reason why the process of oxidative phosphorylation is not optimum at the onset of exercise is thought to be due to the combined influence of mitochondrial inertia and suboptimum O_2 delivery. However, the precise nature of these limiting factors and their relative importance is not entirely understood. Although the magnitude of the phase 2 response (i.e. the projected steady state) rises linearly with the stimulus (exercise intensity), the influence of exercise intensity on the rate of the increase in $\dot{Q}O_2$ (and hence $\dot{V}O_2$) is not known. It is generally accepted though that at exercise intensities above the TAN, O_2 delivery has a greater limiting influence than it does at moderate intensity. At intensities below TAN, O_2 delivery is thought to be more than adequate and the muscles' potential for aerobic metabolism is considered to be the main limiting factor.

Within approximately 2–3 min, and following phase 2, a steady state in $\dot{V}O_2$ is achieved when exercise is of moderate intensity. In this intensity domain, the O_2 cost relative to work rate is approximately $10 \text{ mL} \cdot \text{min}^{-1} \cdot \text{W}^{-1}$, and this assumed O_2 cost of work can be used to calculate the oxygen deficit during the exponential phase 2 (see later). In other words, the O_2 cost of exercise is linearly related to the intensity. However, when exercise is above TAN, the linear power–$\dot{V}O_2$ relationship is disturbed and the O_2 cost of exercise becomes observably elevated over time. This $\dot{V}O_2$ slow component may eventually stabilize within the heavy intensity domain, but nevertheless, the temporal nature of the O_2 cost of exercise prevents the computation of the O_2 deficit since the O_2 requirement at these intensities changes with time.

Why the O_2 cost of exercise should increase with time at these intensities is not precisely understood. Although it has been suggested that it may be due to central factors such as the additional cost of ventilatory work and increases in core temperature, it is now well established that the predominant source of the additional O_2 cost of exercise originates from within the exercising muscle. Despite a similar temporal profile between increases in blood lactate and $\dot{V}O_2$ during heavy and high intensity exercise, a causative relationship between the slow component and lactate production is currently considered unlikely and more likely to be coincidental. Instead, one of the most convincing theories to date proposes a combined influence of fibre type distribution, motor unit recruitment and the matching of O_2 delivery to active muscle fibres. Primarily, this theory is based on the concept that there is a greater energy cost of force production in type II, fast-twitch fibres in comparison to type I, slow-twitch fibres and that there is a strong relationship between percentage type I fibres and the amplitude of the slow component. As well, ensuing heavy intensity exercise and possibly suboptimum O_2 delivery is considered to result in fatigue of already recruited type II fibres, recruitment of additional type II fibres and maybe an increase in the firing frequency of both type I and type II fibres, all of which will result in a total increase in ATP turnover and $\dot{V}O_2$ for a given exercise demand with time.

Assessing the oxygen uptake kinetic response

Practical considerations

Most frequently, a change from one metabolic state to another is replicated in the laboratory using a 'square wave' or 'step' transition during either cycle ergometry or treadmill running. This involves a period of rest or low level exercise followed by a sudden increase in resistance (cycling) or speed and incline (treadmill) to the pre-scribed exercise intensity. During the test, which may last for as long as the study requires, $\dot{V}O_2$ and other variables of interest may be assessed in order to gauge the system's response to the exercise demand.

Since the $\dot{V}O_2$ kinetic response is dynamic and a function of time, it is crucial to carefully preserve the temporal nature of the $\dot{V}O_2$ response during the exercise test. This can be achieved by assessing $\dot{V}O_2$ on a breath-by-breath basis, in contrast to traditional systems that utilize mixing chambers and report $\dot{V}O_2$ on an averaged basis and lose the necessary detail required. The ability to assess $\dot{V}O_2$ on a breath-by-breath basis has been facilitated by the current availability of fast responding O_2 and CO_2 analysers, mass spectrometry and turbine flow meters within custom-made metabolic cart systems. These allow for gas samples to be measured as quickly as every 20 ms, and volume to be assessed with optimum accuracy, and provide the high temporal resolution required. However, breath-by-breath $\dot{V}O_2$ responses are inherently 'noisy'. This means that there is large variance from one breath to the next, and the trace of a typical untrained subject during even steady-state exercise can appear to be extreme-ly erratic. The source of this 'noise' is mostly due to breath-by-breath variance in $\dot{V}E$ (caused by variation in both tidal volume and breathing frequency) and is probably physiological in origin. It does, however, mask the underlying $\dot{Q}O_2$ signal that is of interest. Traditionally, of course, the use of mixing chambers dampens this effect, as does averaging a number of breaths together. Therefore, although the breath-by-breath response is optimum in order to preserve the temporal detail, it comes at a cost of having to deal with the superimposed 'noise' over and above the signal. However, if the magnitude of the change in the signal is sufficiently greater than the magnitude of the noise, then this problem is reduced. Thus the concern is with the signal to noise ratio, rather than simply the noise per se.

In such situations where the signal to noise ratio is poor (such as is often the case with children or diseased individuals for whom the signal is small) it is possible to reduce the magnitude of the noise by averaging the response profiles of a number of identical transitions. This is achieved by interpolating the breath-by-breath signal to a given time frame (usually 1 s), time aligning the transitions, and averaging the data points at each time interval. The technique of averaging as many as 10 transitions to acquire a single $\dot{V}O_2$ profile for analysis is time-consuming, but as will be discussed below, essential.

Quantifying the response

The aim of quantifying the $\dot{V}O_2$ kinetic response is to evaluate the speed of the response (i.e. how long does phase 1 last? How quickly does $\dot{V}O_2$ rise during phase 2? When does the slow component become apparent?) and the magnitude of the re-sponse (i.e. how much does $\dot{V}O_2$ rise during phases 1, 2 and 3?). This may be achieved using non-linear regression and iterative fitting procedures, which basically fit a specified model to the available data as best as possible by choosing the line of best fit that reduces the residual error (within the remits of the specified model). These methods provide response parameters that relate to both the speed of the response

$$\Delta \dot{V}O_2(t) = \Delta \dot{V}O_{2(ss)} \bullet (1-e^{-t/\tau}) \qquad \text{[model 1]}$$

$$\Delta \dot{V}O_2(t) = \Delta \dot{V}O_{2(ss)} \bullet (1-e^{-(t-\delta)/\tau}) \qquad \text{[model 2]}$$

$$\Delta \dot{V}O_2(t) = A_1 \bullet (1-e^{-(t-\delta_1)/\tau_1}) + A_2 \bullet (1-e^{-(t-\delta_2)/\tau_2}) \qquad \text{[model 3]}$$

$$\Delta \dot{V}O_2(t) = A_1 \bullet (1-e^{-(t-\delta_1)/\tau_1}) + S(t-\delta_2) \qquad \text{[model 4]}$$

$$\Delta \dot{V}O_2(t) = A_1 \bullet (1-e^{-(t-\delta_1)/\tau_1}) + A_2 \bullet (1-e^{-(t-\delta_2)/\tau_2}) + A_3 \bullet (1-e^{-(t-\delta_3)/\tau_3}) \qquad \text{[model 5]}$$

Figure 9.3 Models used for the estimation of kinetic parameters. t, Time in seconds; $\Delta \dot{V}O_2(t)$, increase in $\dot{V}O_2$ at time t above the prior control level; $\Delta \dot{V}O_2(ss)$, steady-state increment in $\dot{V}O_2$; τ, time constant which is time to achieve 63% of the $\Delta \dot{V}O_2(ss)$; A_1, A_2 and A_3, τ_1, τ_2 and τ_3, and δ_1, δ_2 and δ_3, amplitudes, time constants, and time delays of each exponential, respectively.

and the $\dot{V}O_2$ amplitude. Three major issues present themselves with regard to such modelling procedures:

(1) The basic pattern of the response must be known in order to apply an appropriate model

A number of models have been proposed to represent the pattern of the kinetic response. Originally, it was considered that the speed of the response could be assessed by measuring the time it took to reach half of the peak exercise $\dot{V}O_2$ achieved during the exercise test (the $t_{1/2}$). This method, however, fails to observe the exponential nature of the response, and subsequently the time constant (τ), which represents the time taken to achieve 63% of the change in $\dot{V}O_2$ from baseline to steady state ($\Delta \dot{V}O_2$), has been used in its place and is solved using model 1 (Fig. 9.3). This model allows a monoexponential to be fit to data from the onset of exercise (i.e. when time = 0), and the time constant is usually referred to as the mean response time (MRT). However, as has been identified above, the phase 1 response that lasts 10–20 s is independent of $\dot{Q}O_2$, which only becomes evident at the mouth after the muscle–lung transit delay. Therefore, there is a delay in time before $\dot{V}O_2$ is representative of the exponential increase in $\dot{Q}O_2$. In order to account for this, a delay term needs to be included in the model (model 2), and phase 1 data eliminated from the modelling process (Fig. 9.4). Although the MRT does not necessarily allow for the accurate determination of the $\dot{Q}O_2$ kinetics, it does provide a useful parameter with which to assess the O_2 deficit in the moderate intensity domain, which is the product of the increase in $\dot{V}O_2$ during the transition ($\Delta \dot{V}O_2$) and the MRT.

The situation becomes slightly more complex when dealing with heavy and very heavy intensity exercise. The true nature of the slow component, as has been discussed, is not entirely understood. Despite this, some authors have chosen to model the slow component as an additional exponential (model 3), suggesting that it represents a delayed and slowly emerging component rather than one that emerges in synchrony with the initial phase 2 primary component. Thus the model includes two exponentials each with an independent delay term and two amplitudes which represent the amplitude of the primary and slow component. With this model, the secondary delay (δ_2) has been interpreted as the time of the onset of the slow component. Other authors have chosen to model the slow component as a linear term (model 4), which has some justification at exercise intensities above CP since at these intensities $\dot{V}O_2$ rises rapidly towards peak $\dot{V}O_2$.

Despite the widespread use of these models, unlike the primary phase 2 component, modelling the slow component with either an exponential or a linear term does not have any sound physiological rationale. In fact, attempts to combine models of both the primary and slow component in one model can negate the accuracy

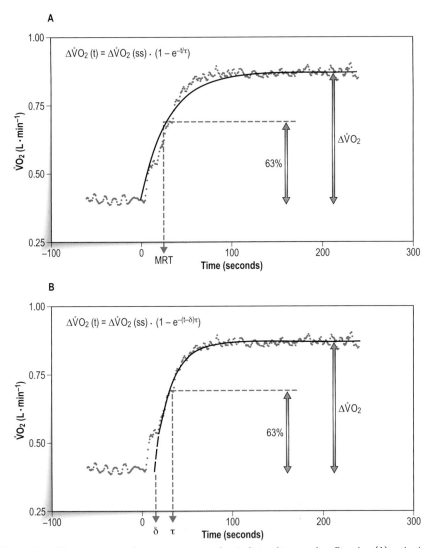

Figure 9.4 The oxygen uptake response to moderate intensity exercise, fit using (A) a single exponential from the onset of exercise ($t = 0$ s), equating to the mean response time (MRT) and (B) a single exponential and delay term to data following phase 1 only. Notice the far better fit to the exponential in B compared with A. See Figure 9.3 for explanation of symbols.

with which the primary time constant and amplitude are estimated. Some authors have therefore chosen to simply quantify the amplitude of the slow component as the change in $\dot{V}O_2$ between the third and sixth minute of exercise. Others have chosen to attempt to objectively identify the onset of the slow component, and model the data of the primary component independently. Each of these methods has its advantages and disadvantages, but to date a model with which to quantify the response to heavy intensity exercise that has a sound physiological basis has yet to be identified.

(2) The signal to noise ratio must be sufficiently good to allow model parameters to be estimated with confidence When a non-linear regression model is applied to 'noisy' data, the iterative procedure attempts to find the 'best' fit. However, if the data are very noisy, it becomes increasingly likely that the model fit may not actually represent the signal, and basically, get the fit wrong. In order to assess how likely this is, it is possible to compute the confidence intervals for the response parameters. Thus, if the model returns a time constant that is 30 s but with a 95% confidence interval of ±25 s, we have poor confidence in the fitting procedure and probably a poor signal to noise ratio. Generally speaking, it is favourable to achieve confidence intervals of at most ±5 s. With athletes who display a very large signal, it is often possible to achieve excellent confidence intervals even with just a single transition. With children, it is inherently difficult to achieve this.

(3) As the phase 1 response is short, involves very few breaths and consequently has limited data points, it is difficult to quantify accurately The phase 1 response is without question an intriguing part of the kinetic response, and holds within it a great deal of information pertaining to ventilatory control and the neural response to exercise. However, simple breath-by-breath analysis of the response is frequently too noisy to allow any confident quantification in terms of both duration and magnitude. Despite this, a number of authors have attempted to model phase 1 with an exponential (model 5), in the same way that phase 2 might be modelled, again, even though there is no physiological justification that phase 1 is exponential in nature. Other authors have either attempted to assess the duration of the response by observing the time at which $PetO_2$, $PetCO_2$ and R shift from baseline, or for the purpose of modelling the phase 2 response, assumed phase 1 to be a constant between subjects. Irrespective of the methods used, caution should always be employed when interpreting data reported on the phase 1 $\dot{V}O_2$ response.

OXYGEN UPTAKE KINETIC RESPONSE IN CHILDREN

Concerns with accurately quantifying the $\dot{V}O_2$ kinetic response due to breath-by-breath noise are magnified with children. Children's smaller working muscle mass means that the $\dot{V}O_2$ amplitude (signal) is small, but unfortunately for reasons not identified, children also display greater breath-by-breath variance than adults (Fig. 9.5). Thus, in order to attain suitable confidence in estimated parameters it is necessary for children to complete a large number of identical transitions. The available data that document age-related changes in $\dot{V}O_2$ kinetics must therefore be interpreted in light of these concerns, especially since few authors have reported the confidence intervals of the parameters investigated. Even so, there are clearly emerging patterns that suggest that the kinetic response to exercise changes during growth and maturation and may be independent of more commonly reported measures of exercise responses.

Defining the domain

As has been identified above, the pattern of the $\dot{V}O_2$ kinetic response differs according to the exercise intensity domain, and in order to make valid intra- and inter-study comparisons it is essential that subjects are exercising at the same exercise intensity relative to the domain demarcator. As with adults, TAN may be identified with children as either the TLAC or the TVENT, the latter being the more attractive choice due

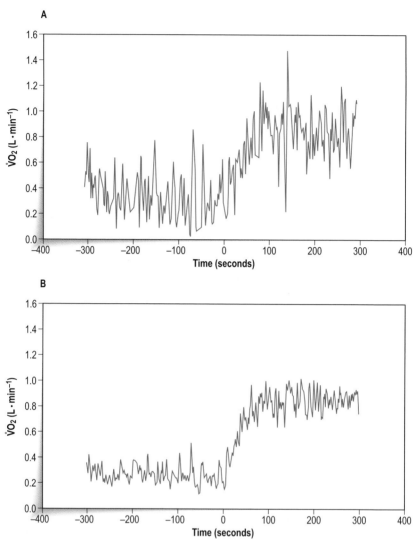

Figure 9.5 Typical breath-by-breath response profile for an 11-year-old child exercising from baseline to 80% of ventilatory threshold. (A) A single transition, where the small amplitude and large breath-by-breath variation make non-linear regression procedures almost meaningless; (B) Eight transitions averaged together, with which reasonable confidence in response parameters may be obtained.

to its non-invasive assessment. However, many studies with children have chosen to set exercise intensities relative to peak $\dot{V}O_2$ alone, or enforced a single exercise intensity across individuals, which is problematic since we know that TAN varies considerably between children with respect to peak $\dot{V}O_2$. In order to set exercise intensities in the moderate domain, it is therefore optimal to set an exercise intensity as a percentage of TAN, such as an exercise intensity equivalent to 80% of TVENT. For the heavy intensity domain, the most correct method would evaluate both TAN and CP and set an exercise intensity equivalent to 50% of the difference between the two demarcators. This, however, imposes considerable practical issues, since the determination of CP is highly labour intensive both in terms of the effort required of the subject and the number of steady-state tests involved. Possibly due to these issues, little is known with regard to CP in children and only one study has evaluated this demarcator in this population. Fawkner & Armstrong (2002a) assessed the CP of a group of 10-year-old boys and girls. They reported that CP occurred at between 70% and 80% of peak $\dot{V}O_2$, similar to values reported for adults, and was strongly related to TVENT. Therefore, with both children and adults, the most practical method for setting exercise intensities within the heavy intensity domain is to set intensities equivalent to some percentage of the difference between TAN and peak $\dot{V}O_2$. Most frequently, heavy intensity exercise is imposed as 40% of the difference between TAN and peak $\dot{V}O_2$ (40% Δ), which has been shown to be below CP in most children (Fawkner & Armstrong 2003a).

Phase 1

Data regarding the duration and magnitude of the phase 1 response in children are presented in Table 9.1. Only two studies have examined the magnitude of the phase 1 response between different aged subjects. Springer et al (1991) in comparing the response of 6- to 10-year-olds and 18- to 33-year-olds reported that 15 s following a transition from rest to 80% of TVENT, phase 1 represented a greater percentage of total change in $\dot{V}O_2$ in the adult group. This was in contrast to an earlier study which found no such difference between 7- to 10-year-olds and 15- to 18-year-olds (Cooper et al 1985), the reasons for these discrepancies possibly being related to the narrower age differences in the earlier study.

Table 9.1 Parameters of the phase 1 oxygen uptake response in adult and child groups

Author	Gender	Age (years)	N	Step change	Time phase 1 (s)	%Δ $\dot{V}O_2$
Cooper et al	M + F	7–18	10	Rest – 75% TVENT	20 ‡	42.5 (8.9)
(1985)		15–18	10	Rest – 20 W	20 ‡	63.5 (5.6)
Springer	M + F	6–10	9	Rest – 80% TVENT	15 ‡	39 (6)
et al (1991)		18–33	9	Rest – 80% TVENT	15 ‡	51 (11)
Hebestreit	M	9–12	9	20 W – 50% peak $\dot{V}O_2$	15.3 (8.5)	
et al (1998)				20 W – 100% peak $\dot{V}O_2$	14.7 (3.8)	
				20 W – 130% peak $\dot{V}O_2$	15.7 (4.0)	
	M	19–27	8	20 W – 50% peak $\dot{V}O_2$	22.5 (6.3)	
				20 W – 100% peak $\dot{V}O_2$	17.4 (3.5)	
				20 W – 130% peak $\dot{V}O_2$	13.3 (2.6)	
Fawkner &	M	10–11	13	BL – 40% Δ	16.7 (3.3)	
Armstrong		12–13			19.5 (3.0)	
(2004a)	F	11	9		20.7 (4.7)	
		13			24.3 (6.1)	

%Δ$\dot{V}O_2$, % contribution to the total change in $\dot{V}O_2$; BL, baseline pedalling; ‡, predetermined set time for duration of phase 1; 40%Δ, 40% of the difference between ventilatory threshold and peak $\dot{V}O_2$. Values are mean (standard deviation).

A more recent study considered the change in the duration of the phase 1 response in children with changing exercise intensities. It was observed that the length of phase 1 in 9- to 12-year-old children was significantly shorter following the transition to 50% of peak $\dot{V}O_2$ than was found with adults (Hebestreit et al 1998). In support of an age-related change in the duration of phase 1, Fawkner & Armstrong (2004a) demonstrated, in a longitudinal study, that the phase 1 response significantly increased in both boys and girls over a 2 year period.

The interpretation of any age- or sex-related differences in phase 1 are made difficult by a lack of data illustrating the change in $\dot{Q}$, SV or HR immediately following the onset of exercise in children. Steady-state information is available, though, which suggests that children compared to adults are characterized by a smaller SV, which is directly related to a smaller heart size. Although this is partially compensated for by a higher HR, children have a lower $\dot{Q}$ for any given $\dot{V}O_2$. During steady-state exercise, the Fick equation is maintained by a proportionally higher arteriovenous O_2 difference in children than adults. However, at the onset of exercise and during the muscle–lung transit delay, the compensatory effect of a higher arteriovenous O_2 difference plays no role in $\dot{V}O_2$, and thus the magnitude of the phase 1 $\dot{V}O_2$ response becomes limited by the SV and HR response. Effectively, the larger the change in SV and HR, the larger the contribution to steady-state $\dot{V}O_2$ that can be made during phase 1. Thus, it could be expected that the $\dot{V}O_2$ amplitude would be equal between adults and children when expressed relative to body surface area (therefore removing the effect of differing SV), but in absolute terms represents a higher percentage of the total change in $\dot{V}O_2$ in adults. This hypothesis is supported by the data of Springer et al (1991) but offers little explanation for why the phase 1 response might be longer in adults than in children. It would be expected that the muscle–lung transit delay is a linear function of growth, but it cannot be ignored that there is simply a shorter distance between the exercising muscles and the lung in children, and this might explain this age-related phenomenon.

Moderate intensity

Phase 2 time constant

A collection of studies have used cross-sectional designs to attempt to identify whether or not the phase 2 $\dot{V}O_2$ time constant (τ) is dependent upon age. The details of these studies are discussed elsewhere (Fawkner & Armstrong 2003b) and they are summarized in Table 9.2. Generally, studies have been inconsistent in their interpretation of age-related differences in the $\dot{V}O_2$ time constant, and Table 9.2 clearly identifies the wide inter-study variance that exists in the reported values for τ. This is most likely to be due to problems with defining exercise intensities, small numbers of study participants, few repeated transitions and the choice of model used. To illustrate this latter problem, and specifically identify the model that best fits the $\dot{V}O_2$ kinetic response to moderate intensity exercise, Fawkner & Armstrong (2002b) modelled the response of thirty 11- to 12-year-old boys and girls to exercise at 80% of TVENT using a range of models previously adopted. The children completed as many transitions as were necessary to achieve confidence intervals in τ of less than ±5 s. Models 1 and 2 were fit to the averaged responses, each with and without the inclusion of phase 1 data (estimated to be 15 s). By comparing the residuals for each model, it was confirmed that, as with adults, model 2 using data following phase 1 is the most appropriate model to apply to children's moderate intensity data (Fig. 9.3). The study also clearly demonstrated the effect that different modelling

Table 9.2 Summary of studies reporting the time constant of oxygen uptake following a transition to moderate intensity exercise during cycle ergometry and treadmill running

Study	Sex	N	Age (years)	Step change	Quantification method	Peak $\dot{V}O_2$ (mL·kg⁻¹·min⁻¹)	Time constant (s)
Freedson et al (1981)	M	28	10.2 (2.3)	BL – 49 W	$t_{1/2}$	47 (4)	34.8 (12.7)
Sady et al (1983)	M	21	10.2 (1.3)	BL – 42 ± 1% $\dot{V}O_2$max	$t_{1/2}$	49 (1)	18.5 (0.75)
	M	21	30.0 (5.6)	BL – 39 ± 1% $\dot{V}O_2$max	$t_{1/2}$	55 (1)	17.5 (0.39)
Cooper et al (1985)	M	5	8 (1)	Rest – 75% TVENT	Model 1, $t > 20$ s	40 (6)	26.5 (3.0)
	M	5	18 (1)			43 (5)	24.3 (2.3)
	F	5	9 (1)			37 (6)	26.5 (4.0)
	F	5	17 (1)			34 (4)	31.6 (6.2)*
Springer et al (1991)	M + F	9	8.2 (1.4)	Rest – 80% TVENT	Model 2, $t > 15$ s	41 (9)	23.9 (4.6)
	M + F	9	28 (7)			45 (7)	26.8 (4.3)
Zanconato et al (1991)	M + F	10	9.0 (1.3)	BL – 80% TVENT	1 min $t_{1/2}$	42 (6)	23.0 (5.3)
	M + F	13	32.6 (4.8)			42 (9)	24.8 (4.7)
Armon et al (1991)	M + F	6	6 – 12	BL – 80% TVENT	Model 1, $t > 0$ s	43 (6)	26 (8)
	M	7	32 (5)			40 (10)	44 (7)*
Hebestreit et al (1998)	M	9	11.1 (1.2)	20 W – 50% peak $\dot{V}O_2$	Model 2, $t >$ phase1	47 (6)	22.8 (5.1)
	M	8	23 (2.6)	20 W – 50% peak $\dot{V}O_2$		53 (7)	26.4 (4.1)
Fawkner & Armstrong (2002b)	M	11	11.6 (0.3)	BL – 80% TVENT	Model 1, $t > 0$ s	50 (6)†	29.5 (3.9)**
	M	12	21.4 (1.6)			50 (6)‡	38.4 (8.7)
	F	12	11.7 (0.4)			44 (6)	30.9 (4.5)*
	F	13	21.9 (1.9)			41 (5)	36.5 (6.3)
	M	11	11.6 (0.3)		Model 1, $t > 15$ s	50 (6)†	29.0 (3.9)**
	M	12	21.4 (1.6)			50 (6)‡	37.8 (9.0)
	F	12	11.7 (0.4)			44 (6)	30.5 (3.9)*
	F	13	21.9 (1.9)			41 (5)	36.3 (6.0)

(continued)

Table 9.2 Continued

Study	Sex	N	Age (years)	Step change	Quantification method	Peak $\dot{V}O_2$ (mL·kg^{-1}·min^{-1})	Time constant (s)
	M	11	11.6 (0.3)		Model 2, $t > 0$ s	50 (6) †	25.9 (3.3)**
	M	12	21.4 (1.6)			50 (6) ‡	33.8 (7.9)
	F	12	11.7 (0.4)			44 (6)	27.8 (4.2)*
	F	13	21.9 (1.9)			41 (5)	32.7 (5.9)
	M	11	11.6 (0.3)		Model 2, $t > 15$ s	50 (6) †	19.0 (2.0)**
	M	12	21.4 (1.6)			50 (6) ‡	27.9 (8.6)
	F	12	11.7 (0.4)			44 (6)	21.0 (5.5)*
	F	13	21.9 (1.9)			41 (5)	26.0 (4.5)
Hamar et al (1991)	M + F	18	14.1 (0.6)	TM 65% $\dot{V}O_2$max	Model 2, $t > 20$ s	54 (5)	20.2 (5.9)
Williams et al (2001)	M	8	12.0 (0.2)	TM 80% T$_{LAC}$	Model 3, $t > 0$ s	52 (2)	10.2 (1.0)
	M	8	30.0 (7.3)			57 (3)	14.7 (2.8)
	M	8	12.0 (0.2)		Model 1, $t > 0$	52 (2)	19.8 (1.2)*
	M	8	30.0 (7.3)			57 (3)	27.2 (2.4)

BL, baseline pedalling; F, females; M, males; MRT, mean response time; $t_{1/2}$, half the time to achieve the peak exercise response; $\dot{V}O_2$, oxygen uptake; $\dot{V}O_2$max, maximal oxygen uptake; TM, treadmill running; T$_{VENT}$, ventilatory threshold; T$_{LAC}$, lactate threshold; values are mean (standard deviation).
* Significant difference between children and adults ($P < 0.05$); ** ($P < 0.01$).
† Significant difference between males and females ($P < 0.05$); ‡ ($P < 0.01$).

techniques have had upon the interpretation of response parameters across the literature (Table 9.2).

Using model 2 following phase 1, a significantly shorter τ in children compared with adults in both males and females has been observed (Fawkner et al 2002). It was therefore suggested that there might be a developmental effect upon the kinetics of $\dot{V}O_2$ at this exercise intensity, and that this may be indicative of a greater potential for oxidative metabolism in children. In fact, close examination of Table 9.2 does suggest that although generally not significant, most of the studies to date support a trend towards a faster τ in children than adults at moderate intensity exercise.

Only two studies have addressed sex differences in the $\dot{V}O_2$ kinetic response to moderate intensity exercise. Cooper et al (1985) reported a significantly slower τ in five teenage girls (15–18 years) than in five teenage boys and five younger (7–10 years) girls and boys. These authors attributed the sex and age difference to the teenage girls' significantly smaller mass-related $\dot{V}O_2$max. Contrary to this study, Fawkner et al (2002) found no sex difference in τ in either children or adults, despite significant sex differences in peak $\dot{V}O_2$ expressed in traditional ratio form or when suitably scaled to body mass. This study also reported no significant relationship between peak $\dot{V}O_2$ and τ in the children or the women, but a significant negative relationship between the two variables in the men. Traditionally, it has been assumed that peak $\dot{V}O_2$ and τ are causally linked, but more recent data have contradicted this. Training studies completed with adults have identified independent training adaptations on peak $\dot{V}O_2$ and τ, and Obert et al (2000) have demonstrated significant differences in $\dot{V}O_2$max between a group of trained and untrained boys and girls, but no significant difference in τ.

Peak $\dot{V}O_2$ is considered to be predominantly limited by $\dot{Q}$, i.e. O_2 delivery. Conversely, it is generally accepted that O_2 delivery plays a minor role in limiting the speed of the kinetic response at moderate intensity, which is limited by the aerobic potential of the exercising muscle. It is therefore not surprising that these two parameters of 'fitness' are not causally linked. In fact, sex differences in peak $\dot{V}O_2$ even in the prepubertal years are explained by sex differences in $\dot{Q}$, but to date there is limited evidence that sex differences in the metabolic profile of the exercising muscle exist. Thus, it appears that certainly in children, sex differences in the kinetic response to moderate intensity do not exist, and that τ is independent of peak $\dot{V}O_2$.

Gain of the primary component

As has been alluded to earlier, it is not only the speed of the $\dot{V}O_2$ kinetic response, but also the magnitude of the response that provides some indications of the efficiency of the integrated systems. The phase 2 amplitude of the response to moderate intensity exercise is equivalent to the difference between the asymptote (the projected steady state) of the exponential and the $\dot{V}O_2$ before the onset of exercise ($\Delta\dot{V}O_2$, Fig. 9.3). The gain of the primary component refers to the O_2 cost of this amplitude, and is often expressed relative to body mass (i.e. mL $\cdot$ min^{-1} $\cdot$ kg^{-1}). When expressed in this way, the gain of the primary component is consistently reported to be higher in children than adults, which supports studies that have frequently reported a higher O_2 cost of steady-state exercise in younger subjects. However, there are concerns with using the simple ratio standard to account for body mass, and alternatively, the gain of the primary component may be expressed relative to exercise intensity (i.e. mL $\cdot$ min^{-1} $\cdot$ W^{-1}). It is generally accepted that the O_2 cost of exercise in the moderate domain equates to approximately 10 mL $\cdot$ min^{-1} $\cdot$ W^{-1} in adults, and is a function of linearity between exercise intensity and O_2 cost at work rates below TAN. With children, the primary gain has been equated to between 11 and 12 mL $\cdot$ min^{-1} $\cdot$ W^{-1} in two studies (Armon et al 1991, Hebestreit et al 1998), although only the earlier of these two studies identified a significant difference between children and adults. Whether or not there is an age-dependent effect on the gain of the primary component during moderate intensity transitions is not known, but remains to be examined further.

Heavy and very heavy intensity exercise

As discussed above, the assessment of the kinetic response to exercise intensities above TAN depends heavily upon the ability to identify the correct relative exercise intensity, and application of an appropriate model. Since the determination of CP is time-consuming and difficult to assess with children, those studies that have attempted to address the response to heavy and very heavy intensity exercise with this population have done so by setting intensities relative to TAN and peak $\dot{V}O_2$. To date, only a small number of studies have explored this exercise response, but there is some consensus with regard to the fundamental age differences in the various components of the response. These studies are summarized in Table 9.3 and discussed in brief below. For more, detail see Fawkner & Armstrong (2003b).

Table 9.3 Summary of studies reporting age differences in the response to heavy and very heavy intensity exercise

Author	Gender	N	Age (years)	Step change	Quantification method	Age interaction	Nature of age interaction
Zanconato	M + F	10	9.0 (1.3)	BL – 50% Δ	1 min $t_{1/2}$	No	N/A
et al (1981)	M + F	13	32.6 (4.8)				
Armon et al	M + F	6	6–12	BL – 25% Δ	Model 4, $\delta_1 =$	Yes	Shorter τ
(1991)	M	7	32 (5)	BL – 50% Δ	δ_2, $t > 0$ s		
				BL – 75% Δ	SC = slope of line between 3 and 6 minutes	Yes	Smaller slope
Williams	M	8	12 (0.2)	TM – 50% Δ	Model 5,	Yes	Shorter
et al (2001)	M	8	30 (7.3)		$t > 0$ s		primary τ
					SC = %	Yes	Smaller %
					$\Delta\dot{V}O_2$tot		$\Delta\dot{V}O_2$tot
Fawkner &	M	13	10.6 (0.3)	BL – 40% Δ	Model 2,	Yes	Shorter
Armstrong	F	9	10.9 (0.2)		phase 1 $< t <$		primary τ
(2004a)					onset of slow component		
	M	13	12.6 (0.3)		SC = %	Yes	Smaller %
	F	9	12.9 (0.3)		$\Delta\dot{V}O_2$tot		$\Delta\dot{V}O_2$tot

BL, baseline pedalling; F, females; M, males; $t_{1/2}$; half the time to achieve the peak exercise response; $\dot{V}O_2$, oxygen uptake; TM, treadmill running; SC, slow component; Δ, difference between ventilatory threshold and peak $\dot{V}O_2$; $\Delta\dot{V}O_2$tot, the difference between the amplitude of the primary component and the end exercise $\dot{V}O_2$; τ, time constant; δ_1, δ_2, time delays of each exponential; values are mean (standard deviation).

Although there are concerns with some of the methodology adopted by Armon et al (1991), these authors made the first valuable contribution to identifying differences in the pattern of the response to heavy intensity exercise between adults and children. They suggested that the response to heavy and very heavy intensity cycling in children could be suitably modelled using a single exponential. In other words, children did not display the slow component response identified in adults. It was further suggested that this was due to children achieving a greater percentage of the final $\dot{V}O_2$ steady state during the primary component (phase 2), a greater O_2 gain during the primary component and a faster primary time constant. This study was later supported during treadmill running, in which the contribution of the slow component (suitably quantified as the difference between the amplitude of the primary component and the end exercise $\dot{V}O_2$) to the total change in $\dot{V}O_2$ was significantly smaller in boys than in men (Williams et al 2001). Again, it was suggested that children's responses could be adequately modelled using the equivalent of just a single exponential, that the gain of the primary component was greater in children, and that the primary time constant was significantly faster in boys than in men.

The proposal that children's responses to heavy intensity exercise might change with age was carefully examined in a 2-year longitudinal study involving 13 pre-pubertal boys and 9 prepubertal girls (Fawkner & Armstrong 2004a). The response to 40% Δ was modelled by first identifying the onset of the slow component, and then modelling with a single exponential (model 2) only the primary component. The slow component was then quantified as in the study of Williams et al (2001). As in previous studies, when the children were younger, the relative slow component was smaller, the gain of the primary response was greater and the primary time constant was faster. Contrary to other studies, however, a slow component was clearly demonstrated in the children at both ages. The same authors demonstrated empirically elsewhere that in fact the slow component does exist in children and should not be modelled as a single exponential process (Fawkner & Armstrong 2004b) (Fig. 9.6).

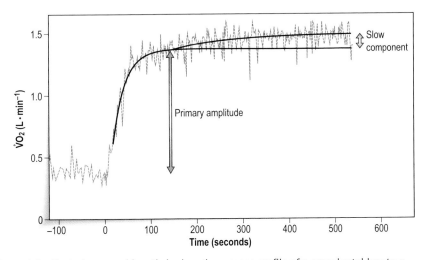

Figure 9.6 Typical averaged breath-by-breath response profile of a prepubertal boy to a transition to 40% of the difference between his ventilatory threshold and peak $\dot{V}O_2$ (heavy intensity). The data have been modelled using a double exponential with independent time delays from the end of phase 1 (model 3). The primary amplitude has been extended to clearly demonstrate the slow component.

Explanations for these age-related changes in the phase 2 response to heavy intensity exercise are difficult to confirm. Referring back to the control theories regarding the dynamics of $\dot{V}O_2$ at the onset of exercise, the primary response is considered to be principally dependent upon the mitochondrial potential to generate the required ATP for exercise, with a possible contribution from the efficiency to deliver O_2 to the site of utilization. Thus, the observed faster primary time constant response in children and higher O_2 cost of exercise during the primary phase suggest that a developmental influence upon the O_2 utilization potential is evident. This supports the literature that suggests that adolescents may have an enzyme profile supportive of a greater rate of pyruvate oxidation than adults (see Chapter 4). It is also interesting to compare these response characteristics to those of subjects who differ in the fibre type profile of the muscle. A greater O_2 cost and faster primary component time constant have been reported in adult subjects with a high ratio of type I to type II muscle fibres (Pringle et al 2003). There is currently limited evidence suggesting that the fibre type profile of the muscle changes during growth and maturation, and this evidence is contradictory (see Chapter 4). This possible explanation therefore remains to be proven, and in fact, the contribution of fibre type profiles and their activation to parameters of the kinetic response to heavy intensity exercise remains a topic of great interest in both the adult and paediatric literature.

It should not be ignored that there is also evidence of a tendency for O_2 delivery (muscle blood flow per unit tissue) to decrease from the ages of 12 through to 16 years (Koch 1980). However, the extent to which O_2 delivery limits the phase 2 response to heavy intensity exercise is clouded by contradictory literature, and it seems most likely that O_2 becomes limiting only when severely restricted by disease or old age. Whether poorer O_2 delivery develops during the transition from childhood into adulthood and limits the kinetic response to heavy intensity exercise remains to be proven.

Smaller slow components in children compared with adults need to be interpreted in light of the above issues regarding the primary component. As has been discussed earlier, the mechanisms underpinning the slow component are not entirely understood, and although it is usually modelled as a discrete component, it is likely that the slow component is a function of the mechanisms controlling energy turnover from the first onset of exercise. To this extent, in each of the studies mentioned previously, the O_2 cost at the end of exercise was equal between the younger and older subjects. Thus the greater relative contribution of the slow component in the older subjects was in fact a function of the smaller primary amplitude rather than a greater slow component per se (this is represented diagrammatically in Fig. 9.7). This pattern is in accordance with the comparison of adults with a high and low percentage of type I fibres. Therefore it seems plausible that the energy cost of steady-state heavy intensity exercise might be independent of age, but that age-related changes in the aerobic contribution to the energy requirements during the transition are evident. Could this greater efficiency of the aerobic system help to explain the low end-exercise blood lactates frequently reported in children? Certainly there may be some indirect link, but to date studies have failed to report any relationship between response parameters to heavy intensity exercise and end-exercise blood lactate in children.

Much of the original supposition that blood lactate and the slow component were causally linked came from training studies with adults that demonstrated a reduction in the slow component with training, coincident with a reduction in end-exercise blood lactate levels. Although a causal link between blood lactate and the slow component has now been generally disregarded, training studies with adults have invari-

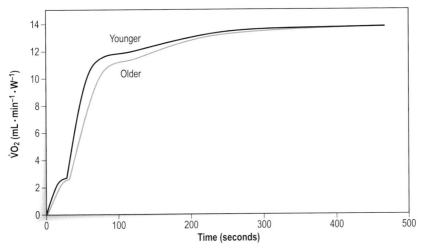

Figure 9.7 Model of the gain of the primary component and oxygen cost at the end of exercise in younger and older subjects.

ably reported training adaptations of the kinetic response to heavy intensity exercise. A reduction in the primary time constant and a reduction in the relative amplitude of the slow component at the same absolute work rates have been reported and this is in agreement with training adaptations in oxidative enzyme activity, O_2 delivery and fibre type recruitment. There is to date no evidence to suggest that the response to heavy intensity exercise in children may equally respond to training. Obert et al (2000) identified no difference between a group of trained and untrained children in the primary time constant or the percentage contribution of the slow component to the total change in $\dot{V}O_2$ when cycling at 90% of their maximal aerobic power. However, longitudinal training studies that are appropriately controlled and that are of sufficient length are required before training adaptations of the $\dot{V}O_2$ kinetic response to exercise in children might be identified.

There are some data to suggest that sex differences in the kinetic response to heavy intensity exercise might exist. A comparison of 25 prepubertal boys and 23 prepubertal girls identified that the boys had a faster primary time constant than the girls and a smaller contribution of the slow component to the total change in $\dot{V}O_2$ (Fawkner & Armstrong 2004c). Interestingly, this was contrary to moderate intensity exercise, where the same research group had reported no such sex differences in the kinetic response. Since the response to exercise is thought more likely to be limited by O_2 delivery at heavy intensity than at moderate intensity, it is reasonable to suggest that these sex differences might be due to the sex differences in SV that are known to exist in the prepubertal years. The girls, however, had higher end-exercise HR values, and as with steady-state exercise, this may have been sufficient to offset any sex difference in SV such that $\dot{Q}$ was equal between the boys and girls. As mentioned previously, there is limited evidence to suggest that sex differences in the metabolic profile of the muscle, specifically fibre types, might exist and therefore explanations for these sex differences are difficult to conclude. Nevertheless, these data support the concept that even in the prepubertal years, sex differences in the response to exercise do exist.

Severe intensity exercise

As with the scarcity of data relating to the slow component with children, there are only a handful of studies that have attempted to investigate the response to exercise at or above maximal intensities, and most of these have utilized somewhat crude analysis techniques (Table 9.4). Early studies demonstrated that children achieved a greater percentage of their peak exercise response after 30 s of either treadmill or cycle exercise compared with adults (Mácek & Vavra 1977, Robinson 1938). Boys exercising at an intensity equivalent to 100% $\dot{V}O_2$max achieved (mean (standard deviation)) 56.4% (7.0%) $\dot{V}O_2$max after 30 s compared with 35.5% (7.0%) $\dot{V}O_2$max in men, had smaller O_2 deficits and lower end-exercise blood lactates (Mácek & Vavra 1980). These data were interpreted as evidence of a faster adaptation of aerobic metabolism in children. There has, however, been some contradictory evidence, since both Hebestreit et al (1998) and Zanconato et al (1991) did not observe any age-related changes in the speed of the response to exercise at 100%, 125% and 130% peak $\dot{V}O_2$. Despite this, though, the study by Zanconato et al (1991) accurately measured the cumulative O_2 cost of the exercise. By collecting gas exchange data for 10 min following the 60 s exercise bout, the O_2 cost per joule of the exercise was found to be significantly greater in children than adults. These authors proposed that their results indicated that children have lower 'anaerobic capacity' than adults – due to a lesser ability for

Table 9.4   Summary of studies reporting age differences in the response to severe intensity exercise

Author	Gender	N	Age (years)	Step change	Quantification method	Age interaction
Robinson 1938	M	8	6.0	TM – exhaustion	% of peak $\dot{V}O_2$ after 30 s	Yes
	M	10	10.5			
	M	52	20–91			
Mácek & Vávra (1977)	M	10	10	TM – exhaustion	% of peak $\dot{V}O_2$ after 30 s	Yes
	M	14	12			
	M	23	15			
	M	6	17			
Mácek & Vávra (1980)	M	10	10–11	BL – exhaustion	% of peak $\dot{V}O_2$ after 30 s	Yes
	M	11	20–22			
Sady (1981)	M	21	10.2 (0.3)	BL – 110% $\dot{V}O_2$max	$t_{1/2}$	Yes
	M	21	30.0 (1.2)			
Zanconato et al. (1981)	M + F	10	9.0 (1.3)	BL – 100% peak $\dot{V}O_2$ for 1 min BL – 125% peak $\dot{V}O_2$ for 1 min	$t_{1/2}$	No
	M + F	13	32.6 (4.8)			
Hebestreit et al (1998)	M	9	11.1 (1.2)	20W–100% peak $\dot{V}O_2$ for 120 s 20W – 130% peak $\dot{V}O_2$ for 75 s	Model 2, $t >$ phase1	No
	M	8	23 (2.6)			

BL, baseline pedalling; F, females; M, males; $t_{1/2}$, half the time to achieve the peak exercise response; $\dot{V}O_2$, oxygen uptake; $\dot{V}O_2$max, maximal oxygen uptake; TM, treadmill running; values are mean (standard deviation).

anaerobic metabolism. Certainly there is some evidence to suggest that children may have reduced muscle glycolytic ability during high intensity exercise (see Chapter 4), but evidence from studies relating to the kinetic response of $\dot{V}O_2$ suggests that it is more likely that children's metabolic profiles are better adapted to aerobic metabolism, rather than that they are limited glycolytically.

SUMMARY

At present, it appears that the $\dot{V}O_2$ kinetic response does undergo maturation with age. At moderate intensity, the kinetic response may be faster in children than adults, and at exercise intensities above T_{AN}, a faster phase 2 response, greater relative $\dot{V}O_2$ during the primary phase and smaller slow component are evident in children. Taken in combination, these data contribute to the understanding that children have a greater potential for aerobic metabolism than adults, and subsequently will depend less upon glycolytic reserves to achieve the same exercise intensity.

There are currently limited data with which to interpret age- and sex-related differences in the $\dot{V}O_2$ kinetic response to exercise, and to fully understand and support the interpretation of this response in children. This is unfortunate, since parameters of the $\dot{V}O_2$ kinetic response contain valuable information with regard to metabolic and cardiorespiratory responses to exercise that may have important relevance to evaluating athletic ability and the capacity to carry out day-to-day activities in children. To date the data focus entirely on the healthy child, but the consequences of a slow kinetic response brought upon by disease will have critical implications regarding exercise tolerance and the ability to carry out everyday activities in some children. However, until the response is more clearly understood and we are able to confidently compute relevant response parameters, the ability to utilize these exercise testing modalities for assessment of athletic potential and exercise tolerance in the diseased state is limited.

KEY POINTS

1. The $\dot{V}O_2$ kinetic response is representative of the body's ability to adjust to a change in energy demand due to exercise. It is an outcome of the combined efficiency of the cardiovascular, pulmonary and metabolic systems.
2. At the onset of exercise, $\dot{V}O_2$, which is representative of oxygen uptake at the muscle, does not increase in direct synchrony with the demand for energy, but lags behind, increasing exponentially, such that the additionally required ATP must be generated through anaerobic sources. The O_2 cost of the energy derived anaerobically is termed the O_2 deficit.
3. The speed with which $\dot{V}O_2$ responds to the change in exercise intensity may be quantified as the time constant, τ, which is the time to achieve 63% of the change in $\dot{V}O_2$.
4. In the moderate intensity domain, $\dot{V}O_2$ achieves a steady state within approximately 2–3 min. In the heavy intensity domain, $\dot{V}O_2$ continues to increase and may eventually achieve a steady state; this is termed the slow component.
5. Data that detail the $\dot{V}O_2$ kinetic response to exercise in children are sparse, and data should be considered with some degree of caution due to the methodological issues involved in assessing the kinetic response with children.
6. Children may display a smaller and shorter phase 1 than adults.

7. The phase 2 response is faster in younger compared with older children and adult subjects, although the data are more consistent at exercise intensities above the anaerobic threshold.
8. The O_2 cost of exercise during phase 2 is greater in younger children, i.e. aerobic metabolism contributes to a greater extent during the transitional phase than do alternative anaerobic sources.
9. The slow component response is attenuated in younger children.
10. There are no sex differences in the $\dot{V}O_2$ kinetic response at moderate intensity, but girls appear to have slower phase 2 kinetics and larger slow components than boys when exercising at heavy intensity. Whether this is a function of sex differences in O_2 delivery or potential for aerobic metabolism is not known.
11. The body of evidence suggests that there is an age-dependent effect on the $\dot{V}O_2$ kinetic response and slow component, and this might be indicative of children having a greater potential for aerobic metabolism than adults.

References

Armon Y, Cooper D M, Flores R et al 1991 Oxygen uptake dynamics during high-intensity exercise in children and adults. Journal of Applied Physiology 70:841–848

Cooper D M, Berry C, Lamarra N et al 1985 Kinetics of oxygen uptake and heart rate at onset of exercise in children. Journal of Applied Physiology 59:211–217

Fawkner S G, Armstrong N 2002a Assessment of critical power in children. Pediatric Exercise Science 14:259–268

Fawkner S G, Armstrong N 2002b Modelling the $\dot{V}O_2$ kinetic response to moderate intensity exercise in children. Acta Kinesiologiae Universitatis Tartuensis 7:80–84

Fawkner S G, Armstrong N 2003a The slow component response of $\dot{V}O_2$ to heavy intensity exercise in children. In: Reilly T, Marfell-Jones M (eds) Kinanthopometry viii. Routledge, London, p 105–113

Fawkner S G, Armstrong N 2003b Oxygen uptake kinetic response to exercise in children. Sports Medicine 33:651–669

Fawkner S G, Armstrong N 2004a Longitudinal changes in the kinetic response to heavy-intensity exercise in children. Journal of Applied Physiology 97:460–466

Fawkner S G, Armstrong N 2004b Modelling the $\dot{V}O_2$ kinetic response to heavy intensity exercise in children. Ergonomics 47:1517–1527

Fawkner S G, Armstrong N 2004c Sex differences in the oxygen uptake kinetic response to heavy-intensity exercise in prepubertal children. European Journal of Applied Physiology 93:210–216

Fawkner S G, Armstrong N, Potter C R et al 2002 $\dot{V}O_2$ kinetics in children and adults following the onset of moderate intensity exercise. Journal of Sports Sciences 20:319–326

Freedson P S, Gilliam T B, Sady S P et al 1981 Transient $\dot{V}O_2$ characteristics in children at the onset of steady-rate exercise. Research Quarterly for Exercise and Sport 52:167–173

Hamar D, Tkac M, Komadesl L et al 1991 Oxygen uptake kinetics at various intensities of exercise on the treadmill in young athletes. In: Frenkl R, Szmodis I (eds) Children and exercise pediatric work physiology xv. National Institute for Health Promotion, Budapest, p 187–201

Hebestreit H, Kreimler S, Hughson R L et al 1998 Kinetics of oxygen uptake at the onset of exercise in boys and men. Journal of Applied Physiology 85:1833–1841

Koch G 1980 Aerobic power, lung dimensions, ventilatory capacity and muscle blood flow in 12–16-year-old boys with high physical activity. In: Berg K, Eriksson BO (eds) Children and exercise IX. University Park Press, Baltimore, p 99–108

Mácek M, Vavra J 1977 Relation between aerobic and anaerobic energy supply during maximal exercise in boys. In: Lavellée H, Shephard R J Frontiers of activity and child health. Pelican, Quebec, p 157–159

Mácek M, Vávra J 1980 The adjustment of oxygen uptake at the onset of exercise; a comparison between prepubertal boys and young adults. International Journal of Sports Medicine 1:70–72

Obert P, Cleuziou C, Candau R et al 2000 The slow component of O_2 uptake kinetics during high-intensity exercise in trained and untrained prepubertal children. International Journal of Sports Medicine 21:31–36

Pringle J S, Doust J H, Carter H et al 2003 Oxygen uptake kinetics during moderate, heavy and severe intensity 'submaximal' exercise in humans: The influence of muscle fibre type and capillarisation. European Journal of Applied Physiology 89:289–300

Robinson S 1938 Experimental studies of physical fitness in relation to age. Internationale Zeitschrift für Angewandte Physiologie, Einschliesslich Arbeitsphysiologie 10:251–323

Sady S P 1981 Transient oxygen uptake and heart rate responses at the onset of relative endurance exercise in prepubertal boys and adult men. International Journal of Sports Medicine 2:240–244

Sady S P, Katch V I, Villanacci J F et al 1983 Children-adult comparisons of $\dot{V}O_2$ and HR kinetics during submaximal exercise. Research Quarterly for Exercise and Sport 54:55–59

Springer C, Barstow T J, Wasserman K et al 1991 Oxygen uptake and heart rate responses during hypoxic exercise in children and adults. Medicine and Science in Sports and Exercise 23:71–79

Williams C A, Carter H, Jones A M et al 2001 Oxygen uptake kinetics during treadmill running in boys and men. Journal of Applied Physiology 90:1700–1706

Zanconato S, Cooper D M, Armon Y 1991 Oxygen cost and oxygen uptake dynamics and recovery with 1 min of exercise in children and adults. Journal of Applied Physiology 71:993–998

Further reading

Barstow T J, Scheuermann B W 2005 $\dot{V}O_2$ kinetics. Effects of maturation and ageing. In: Jones A, Poole D C (eds) Oxygen uptake kinetics in sport, exercise and medicine. Routledge, London and New York, p 331–352

Barstow T J, Jones A M, Nguyen P H et al 1996 Influence of muscle fiber type and pedal frequency on oxygen uptake kinetics of heavy exercise. Journal of Applied Physiology 81:1642–1650

Gaesser G A, Poole D C 1996 The slow component of oxygen uptake kinetics in humans. Exercise and Sports Sciences Reviews 24:35–71

Jones A M, Poole D C 2005 Oxygen uptake kinetics in sport, exercise and medicine. Routledge, London

Whipp B J, Rossiter H B, Ward S A 2002 Exertional oxygen uptake kinetics : a stamen of stamina. Biochemical Society Transactions 30:237–247

Chapter 10

Responses to training

Keith Tolfrey

LEARNING OBJECTIVES

After studying this chapter you should be able to:

1. examine the impact that outcome goals have on exercise training characteristics
2. describe the primary components of an exercise training programme (e.g. intensity) and examine the interrelationships between them
3. compare and contrast cross-sectional and longitudinal (prospective) research designs whilst examining the effect this has on our understanding of the relationship between exercise training and physiological parameters
4. identify studies that have provided evidence that resistance exercise training can be a safe form of exercise for most young people
5. describe the factors that need to be considered when designing a safe and effective resistance training programme
6. critically evaluate the evidence that shows prepubertal children are able to demonstrate significant gains in muscular strength following resistance exercise training
7. differentiate between the underlying mechanisms for increases in muscular strength in prepubertal children and adolescents

8. determine whether there is a critical period during childhood when improvements in peak oxygen uptake (peak $\dot{V}O_2$) may be optimized
9. evaluate the quantity and quality of evidence supporting a blunted aerobic training response in prepubertal children
10. identify the factors that are likely to underpin the smaller gains in peak $\dot{V}O_2$ reported prior to puberty
11. discuss the impact of age, biological maturity, and participant sex on aerobic trainability
12. compare and contrast data pertaining to anaerobic adaptations relative to muscle strength and peak $\dot{V}O_2$
13. evaluate the significance of studies using the muscle biopsy technique with young people when considering changes in anaerobic metabolism
14. critically appraise where future research projects might focus when considering physiological trainability in young people.

INTRODUCTION

Although physical inactivity in many young people is a worrying trend and is probably the primary cause of several serious health problems, it is also clear that some children and adolescents exercise on a regular basis in an effort to attain specific goals (i.e. they engage in exercise training). The goals may vary from those that are based on improving sports performance to those that emphasize gains in physical health, recognizing that the two goals are not entirely independent. In reality, the number of young people who use exercise training to improve their health on a totally volitional basis, excluding volunteers for research projects, is probably very low indeed. Most diseases or health problems, regardless of whether there is any evidence of childhood origins, do not have visible symptoms this early in life. Therefore, ill-health is probably an abstract concept for most young people, and their parents for that matter. In contrast, with the ever increasing number of competitive sports that are available to young people, the numbers who use exercise training to improve their chances of sporting success are probably considerably higher.

Whether the goal is performance- or health-related, it should be recognized that most studies focus on alterations in physiological parameters rather than sports performance or physical health per se. That is, the researcher who takes blood samples from young people to determine concentrations of high-density lipoprotein cholesterol (HDL-C) before and after an exercise training intervention is rarely able to study or even predict the incidence of coronary heart disease or arteriosclerosis in the participants who volunteer to complete the study. In a similar vein, evidence that completing an aerobic exercise training programme increases peak oxygen uptake (peak $\dot{V}O_2$) does not necessarily translate into improved cross-country running times. Nevertheless, results from these studies do provide a better understanding of the relationship that exercise or energy expenditure shares with a variety of physiological parameters before reaching full biological maturity. It may be possible to use this knowledge to design and implement future exercise programmes that are safe for young people to use, but also result in adaptations to targeted physiological systems that could logically result in significant sports performance or health-related goals.

Physiological outcome parameters in exercise training studies with young people have included stroke volume; cardiac output; heart rate; blood pressure; oxygen uptake; muscular strength, endurance, and power; lactic acid (blood lactate); lipid-lipoproteins; insulin resistance; glucose tolerance; bone mineral density and content;

and adipose tissue, to list but a few. This chapter will focus primarily on muscle strength, peak oxygen uptake (peak $\dot{V}O_2$), and short-term power output (including anaerobic metabolism). Although it is recognized that power output is not physiological in itself, it is the most common way in which adaptations to the anaerobic energy pathways have been expressed in the literature.

RESEARCH DESIGNS

Before exploring these three main parameters, a generic overview of some exercise training programme characteristics/principles and basic research design issues is necessary to understand the unique nature of working with this special population in this important area. First, the only way to establish a cause and effect relationship between exercise and physiological parameters is through longitudinal (prospective) designs. This does not mean that cross-sectional analyses do not provide some significant insights, but the link between exercise training and physiological adaptation remains forever speculative. A strength of the cross-sectional approach is that it may be possible to study young people who have been engaged in exercise, although normally a particular sport, for prolonged periods of time (years) that far outreach those that are usually seen in longitudinal designs (months or just weeks). Moreover, it is less time-consuming and arduous for both researcher and participant from a data collection standpoint. Unfortunately, longitudinal studies are often relatively short and involve quite small samples of participants who usually volunteer, thus introducing potential bias. Without a well-matched control group, neither research design is likely to procure any meaningful information. Where possible, participants should be randomly assigned to control and experimental groups, although pair matching using the primary outcome parameter may be preferable given that sample sizes are often so small that random allocation may still result in pre-intervention between-group differences. Any extraneous factors that may affect the primary outcome variable, in addition to the exercise intervention, should be either controlled or at least measured so that they may be accounted for using appropriate statistical techniques (e.g. analysis of covariance or partial correlations). In a well-designed study, the control group should allow the identification of an independent exercise effect in the experimental group that is free from the influence of growth, development and biological maturation.

If the aim of a study is merely to identify a causative link between exercise and an outcome parameter, then it may be prudent to allow the young people to engage in a variety of activities that require no quantification – as long as it is clear that they do more than the controls. The identification of a possible dose–response relationship is, however, only possible through the careful standardization and quantification of the exercise training programme and measurement of physiological parameters using reliable and valid methods. It has been common to use findings from the literature on adults to assist in the design of exercise programmes with young people, but the principles are much the same. That is, the total exercise volume is manipulated by varying the intensity, duration, frequency and programme length. It is well recognized that the interplay between exercise intensity and duration is the primary determinant of exercise volume in most research studies, although the impact of the remaining facets is also important. Exercise training principles such as overload, progression, specificity, and detraining would appear to apply equally as well to young people as they do to adults. It should be recognized at this early stage that the systematic manipulation of the exercise training principles and characteristics identified above

has not yet been achieved when working with young people or a specific physiological parameter. Therefore, what is not known in this field of study far outweighs
what is known currently.

MUSCLE STRENGTH

When children and adolescents complete a resistance training programme they will
almost certainly increase their muscle strength from the baseline (pre-training) value.
The following section will substantiate such a bold statement and will also reveal that
numerous essential factors must be satisfied for it to have any credence. The component parts of a training programme will determine the extent to which a child or
adolescent increases their strength. That is, the resistive load, the number of times
the load is moved before a rest is taken (repetitions), the number of sets (groups of
repetitions), session frequency (how many per week), and total programme length
(weeks). A feature of resistance exercise research with adults is that individual components of the training programme have been manipulated in order to identify the
effect that this might have on muscle strength or, in some cases, muscle size. Thus,
considerable discussion has centred on developing the 'optimal' combination of load,
repetitions, sets and weekly frequency. It is unlikely that a single, optimal resistance
training programme exists because study goals vary so widely. However, given how
difficult it can be to get young people to engage in regular physical activity, it may be
prudent to identify the minimum amount of resistance training that is still associated
with meaningful gains in muscle strength. For example, is it necessary to train three
times a week or would just two sessions suffice? Should young people be working
with relatively light loads and high repetitions (e.g. 15 to 20) or heavier loads and low
repetitions (e.g. 6 to 10)? These questions will be covered in the following subsections.

Safety

Before highlighting some of the main outcomes of research in this field, it is worth
focusing on initial concerns that resistance exercise training is something that is best
left alone until the body has reached full physical maturity, or at least until adolescence. There is no doubt that children can sustain injuries when attempting to
improve their strength through resistance training. However, it is also clear that the
majority of these problems have occurred through inappropriate practice when the
resistive load has been too high and/or the exercise has been conducted without
qualified supervision. This is not a unique feature of resistance training in the young;
the likelihood of injury for adults in the same situation would also be high. The fact
that the majority of research studies with children have not reported any injuries
sustained by the study participants is not evidence in itself because few have been
designed specifically to identify this outcome. However, a study by Rians et al (1987)
used a prospective design to evaluate whether a closely supervised circuit training
programme was safe for 18 prepubertal boys (stage one of secondary sexual characteristics). The boys used eight hydraulic resistive machine stations three times a
week for 14 weeks. During each session, as many lifts as possible were completed
within 30 s at each work station with 30 s of rest between stations – the resistance
exercise lasted for 30 min. The contractions were only concentric and the load was
increased progressively over the 14 weeks. Compared with 10 maturity-matched
controls, the concentric work output at the end of the training programme had

increased substantially in the trained group (~sixfold difference between groups). Injury surveillance, completed by a doctor, revealed one strength training injury during a shoulder press over the 14-week intervention. Whilst resting the shoulder for three sessions, the boy continued to exercise his other muscle groups using the remaining machines. Numerous other musculoskeletal 'complaints' were made by the boys, but they were all resolved by improvements in technique. Biphasic scintigraphy suggested that muscle was not damaged by the training and this was confirmed when non-fractionated, phosphocreatine concentrations were not elevated at any stage of the study. Although the epiphyseal plates in the tibia, ulna and radius of three boys appeared to be abnormal at various stages of the study, Rians et al (1987) concluded that the resistance exercise programme was unlikely to be the cause. Of course, this study cannot be used as evidence that 'any' resistance training programme is safe, but a search of the literature reveals others that support these results when a variety of programmes with different characteristics and participants have been examined. A number of influential groups including the American Academy of Pediatrics, the National Strength and Conditioning Association, the American College of Sports Medicine and the British Association of Sport and Exercise Sciences have all since published guidelines or recommendations for strength training in young people after concluding that it is a safe form of exercise provided it is closely monitored and the exercise programmes are designed appropriately.

Increases in strength

A meta-analysis by Falk & Tenenbaum (1996), which included 54 effect sizes (ES) from nine studies with participants who were described as children, reported that the overall weighted mean (standard deviation) ES was 0.57 (0.12). After discarding the three studies with extreme ES, the majority of studies in this analysis showed that gains in muscle strength varied between 14% and 30% above that which would be expected from normal growth and development. Although it was not possible to determine whether age affected the strength gains identified in the meta-analysis, the authors did indicate that adolescents probably experience greater absolute increases than children following similar training programmes, but the relative improvements are larger in the youngest age groups because of the lower baseline strength. Insufficient data were available in this quantitative review to determine whether muscle strength trainability is dependent upon sex, maturity or training intensity.

Using the same analytical review technique, Payne et al (1997) examined the effect of resistance training in children and youth. Twenty-eight studies met the criteria for inclusion in this meta-analysis, resulting in 252 valid ES. The main conclusion was that, regardless of participant or study characteristics, resistance training resulted in significant improvements in muscular strength with a mean (standard deviation) ES of 0.75 (0.57). Using the average age at peak height velocity (PHV) from the literature to categorize the young people into 'younger' or 'older' groups resulted in similar ES (0.75 vs. 0.69, respectively). The relatively small number of ES ($n = 11$) for the older group means that further evidence is warranted before it can be assumed that neither age nor maturity influence strength gains following resistance training. The mean ES (0.81) for girls was higher than for boys (0.72), but the number of ES available for girls was quite low ($n = 23$). Although the authors speculated that this might be related to differences in maturation between girls and boys included in their analyses, they did not provide any further evidence from the individual studies to support this.

Furthermore, an alternative hypothesis linking baseline strength measurements to the magnitude of change is more plausible given that untrained girls are normally weaker than their male counterparts. Despite the larger number of ES in this study compared to Falk & Tenenbaum's (1996) study, it was still not possible to delineate the effects of training intensity on strength gains in children and youth.

Changes in muscle size

Where training-induced increases in strength have been demonstrated, the majority of studies have shown that muscle hypertrophy does not occur before puberty. Although testosterone, growth hormone (GH), insulin-like growth factor I (IGF-I), and insulin all influence muscle hypertrophy during normal growth and maturation, their interaction with resistance training is not clear. The consensus within the literature suggests that until concentrations of testosterone increase during puberty, muscle hypertrophy is not likely to occur following a resistance training programme. It is possible that muscle size measurements have lacked sensitivity and the stimulus for change has been insufficient in many cases. Most studies have used quite basic anthropometric measurements (limb girths and skinfolds) which may be open to considerable variation and are not able to isolate the muscle tissue. For example, Faigenbaum et al (1993) measured the circumferences of the chest, waist, thigh, and upper arm before and after a biweekly resistance training programme spanning 8 weeks in which the average increase in muscular strength was ~61% after normal growth and development had been accounted for. All four of the circumference measurements changed by less than 2.5% and mirrored the response seen in the maturity-matched, randomly allocated control girls and boys. It is perhaps not surprising that changes that reflect muscle size were not detected after only 8 weeks; given that adults do not normally experience meaningful increases in muscle size in the early stages of a resistance training programme, there is little reason to suggest that children with relatively low concentrations of testosterone will be any different. In contrast, a study of two prepubertal monozygotic twin boys resulted in a significant increase in anatomical cross-sectional area (ACSA) of the quadriceps measured using magnetic resonance imaging (MRI) following 10 weeks of unilateral isometric knee extensor training (Mersch & Stoboy 1989). Muscle hypertrophy in the trained leg varied from 4.0% to 9.2% depending on which segment of the quadriceps was measured; this is probably linked to the well-known observation that muscle tension varies over the range of movement when moving a fixed external load or it varies across the muscle length during an isometric contraction. This variation in muscle hypertrophy has been reported in other studies with adults and highlights that if the relatively small increases in muscle size that may occur in children are to be detected, then several measurements over the length of the muscle may be required. It has not escaped notice that data from only two boys need to be further substantiated.

Fukunaga et al (1992) used ultrasonography measurements of the upper arm to conclude that it may be possible for children (skeletal age 6.2–10.7 years) to experience increases in ACSA following isometric elbow flexion training. On average, the increase in ACSA was 10.4% compared with only 5.0% in maturity-matched controls. Unfortunately, they did not give specific details of the ultrasound measurements and surprisingly the changes in elbow extensor strength and size were greater than those reported for the flexors. It was not surprising that skeletal age only explained 13% of the variance in ACSA change given that all of the children in this study were probably still prepubertal. Despite the findings from these two studies, it is still clear that even if the muscle can increase in size, the magnitude of this change is going to be relatively small compared to the substantial increases in strength that are possible.

If we assume that children need more testosterone to facilitate an increase in muscle size, it would make sense that adolescent boys, who experience a large increase in this androgen at the onset of puberty, should find that muscle hypertrophy parallels improvements in strength. However, a search of the literature reveals that this is not well supported by empirical data. The paucity of evidence may reflect that the majority of research in this field has been with children, that the adolescents normally only train for up to 12 weeks, or that studies have simply not included an assessment of muscle size.

Using soft-tissue radiography, Vrijens (1978) measured ACSA of the thigh and upper arm before and after an 8-week isotonic (constant external resistance) training programme in 12 adolescent boys (16.7 years). The average increase of 25% in arm strength appeared to be due in part to a 14.3% increase in upper arm ACSA; however, a similar increase in leg strength saw an increase of only 4.6% in thigh ACSA. The larger increase in arm ACSA may have been dependent on the pre-training size or it is possible that the tissue scan was made at a point along the muscle length where the increase was at its greatest in the arm, but not the thigh. Insufficient detail is given in the paper to determine exactly where these measurements were made. The changes in ACSA are still quite small considering the boys were likely to be approaching full physical maturity; this probably reflects the low volume of resistance exercise that the boys completed.

In one of the only other published studies to measure changes in both size and strength in adolescent twins (14.9 years) following resistance training, Komi et al (1978) found that a 20% increase in maximum isometric knee extension force was not matched by a change in thigh girth (1.6%). Changes in limb girths reported in Vrijens' (1978) study were much smaller than the radiographic scans (upper arm 3.9% and thigh 2.0%), again suggesting that this method is not sensitive enough to detect more subtle changes in the underlying muscle. Moreover, any conclusions based on data from only six participants are open to question.

The large increase in circulating hormones and growth factors at the onset of puberty stimulates a period of rapid growth and development in lean tissue in boys. It is conceivable that this stimulus might be so strong that it could override the influence of any other external factors on muscle size including resistance training. As pubertal changes in girls are different, it would be interesting to see if resistance training during a period of rapid growth in boys and girls resulted in a differential outcome. This hypothesis does not appear to have been tested in the literature, but there is some support for it when considering peak $\dot{V}O_2$ measurements in twins.

Neurological changes

In the absence of muscle hypertrophy, the logical assumption has been that neurological mechanisms must underpin the increases in strength discussed earlier. However, direct evidence of this in young people is scant. In the previously mentioned study with adolescents, Komi et al (1978) used integrated electromyographic activity (iEMG) of the rectus femoris to assess whether changes in muscle strength following a 12-week resistance training programme could be ascribed to neural adaptations. In an effort to place the electrode pairs in the same place on repeat testing, each site on the skin was marked by a drop of 20% silver nitrate solution. The maximum iEMG in the trained leg increased on average by 37.8% whereas the changes in the untrained leg and the control member of the twin pair were only 0.6% and 3.3%, respectively. The authors postulated that this increase was a consequence of the training and that it suggested a reduction of inhibitory inputs to the active alpha-motor neurons resulting in a greater flow of activation reaching the muscle site. Although it did not reach statistical significance, the iEMG/tension curve shifted to the right over the 12-week training period in five of the six trained twins, which was interpreted as a more economic use of the rectus femoris. It is difficult to understand how or why the increase in iEMG was almost double the improvement reported in knee extension force; no explanation was forwarded in the paper.

Ozmun et al (1994) also used iEMG, but over the biceps brachii in eight prepubertal children who completed an 8-week elbow flexion, constant external resistance training programme. Both isokinetic (27.8% vs. 15.5%) and isotonic (22.6% vs. 3.8%) strength increased in the trained group compared to a maturity-matched, randomly assigned control group. The bigger difference between the trained and control participants for the isotonic strength measurement, compared with isokinetic, was said to be a learning effect or due to the specificity of the training. However, after initial tests revealed differences between trial one and trials two, four and five, trial one was discarded for all subsequent ANOVA analyses to counter a potential learning effect. The 16.8% increase in iEMG amplitude for the trained group compared with a 6.0% reduction for the controls could reflect an enhancement in motor unit recruitment, improvement in the firing rate of activated motor units, or alteration of EMG firing patterns according to Ozmun and colleagues (1994). The iEMG amplitude of the trained group was ~21% lower than the controls' prior to the intervention whereas the post-intervention values were almost identical, suggesting that the baseline values should have been included in the analyses as covariates and that changes may reflect regression to the mean. Ozmun also acknowledged that the iEMG electrode placement could have altered between the pre- and post-intervention measurements, thus introducing a source of variability to the results that could not be quantified. However, there is no reason to believe that this source of error would not be randomly distributed between the trained and control groups.

In what has, to date, become the most frequently cited resistance exercise training programme with children, Ramsay et al (1990) sought to identify specifically whether changes in muscular strength following resistance training were due to hypertrophy or neurological function. The 13 boys who were randomly assigned to 20 weeks of training increased their muscular strength above the growth experienced by the maturity-matched controls; these changes were demonstrated no matter how strength was measured (one repetition maximum (1 RM), isokinetic, isometric). Mid-upper-arm and thigh muscle ACSA changes assessed using computerized axial tomography scans did not differ between the experimental and control boys. A rather unique feature of this study was the use of percutaneous electrical stimulation to evoke muscle contraction in the elbow flexors and knee extensors. That is, a brief electrical stimulus was applied to the muscle in order to evoke a contraction. It was possible to assess twitch torque (TT), time to peak torque (TPT), half-relaxation time (HRT), and percent motor unit activation (%MUA) using this technique. It should be recognized that these methods may be rather uncomfortable or even painful for some individuals; hence they are rarely used with young children. When the pre-intervention %MUA values for all boys were pooled, the value for elbow flexors was 89% and for knee extensors 78%. The training resulted in 13.2% and 17.4% increases, respectively, but this was not statistically significant, perhaps signalling a heterogeneous response within the group. The increases in %MUA were less than the improvements measured in isometric strength, implying that this factor may only partially explain this adaptation. The evoked TT of the elbow flexors and knee extensors both increased after training (~30%). However, no changes in TPT or HRT were reported. Evoked TT changes may be indicative of the intrinsic force-producing capacity of muscle, but the single twitch used in this study, as opposed to very painful tetanic stimulation, is unlikely to induce maximal activation of the muscle. Therefore, the authors wrote that:

> We cannot state for certain that the observed increases in twitch torque reflect training induced increases in intrinsic force-producing capacity of the elbow flexor or knee extensor muscles. The functional significance of the observed increases in twitch torque in the present study remains to be determined. (Ramsay et al 1990, p. 612)

It was suggested that the TT improvements probably meant a change in the excitation–contraction coupling. Some of the strength adaptations occurred early and others late in the 20-week study period. The temporal patterns of change were used to indirectly assess relative levels of baseline conditioning in the different muscle groups. It appears as though gains in strength in the legs may lag behind those seen in the arms because of the daily weight-bearing role of the legs. Given that the TT changes were only detected beyond the midpoint of the study, it was suggested that if intrinsic muscle adaptation can be induced by training, then it is only likely to happen after at least 10 weeks of training with a specific, heavy load (refer to the Ramsay study for resistance training programme details, p. 606). Finally, although modifications in motor unit coordination, recruitment and firing frequency were all mentioned as possible factors, none of these were measured directly in this study.

Characteristics of resistance training

Although it is not the intention to review the many combinations and permutations that can arise by manipulating the components of a resistance training programme, this section will highlight some of the main points that have some scientific foundation within the literature. As it is not within the scope of this chapter to identify all of the research studies and groups who have reported their findings in the literature, the following section highlights some of the major results that have been presented by Faigenbaum and his associates over the last 12 years. A search of the literature using any of the computer-based search engines will provide further details of the individual studies by Faigenbaum and his colleagues.

For fear of injuring children and adolescents alike, most practitioners and researchers have avoided using the 1 RM as a tool for assessing muscle strength. If conducted inappropriately, there is no doubt that lifting the heaviest weight that a muscle is capable of could damage not only the muscle, but also other surrounding tissues. A systematic evaluation of maximal strength testing using the 1 RM with children ranging from 6 to 12 years of age has recently provided evidence that it may be a safe practice. However, it is important to note that this research involved supervision of the children by qualified professionals, the children were medically screened for signs of contraindications, and the 1 RM was performed using child-sized resistance training machines for the chest press (not bench press) and leg press/extension.

Several studies have demonstrated that, like most physiological parameters, the benefits of resistance training soon revert to an untrained level in the absence of a training overload stimulus in young people. The time that it takes to lose most of the training-induced gains varies depending on the muscle and the initial magnitude of the increase. For example, muscles that are used on a daily basis in postural or weight-bearing roles may retain the increased strength for longer following the end of a training programme.

By comparing a high load–low repetition (6–8 repetitions at ~80% of 1 RM) with a moderate load–high repetition (13–15 repetitions at ~69% of 1 RM) programme, it was shown that lifting a lighter load more often may result in greater gains in both muscle strength and endurance in 5- to 11-year-old girls and boys who trained twice weekly over 8 weeks. Although the final lift of each set, in both conditions, represented momentary muscular fatigue, it is not clear if this results in comparable total exercise volumes when comparing the heavy–low and moderate–high protocols. Therefore, perhaps this outcome should not be all that surprising given that the total exercise volume appears to be considerably higher in the most efficacious programme (i.e. moderate load–high repetition). Thus, future studies should attempt to equate the exercise volume whilst manipulating the number of repetitions.

Finally, it is clear that meaningful increases in muscle strength are possible in young people when they complete at least two training sessions per week. Although a dose–response relationship between training frequency and strength gains may exist, direct evidence of this does not appear to be available. If resistance exercise training is going to fit in with an assortment of other physical and non-physical activities that young people are engaged in during a typical week, then the rationale for more than two weekly sessions is not compelling. In contrast, the efficacy of a single training session per week is dependent, to a degree, upon the volume of exercise that can be accommodated within the time that is available. Furthermore, the amount of prior resistance exercise experience that an individual has will also influence any increases that might be experienced. Table 10.1 includes the characteristics of a resistance exercise training programme that should result in significant gains in muscle strength with most normal, previously untrained young people. Of course, a variety of other protocols may also be effective, but the details in this table have received the most support in the literature to date.

Table 10.1   Resistance exercise training prescription for young people

Characteristic	Prescription
Frequency	2 times per week
Load	12 to 15 RM per set
Sets	1 to 3 (1 for learning technique)
Type	Child-sized equipment wherever possible

RM, repetition maximum.
Note: The rest period between multiple sets should reflect the goals of the programme.

AEROBIC FITNESS

It is well recognized that adults are able to increase cardiorespiratory (or aerobic) fitness, or maximal oxygen uptake ($\dot{V}O_2max$), given an appropriate exercise stimulus over a period of time. The relative increase in $\dot{V}O_2max$, usually 15–30%, is dependent upon the overall training characteristics (mode, frequency, intensity, duration and programme length) and the initial baseline capacity. The data supporting an improvement in this population are unequivocal. However, the relationship between exercise training and adaptations in aerobic metabolism may not be quite as clear-cut in children who have yet to reach puberty. Several important reviews (see Further reading section) have provided convincing evidence that adolescents experience significant improvements in aerobic power following an exercise training programme that satisfies criteria in adults. Therefore, this section of the chapter will concentrate on studies that have included prepubertal girls and boys given that these results are more controversial.

Golden period?

In what may now be regarded as a classic paper, Katch (1983) proposed a physical conditioning hypothesis called the 'trigger hypothesis'. He stated that during puberty in most children there is a critical period, the trigger point, below which the effects of exercise training will be negligible, or will not occur at all. The mechanism underpinning this theory relates to changes in hormonal status that

> *initiate puberty and influence functional development and subsequent organic adaptations. (Katch 1983, p. 241)*

The specific importance of androgens and growth hormone were highlighted. It is clear that although a variety of different mechanisms have been suggested to explain alterations in aerobic function following exercise training in young people, very few of these are supported with data that have been collected from measurements involving children or adolescents (Rowland 2005). This is not a criticism of the extant literature, but a consequence of the ethical standards that constrain the work to ensure that young people do not experience unnecessary pain or anxiety in the pursuit of advancing scientific knowledge.

A popular hypothesis has emerged that suggests a critical period exists in which young people may be particularly susceptible to increases in aerobic power via endurance training. Alternatively, children who have yet to reach this stage may not be aerobically trainable (Katch 1983). The effects of long-term training (5 years) were studied in three groups of Japanese boys in relation to changes in stature (Kobayashi et al 1978). The seven boys in group 1 were engaged in a variety of school-based activities including endurance running, football and swimming four or five times a week for up to 1.5 hours a day. Their individual growth curves for peak $\dot{V}O_2$ and height were compared with normal controls (group 2, $n = 43$) and six highly trained boys (group 3). Peak $\dot{V}O_2$ increased very little during the years prior to PHV, but a 'striking' increase for six boys in group 1 and many of the boys in group 2 was reported to be closely related to the age at PHV. The increases in peak $\dot{V}O_2$ were attributed to training rather than normal increases as a consequence of ageing and the growth spurt (PHV) for groups 1 and 3 because they outstripped those seen in the controls (group 2). A limitation of this study was that measurements of peak $\dot{V}O_2$ for the controls were started after the age of PHV, precluding a direct comparison with the trained children (group 1) during the prepubertal period. Furthermore, the sample sizes for the trained groups were relatively small. However, supportive evidence was provided by

Mirwald et al (1981) from biennial measurements of 25 boys from 7 through to 17 years of age. Although peak $\dot{V}O_2$ was always higher in the 'active' boys ($n = 14$) compared to those grouped as 'inactive' ($n = 11$) using responses to a questionnaire, the difference reached statistical significance at PHV. The boys who were included in the analyses for this study had to be classified as active or inactive on five of the six assessments including the final measurement at 17 years of age. It is not clear how the 106 boys who were present for the final assessment, but did not meet the criteria for inclusion in the analyses, had altered their physical activity status during the 10 years. The authors suggested that genetics may underpin a synergistic relationship between physical activity and a high peak $\dot{V}O_2$. In addition, within-group heterogeneity and changes in testosterone during adolescence were factors that were explored as underlying mechanisms.

In contrast, two separate investigations involving sets of identical male twins failed to demonstrate acceleration in the development of aerobic power during the pubertal years (Danis et al 2003, Weber et al 1976). In both studies one of the twins completed an aerobic exercise programme whilst the twin brother acted as the non-trained control. In the earlier study the boys trained for 10 weeks, whereas the latter programme lasted 6 months. Peak $\dot{V}O_2$ increased significantly as a result of training in the prepubertal boys, but was unchanged relative to the matched controls in the pubertal boys. These authors suggested that the training stimulus may not have been strong enough to override the maturity-induced acceleration in the development of cardiorespiratory capacity. Interestingly, the findings from these two studies are at odds with a commonly held supposition that it is more mature young people who are more inclined to improve following training and not those who have yet to reach puberty (Katch 1983). It would appear that more research is needed to determine whether a 'golden' trainability period exists, where the interaction between an external stimulus is amplified by endogenous physiological changes that occur during the natural process of growth, maturation and development.

Blunted response

It is clear that children are unlikely to experience changes in cardiorespiratory function on the same scale as adolescents or adults following exercise training. Most studies report changes in peak $\dot{V}O_2$ that are less than 10% (~6% on average) and those that report changes greater than 15% are exceptional. In some early studies, the omission of matched controls or a control period in repeated measures designs precluded valid conclusions beyond those that may be assigned to growth and maturation. Due to inherent difficulties in getting children to comply with structured exercise training programmes, sample sizes often fell short of what would be required to make a definitive statement. In the absence of an appropriate exercise overload stimulus, large changes in peak $\dot{V}O_2$ should not be expected regardless of who completes the training. Many studies have failed to monitor the training volume adequately and/or they have not been able to account for the impact of other extraneous variables. Therefore, when attempting to identify a consensus within this literature, it is important that careful attention is paid to the specific details of individual studies. Nevertheless, although numerous methodological flaws blighted many of the early studies, more recent studies have avoided these deficiencies, yet they continue to find smaller changes in children compared with adults.

Baseline influence

The pre-training (baseline) level of fitness (peak $\dot{V}O_2$) has been identified as a potential determinant for the amount of change that children are likely to experience following a training programme. Those with a relatively high baseline are more inclined to demonstrate a blunted response to the exercise stimulus because, it has been argued, they are already close to their upper limit (ceiling effect). Many of the well-designed studies provide some support for this, probably because research projects that are advertised in the community or are run in schools on a voluntary basis attract participants who may already possess some of the positive attributes that the research team are seeking to improve. A limitation to this theory is that young endurance trained athletes who have often been training and competing for many years, rather than just 3–12 months, have peak $\dot{V}O_2$ values that are far in excess of those reported by most healthy untrained, yet active children. In contrast, children who are unfit to begin with should have the most to gain from an exercise training programme. The 14 girls who completed 12 weeks of stationary cycling for 30 minutes, three times a week for 12 weeks in the study of Tolfrey et al (1998) experienced a 7.9% increase in peak $\dot{V}O_2$ compared with a 3.8% reduction in the maturity-matched control group of girls. However, the combined effect of these diametrically opposite changes resulted in post-training peak $\dot{V}O_2$ values that were very similar between the two groups of girls (Fig. 10.1). Spearman rank order correlations between the baseline and per cent change values in this study support the contention that the efficacy of endurance exercise training is partially attributable to what the participants start with.

Initial levels of habitual physical activity (HPA) may be more important than peak $\dot{V}O_2$ when assessing the influence of exercise intervention on cardiorespiratory fitness. Although the mean change in peak $\dot{V}O_2$ in 37 children was not different between individuals who participated in sports teams and those who did not, a significant but weak negative relationship with baseline HPA has been reported (Rowland & Boyajian 1995). After controlling for changes in HPA over the duration of the

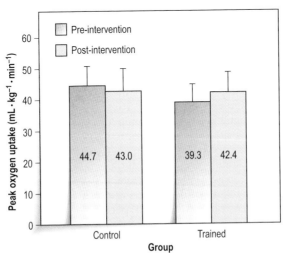

Figure 10.1   Changes in peak oxygen uptake for girls following 12 weeks of aerobic exercise training against a maturity-matched control.

intervention period, Tolfrey et al (1998) found that peak $\dot{V}O_2$ did not increase in young girls and boys. Whether it is possible to measure HPA with sufficient precision to identify its effect on peak $\dot{V}O_2$ within just 12 weeks is questionable. However, future intervention studies that are designed using a longer-term lifestyle model should certainly include some means of controlling for this potential covariate.

Effects of exercise intensity

An intriguing hypothesis is that the exercise intensity shown to be effective for adults may not be intense enough for improvements in young children. Moreover, it is increasingly recognized in studies with adults that if the aim is to increase peak $\dot{V}O_2$ specifically, then athletes have to train at intensities that will induce the highest level of oxygen consumption in a relatively short period of time (i.e. 'severe' or supramaximal intensity). Interestingly, several early studies that failed to report an increase in peak $\dot{V}O_2$ with exercise training consisted of short-duration interval runs or sprints consistent with how most young children play. The weakness in these studies lay not in the chosen intensity, but in the total exercise volume. Although the children trained hard, they may not have completed enough sprints or failed to maintain the intensity for long enough. Moreover, many of these early studies did not last for more than a few weeks.

In what appears to be the only study that has systematically manipulated exercise intensity in a bid to identify if a training threshold exists, Massicotte & MacNab (1974) trained three separate groups of nine boys (11–13 years) for 6 weeks with the heart rate (HR) at 170–180, 150–160 and 130–140 bts · min⁻¹ and compared them to a matched control group who did not train. The strength of this study is that the boys were matched for baseline peak $\dot{V}O_2$ and then randomly assigned to the four experimental groups. Furthermore, the exercise intensity was closely monitored in each boy at the start of each week to ensure that the exercise was effective in raising the HR to the desired intensity. The results showed that only the boys who exercised above 170 bts · min⁻¹ (at least 88% maximum HR (HRmax)) demonstrated an increase in peak $\dot{V}O_2$ (11%). Although the boys in the middle intensity group were exercising, on average, between ~76% and 81% of peak HR, their peak $\dot{V}O_2$ increased by only 1%. On the surface, this well-controlled and carefully monitored study appears to provide strong support for the theory that children need to exercise at higher intensities than most that are reported in the literature. However, a major weakness in the study design is that the three training groups were not matched for total exercise volume. That is, they all exercised for 12 minutes, three times a week over the 6-week training period. In order to equate the volume, the investigators should have manipulated both the exercise duration and intensity.

It has been shown that it is possible for prepubertal children to increase their peak $\dot{V}O_2$ following high intensity sprint running programmes (Baquet et al 2002, Rotstein et al 1986). In the earlier study, 16 boys aged 10 years completed an interval style training programme spanning 9 weeks. Each training session (3 per week) consisted of a series of 600 m, 400 m and 150 m runs (total distance per session ranged from 4.7 to 6.5 km) at an intensity that was described as suitable for each participant's physical conditioning. The intensity was adjusted periodically to achieve a progressive overload. Peak $\dot{V}O_2$ increased from 54.2 to 58.6 mL · kg⁻¹ · min⁻¹ (8.1%) in the trained boys compared with only 2.1% (57.1–58.3 mL · kg⁻¹ · min⁻¹) in the 12 age- and activity-matched controls.

The 33 prepubertal girls and boys in the Baquet study completed a 7-week high intensity intermittent training programme with the explicit intention of improving peak $\dot{V}O_2$. The training programme consisted of a series of sprints lasting between 10 and 20 s that were run at 110–130% of the maximal aerobic speed. Each child trained twice a week, in addition to attending their regular physical education classes, and the total exercise time per session was 30 minutes. The training resulted in an 8.2% increase in peak $\dot{V}O_2$ compared with a 1.9% reduction in the 20 maturity-matched control participants. These studies show that it is possible for prepubertal children to experience a significant change in peak $\dot{V}O_2$ even when the overload stimulus does not conform to the traditional submaximal, continuous exercise format. The authors suggested that this type of exercise might better reflect the type of exercise that younger people are more inclined to choose for themselves. Moreover, it does seem to fit with the training theory that has tended to dictate the programmes that endurance-based adult athletes use. It would be interesting to see if the children would maintain their enthusiasm for such high intensity exercise over a longer period than the 7 weeks used in this study and also to study the impact of manipulating the duration of each sprint to increase exercise volume.

Effects of sex

The majority of studies reported to date have recruited boys as participants. On numerous occasions mixed sex groups have trained together, but the data have been pooled for the analyses, possibly to increase the sample size to maximize the statistical power of the study. On the basis of a 6.3% and 7.4% increase in peak $\dot{V}O_2$ for girls and boys, respectively, following a 12-week, school-based training programme, Rowland & Boyajian (1995) concluded that training was not sex-specific. The results of this study may have been confounded by the inclusion of eight (six girls and two boys) circumpubertal participants because larger increases in peak $\dot{V}O_2$ for pubertal children are well documented.

The 27.4% increase for seven cross-country runners over a 12-week training period observed by Brown et al (1972) may have been biased by differences in maturational status between the runners and by relatively low baseline values for several of the girls. In addition, it was not possible to partition the effects of training from normal patterns of growth as changes in peak $\dot{V}O_2$ were not measured in the control group. The application of these results to other children may be problematic as the peak $\dot{V}O_2$ values were comparable to champion Swedish female middle-distance runners. The girls in Tolfrey et al's (1998) study appeared to benefit more from the training than the boys, but once between sex differences in HPA and body fat were included as covariates in the analyses, no sex effect was apparent. The authors also concluded that baseline differences in peak $\dot{V}O_2$ between the girls and boys meant that the comparison was not like-for-like.

In a similar vein, Baquet and colleagues (2002) reported that the 9.5% increase in peak $\dot{V}O_2$ for 13 boys was not different to the 7.2% improvement experienced by 20 girls who also completed the high intensity intermittent training described earlier. There are no data at present that suggest girls and boys will respond to an endurance exercise training programme in a different manner. However, it should be noted that very few studies have sought to examine this research question systematically.

ANAEROBIC PERFORMANCE

Few studies have examined the influence of exercise training on anaerobic energy pathways, or activities that rely on them, with young people. This might be because this parameter does not share the strong causative relationship with health that has been shown for aerobic fitness (e.g. peak $\dot{V}O_2$). However, anaerobic capacity or power impacts on performance in numerous sports and is, therefore, of great interest to coaches, athletes and physical educators (see Chapter 5). In a recent review Rowland (2005) indicated that anaerobic trainability in young people is not easy to define because of the complex interplay between metabolism, power production and athletic performance. He concluded by stating that:

> Clearly, over-simplistic considerations of anaerobic trainability are to be avoided. (Rowland 2005, p. 205)

Short-term power output

A 3.4% increase in mean power (MP), determined in a 30 s Wingate test, was found in 17 primary school children who completed 18 maximal effort sprint cycling training sessions in 6 weeks (Grodjinovsky et al 1980). The 19 boys who were randomly assigned to the sprint running programme of equal exercise volume in the same study increased MP by 3.7% compared with 14 non-trained controls who experienced a 4.9% reduction over the intervention period. Similar changes in peak power (PP) were reported for the three groups of boys, but only the 3.9% increase for those who completed the cycle training reached statistical significance.

Increases of a similar magnitude were published by Sargeant et al (1985), who measured maximal power (Pmax) using an isokinetic cycle ergometer in 15 peripubertal boys who had 8 weeks of supplementary physical education (PE) (150 min per week); the comparison was with 11 boys who only experienced the normal 150 min of PE per week over the same period. When changes in total body mass were taken into consideration, Pmax $(W \cdot kg^{-1})$ increased by 4.5% on average in the trained boys whereas the change in the controls was only 1.2%. Using basic anthropometry, it was estimated that changes in the controls' lean body mass (LBM, 2.5%), total leg (plus bone) volume (LV, 2.5%) and upper leg (plus bone) volume (ULV, 3.0%) were directly proportional to the overall increase in body size due to normal growth. In contrast, the trained boys demonstrated much larger changes over the 8-week intervention period (LBM 4.8%, LV 8.0% and ULV 9.7%) than could be attributed to the combined effect of growth and the additional PE class time. Therefore, a possible mechanism for the improved ability to generate power shown in this study was an increase in active muscle mass (hypertrophy). Although physical maturation was not measured, the average age of the boys (~13.7 years) suggests that they had already experienced the increase in circulating testosterone that is a feature of puberty in boys. Larger increases in both PP (14.2%) and MP (10.0%) were presented by Rotstein et al (1986) with the 16 boys described in the previous section appraising aerobic adaptations to exercise training.

It has been shown that high intensity exercise training can stimulate changes in peak $\dot{V}O_2$ (e.g. Baquet et al 2002, Rotstein et al 1986). In a similar vein, a study by Obert et al (2001) that used predominantly aerobic interval running resulted in 18% gains in Pmax from a force–velocity test, even after changes in lower limb muscle mass had been accounted for using dual energy X-ray absorptiometry (DEXA) in the 17 prepubertal girls and boys. As no changes were noted in the optimal velocity (Vopt) over the 13-week training programme, the authors concluded that increases in optimal force

(Fopt) generation must have been responsible for the improvement in Pmax. No changes in Pmax, Vopt or Fopt were seen in the 16 maturity-matched control girls and boys.

Although all of the aforementioned studies reported increases in a variety of short-term power output parameters, considerable inter-study variation in the magnitude of this effect was also evident. This is likely to be a combined function of differences in the training programmes, participant characteristics and the methods used to assess short-term power output (i.e. force–velocity test, Wingate anaerobic test, isokinetic cycle ergometry, and sprints on a non-motorized treadmill, see Chapter 5).

Anaerobic metabolism

Due to the invasive nature of measuring metabolic responses directly (i.e. enzyme activity and muscle fibre histology), data related to exercise training in young people are very rare. In a frequently cited study, eight 11- to 13-year-old boys trained 34 times over a 4-month period. The boys completed 5–10 min of callisthenics, 15–25 min of interval running, and played basketball and football in each of the 60 min training sessions (Eriksson et al 1973). In addition, they all attended a 7-day training camp where they skied twice a day. Small samples of muscle were taken from each boy, using the needle biopsy technique, for the quantification of adenosine triphosphate (ATP), phosphocreatine (PCr), muscle glycogen and glucose 6-phosphate (G6P). Although biopsies were taken before and after the training period at rest and following submaximal and maximal exertion exercise, most of the significant training induced adaptations occurred in the resting condition. For example, ATP increased from 4.3 to 4.8 mmol $\cdot$ kg^{-1} (wet weight of muscle, ~12%) and PCr from 14.5 to 20.2 mmol $\cdot$ kg^{-1} (~39%), but depletion patterns for both of these phosphates were not altered by exercise training. The average muscle glycogen concentration at rest increased by ~32% (53.9–71.0 mmol $\cdot$ kg^{-1}), whereas G6P doubled following training (0.2–0.4 mmol $\cdot$ kg^{-1}). As a consequence of these changes, both muscle and blood lactate concentrations were higher after maximal exertion exercise when comparing the post-training values with those in the untrained state (8.8–13.7 mmol $\cdot$ kg^{-1}, ~56% and 4.7–5.9 mmol $\cdot$ L^{-1}, ~26%, respectively). Within the same publication, Eriksson and colleagues (1973) also reported the findings from a study involving five different 11-year-old boys who had completed a 6-week training programme. The programme consisted of cycling for at least 20 minutes, three times a week at an intensity of approximately 90%+ HRmax. Muscle biopsies were taken at rest before, after 2 weeks, and following the training period to assess changes in phosphofructokinase (PFK) and succinate dehydrogenase (SDH) activity. The activities of PFK increased from 8.4 to 12.5 to 15.4 µmol $\cdot$ g^{-1} $\cdot$ min^{-1} (~83% over the 6 weeks) and SDH from 5.4 to 5.8 to 7.0 µmol $\cdot$ g^{-1} $\cdot$ min^{-1} (~30% over the 6 weeks). The small initial increase in SDH was explained partly by a rubella infection in one of the boys which affected his peak $\dot{V}O_2$ over the first 2 weeks of the study. By combining the results from these two separate studies, the authors surmised that the training had increased the glycolytic potential and capacity of skeletal muscle in the young boys. It was also argued that the increased glycolytic and oxidative capacity of skeletal muscle induced by the training combined to produce a greater muscle lactate production. The conclusion from these results was that marked local adaptations take place in skeletal muscle of boys following training and that these changes are similar to those observed in adults, although some differences in the training response also seem to exist. The researchers who conducted this work conceded that the results were based upon a very small sample of boys. A further critical weakness is that comparisons were made between two separate studies rather than within the same group of boys and, in the absence of a non-training matched control group, it was not possible to account for any changes that might have occurred as a result of just normal growth and development.

In another study where muscle biopsies were taken either side of a training programme, six healthy adolescent boys, aged 16–17 years performed interval runs varying from 50 to 250 m and some occasional stair running four times a week for 3 months (Fournier et al 1982). Muscle fibre size and distribution (per cent of type I and type II fibres) were not affected by the training, but PFK activity increased from 28.1 to 33.9 $\mu mol \cdot g^{-1} \cdot min^{-1}$ (~21%). Interestingly, peak $\dot{V}O_2$ ($mL \cdot kg^{-1} \cdot min^{-1}$) increased by ~6% despite the high intensity mode of exercise (sprinting), again suggesting that both continuous moderate to heavy intensity and severe (supramaximal) intensity are effective forms of exercise training when considering this marker of cardiorespiratory fitness in young people. The sample size problems highlighted in the Eriksson study are also pertinent here. It is also important to recognize that although the authors indicated that the changes in PFK and peak $\dot{V}O_2$ were not due to growth, because the changes in stature and body mass did not change to any great extent, this study did not include a matched control group. Of course, studies with participants who are no longer growing and who are 16–17 years of age may not be as revealing as those that include much younger participants who are still experiencing substantial changes in growth, maturation and development. However, the invasive nature of these latter studies would normally preclude younger people.

SUMMARY

Muscle strength

Appropriately supervised and progressively designed resistance exercise training programmes can be safe and effective in increasing strength in both prepubertal children and adolescents. The majority of evidence suggests that prior to puberty, increases in muscle strength are neurological in origin because muscle fibres do not appear to hypertrophy. Whether this is partially a function of imprecise measurement techniques has yet to be explored fully. Recent evidence has shown that the 'gold standard' for strength testing, the 1 RM, may be applicable to young people, but this should only be used by experienced and well-qualified practitioners. By manipulating some of the primary components of a resistance exercise programme it has also been possible to provide some support for a low resistance, high repetition approach to training in the young, especially when they have little or no experience of this type of exercise. Finally, as with most forms of exercise training, it would be prudent to mix resistance exercise with other modes of physical activity to maintain motivation, fun, and interest – critical factors when considering a lifespan approach to exercise and health. Therefore, the twice weekly recommendation is most welcome and fits well with a number of physical activity models in the literature that are geared towards young people.

Aerobic fitness

Although it is generally acknowledged that adolescents will demonstrate significant increases in peak $\dot{V}O_2$ following exercise training, the number of well-controlled studies with this segment of the population is still quite small. Moreover, it is not clear whether a 'golden response' period exists prior to adulthood where improvements in cardiorespiratory parameters might be optimized through exercise training. Although many more investigations have included prepubertal boys than girls, the results from some of the early studies and those that were not well controlled or designed have clouded the picture somewhat. However, it would appear that if the exercise volume is sufficient, young children will experience a significant improvement in aerobic fitness. An intriguing question that requires further exploration is how pre-adolescents will respond to severe (i.e. above peak $\dot{V}O_2$) intensity exercise over a prolonged period (i.e. more than 12 weeks). Of course, overtraining and an increased susceptibility to injury would need to be given very careful consideration if severe exercise intensities were used. Current evidence is not yet strong enough to confidently discount a differential sex response to aerobic exercise training. I have focused on peak $\dot{V}O_2$, primarily because this parameter is most commonly measured when considering aerobic fitness and because of its well-documented links with adult morbidity and mortality. However, numerous studies have also included other markers of fitness (and sports performance) at submaximal and maximal exercise intensities including fixed blood lactate concentrations, lactate inflection points, ventilatory threshold, exercise economy and the running speed corresponding to maximal oxygen uptake ($\dot{V}O_2$max), all of which are increasingly prominent in the literature pertaining to adult endurance athletes and performance.

Anaerobic metabolism

Due to the paucity of information available and some necessary ethical limitations, it is very difficult to state unequivocally that anaerobic adaptations will occur in young people following exercise training. Guidelines to characterize training programmes in this area do not appear to have been published, certainly not any that are based on a strong empirical foundation. There is not enough information to determine whether differences in maturity, age or sex of young people will influence anaerobic trainability. Therefore, there is considerable scope for further research in this exciting field of paediatric exercise physiology.

KEY POINTS

1. Exercise training goals will determine the programme characteristics (e.g. intensity, duration, frequency).
2. The interplay between exercise intensity, duration, frequency and programme length dictate total exercise volume.
3. Studies that have adopted a longitudinal research design are the only ones that are able to examine whether a cause and effect relationship exists between exercise training and physiological adaptation. Few well-designed, random, controlled trials with young people that focus on exercise training are available.
4. Resistance training can be a safe and effective mode of exercise when programmes are well designed, are supervised by knowledgeable staff, and consider carefully the physical attributes that make young people so unique.
5. Both prepubertal children and adolescents demonstrate large gains in muscle strength following a resistance training programme that adheres to the standard principles of exercise training (e.g. overload, progression, specificity).

6. Studies that have demonstrated improvements in muscle strength in young people have found that muscle hypertrophy does not appear to occur prior to puberty, but an increase in muscle size is more likely during adolescence. In the absence of muscle hypertrophy, it has been suggested that neuromuscular adaptations underpin increases in strength in young children; direct evidence supporting this, however, is sparse.

7. Data supporting a 'golden trainability period' for peak $\dot{V}O_2$ are equivocal. It is possible that this reflects weaknesses in study design.

8. Regardless of the training programme characteristics, it is clear that children and adolescents demonstrate a marked reduction in the trainability of peak $\dot{V}O_2$ compared with adults. This is more pronounced in younger and less mature children.

9. The blunted aerobic training response seen in children is probably related to several factors, but exercise volume and the anabolic milieu are primary considerations.

10. There is insufficient empirical evidence to show how anaerobic adaptations following exercise training might be affected by age, biological maturity, participant sex, or manipulation of the exercise volume.

11. Data from studies that have used the highly invasive muscle biopsy technique have provided unique findings. However, the research design limitations of these studies must be considered before extrapolating the findings to young people in general.

12. Without question, there is considerable scope for further research into exercise training and its impact on physiological systems in young people. We know very little about girls who train, long-term exercise programmes (i.e. greater than 12 months), and the use of exercise to ameliorate certain health problems (e.g. obesity).

References

Baquet G, Berthoin S, Dupont G et al 2002 Effects of high intensity intermittent training on peak $\dot{V}O_2$ in prepubertal children. International Journal of Sports Medicine 23:439–444

Brown C H, Harrower J R, Deeter M F 1972 The effects of cross-country running on pre-adolescent girls. Medicine and Science in Sports 4:1–5

Danis A, Kyriazis Y, Klissouras V 2003 The effect of training in male prepubertal and pubertal monozygotic twins. European Journal of Applied Physiology 89:309–318

Eriksson B O, Gollnick P D, Saltin B 1973 Muscle metabolism and enzyme activities after training in boys 11–13 years old. Acta Physiologica Scandinavica 87:485–497

Faigenbaum A D, Zaichkowsky L D, Westcott W L et al 1993 The effects of a twice-a-week strength training program on children. Pediatric Exercise Science 5:339–346

Falk B, Tenenbaum G 1996 The effectiveness of resistance training in children: a meta-analysis. Sports Medicine 22:176–186

Fournier M, Ricci J, Taylor A W et al 1982 Skeletal muscle adaptation in adolescent boys: sprint and endurance training and detraining. Medicine and Science in Sports and Exercise 14:453–456

Fukunaga T, Funato K, Ikegawa S 1992 The effects of resistance training on muscle area and strength in prepubertal age. Annals of Physiology and Anthropology 11:357–364

Grodjinovsky A, Inbar O, Dotan R et al 1980 Training effect on the anaerobic performance of children as measured by the Wingate anaerobic test. In: Berg K, Eriksson B O (eds) Children and exercise IX. University Park Press, Baltimore, p 139–145

Katch V L 1983 Physical conditioning of children. Journal of Adolescent Health Care 3:241–246

Kobayashi K, Kitamura K, Miura M et al 1978 Aerobic power as related to body growth and training in Japanese boys: a longitudinal study. Journal of Applied Physiology 44:666–672

Komi P V, Viitasalao J T, Rauamaa R et al 1978 Effect of isometric strength training on mechanical, electrical and metabolic aspects of muscle function. European Journal of Applied Physiology and Occupational Physiology 40:45–55

Massicotte D R, MacNab R B J 1974 Cardiorespiratory adaptations to training at specified intensities in children. Medicine and Science in Sports 6:242–246

Mersch F, Stoboy H 1989 Strength training and muscle hypertrophy in children. In: Oseid S, Carlsen K H (eds) Children and exercise XIII. Human Kinetics, Champaign, IL, p 165–182

Mirwald R L, Bailey D A, Cameron N et al 1981 Longitudinal comparison of aerobic power in active and inactive boys aged 7.0 to 17.0 years. Annals of Human Biology 8:405–414

Obert P, Mandigout M, Vinet A et al 2001 Effect of a 13-week aerobic training programme on the maximal power developed during a force-velocity test in prepubertal boys and girls. International Journal of Sports Medicine 22:442–446

Ozmun J C, Mikesky A E, Surburg P R 1994 Neuromuscular adaptations following prepubescent strength training. Medicine and Science in Sports and Exercise 26:510–514

Payne V G, Morrow J R, Johnson L et al 1997 Resistance training in children and youth: a meta-analysis. Research Quarterly in Exercise and Sport 68:80–88

Ramsay J A, Blimkie C J, Smith K et al 1990 Strength training effects in prepubescent boys. Medicine and Science in Sports and Exercise 22:605–614

Rians C B, Weltman A, Cahill B R et al 1987 Strength training for prepubescent males: is it safe? American Journal of Sports Medicine 15:483–489

Rotstein A, Dotan R, Bar-Or O et al 1986 Effect of training on anaerobic threshold, maximal aerobic power and anaerobic performance of preadolescent boys. International Journal of Sports Medicine 7:281–286

Rowland T W 2005 Children's exercise physiology, 2nd edn. Human Kinetics, Champaign, IL, p 197–219

Rowland T W, A Boyajian 1995 Aerobic response to endurance exercise training in children. Pediatrics 96:654–658

Sargeant A J, Dolan P, Thorne A 1985 Effects of supplementary physical activity on body composition, aerobic, and anaerobic power in 13-year-old boys. In: Binkhorst R A, Kemper H C G, Saris W H (eds) Children and exercise XI. Human Kinetics, Champaign, IL, p 135–139

Tolfrey K, Campbell I G, Batterham A M 1998 Aerobic trainability of prepubertal boys and girls. Pediatric Exercise Science 10:248–263

Vrijens J 1978 Muscle strength development in pre- and post-pubertal age. Medicine and Sport 11:152–158

Weber G, Kartodihardjo W, Klissouras V 1976 Growth and physical training with reference to heredity. Journal of Applied Physiology 40:211–215

Further reading

Bar-Or O, Rowland T W 2004 Pediatric exercise medicine. Human Kinetics, Champaign, IL, p 46–60

Faigenbaum A, Westcott W 2000 Strength and power for young athletes. Human Kinetics, Champaign, IL

Mahon A D 2000 Exercise training. In: Armstrong N, van Mechelen W (eds) Paediatric exercise science and medicine. Oxford University Press, Oxford, p 201–222

Van Praagh E (ed) 1998 Pediatric anaerobic performance. Human Kinetics, Champaign, IL, p 191–268

Chapter 11

Exercise and environmental conditions

Craig A. Williams

CHAPTER CONTENTS

LEARNING OBJECTIVES

After studying this chapter you should be able to:
1. describe the key thermoregulatory factors in relation to physical and physiological changes in children
2. discuss the effects of growth, maturation and sex on the key thermoregulatory factors
3. describe children's physiological responses to hot and cold environmental temperatures
4. explain the effects of acclimatization and acclimation for children
5. detail the key factors related to fluid and electrolyte balance in children

INTRODUCTION

As a homeothermal mammal, humans have evolved to maintain a constant body temperature between a range of 36–38°C, unlike mammals such as reptiles, which are poikilothermal. Although the body maintains this constancy of temperature, it is subject to frequent fluctuations outside this range. These fluctuations can occur due to a number of factors: diurnal rhythms (resulting in a higher temperature in the evening and lower temperature in the early hours of the morning), ovulation in women (higher temperatures in the second half of the menstrual cycle), exercise, hot baths, illness (e.g. fevers), drugs and food in the stomach. Therefore, although this constancy of temperature (36–38°C) is based on average values, it is important to appreciate the range of temperature which humans and in particular children can tolerate.

CONCEPT OF HEAT BALANCE

Thermal balance follows the law of the conservation of energy, which states that if a system is in balance then the products of heat gain or loss must be equal to zero. If the heat production increases to such an extent that it is greater than the ability of the body to transfer and lose heat, then the heat balance will be positive and therefore body temperature will rise. The concept of thermal balance also known as body temperature balance, as shown in Figure 11.1, can be represented as an equation such that:

$$M \pm R \pm K \pm C - E \pm W \pm S = 0 \text{ or } \textit{thermal balance} \tag{11.1}$$

where M = metabolism, C = convection, E = evaporation, W = work, S = heat storage, R = radiation, K = conduction.

Metabolism

Metabolism is a product of both anaerobic and aerobic processes and can be estimated by measuring oxygen uptake ($\dot{V}O_2$) and converting the resulting $\dot{V}O_2$ into its

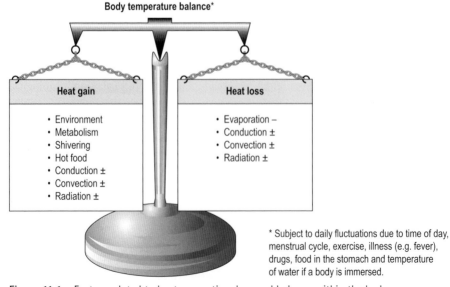

Body temperature balance*

Heat gain	Heat loss
• Environment	• Evaporation –
• Metabolism	• Conduction ±
• Shivering	• Convection ±
• Hot food	• Radiation ±
• Conduction ±	
• Convection ±	
• Radiation ±	

* Subject to daily fluctuations due to time of day, menstrual cycle, exercise, illness (e.g. fever), drugs, food in the stomach and temperature of water if a body is immersed.

Figure 11.1   Factors related to heat generation, loss and balance within the body.

kilocalorie (or joule) equivalent. In the above equation metabolism is not strictly a source of heat exchange but because it is the only way the body can internally produce heat, it is an important variable in the thermal balance equation. For example, a 12-year-old child who has a resting $\dot{V}O_2$ of 0.3 L · min^{-1} at a respiratory quotient (RQ) of 0.84 would produce 1.5 kcal · min^{-1} (0.3 L · min^{-1} × 4.85 kcal · min^{-1}). How these values are then related to different body sizes so comparisons with adults can be made will be discussed later.

Conduction

Conduction is the process of heat balance when two surfaces are in direct contact with one another. The greater the difference in temperatures or thermal gradient between the two surfaces the greater the heat transfer from one surface to the other. The equation for conduction is a function of several components

$$K = (k/d) \, (T_1 - T_2) \, A_k \tag{11.2}$$

where K = conduction, k = coefficient of thermal conductivity, d = thickness of substance, $T_1 - T_2$ = temperature gradient, A_k = area of contact.

The exchange of heat between two surfaces is directly related to the thermal conductivity coefficient; therefore metals, which have a higher coefficient, are excellent conductors, but wood with a lower coefficient is not. This principle can be equally applied to still air and water. At the same temperature, water will provide a greater level of thermal stress to a human body (this example excludes any influence of clothing) than still air. For the inclusion of clothing there is an inverse relationship with conduction and the thickness of an insulating product. When the skin is in contact with a hotter surface, conduction will occur; usually this is not a problem as human behaviour usually dictates that contact with very conductive materials is limited by removing contact between the two. Overall conductive heat loss forms only a small percentage of the heat balance equation because it is subjected to behavioural actions. When children come in contact with cold surfaces, for example a cold bench or floor, they will attempt either to remove themselves from that environment or to generate some heat by becoming more active.

Evaporation

Evaporation is preceded by a minus symbol because it always results in heat loss and therefore is a cooling mechanism. Evaporation is the most important heat loss mechanism when exercising in the heat. It is important to remember that it is the mechanism of sweat evaporating that results in heat loss not in the actual production of the sweat. For evaporation to occur, heat must be supplied to convert water into a gas. This process is known as the latent heat of vaporization and equals 0.58 kcal · mL^{-1} of sweat. Because human sweat contains electrolytes the latent heat value is slightly lower. Other factors that will affect evaporation are the respiratory rate, relative humidity and the intensity of exercise. Heat sweat losses from the skin can be estimated from:

$$E = 40 \, h_D \, (P_{ws} - \phi P_{wa}) / R_w \, T \tag{11.3}$$

where E = heat loss from sweat, h_D = transfer coefficient $(L \cdot min^{-1})$, ϕ = fractional relative humidity, P_{ws} = water pressure vapour at skin temperature (mmHg), P_{wa} = water pressure vapour at ambient temperature, R_w = aqueous gas constant, T = average skin and ambient temperature (K).

The above equation ignores the evaporation losses by respiration and although these are much smaller than losses through sweat, in certain environmental conditions they can be important, for example at altitude or in extremely cold environments. It is possible to estimate evaporative losses by measuring body mass before and after exercise. Corrections for fluid intake and respiratory water loss and the monitoring of urine loss are also needed. In a study by Falk et al (1992c), the mean (standard deviation) sweat rate of prepubertal, midpubertal and late pubertal boys was estimated as 9.78 (0.54), 10.02 (0.51) and 10.75 (0.9) $mL \cdot kg^{-1} \cdot min^{-1}$ during three 20 min cycling bouts at an intensity requiring 50% of their predetermined $\dot{V}O_2max$ in a climatic chamber heat of 41–43°C and 18–22% relative humidity (RH).

Convection

Convection is a movement orientated process, such that a convective current occurs between two surfaces. Convection can be determined as:

$$C = k_c (T_1 - T_2) A_c \qquad (11.4)$$

where C = convection, K_c = surface coefficient of convection heat exchange, A_c = area of convection heat exchange.

Convection is a direct function of the temperature gradient between the two surfaces, the surface area and the surface coefficient. An example of convection occurs when running on a cool day when the heat from the body conducts this heat to the cooler air layers surrounding the skin's body surface. The air surrounding the skin then becomes less dense and rises, only to be replaced by colder air. Factors such as the speed at which the child or adult is travelling (e.g. during cycling) or the velocity of the wind will have a large influence on the convective currents. The effects of the velocity of the wind and the ambient temperature have been integrated into a formula known as the wind-chill index. This index is useful as it establishes a heat loss value that enables people who work or exercise in outdoor conditions, such as mountaineers, to take measures to safeguard against the cooling effect on the body. The index is determined as:

$$K_o = (100 V + 10.5 - V)^{0.5} \times (33 - T) \qquad (11.5)$$

where K_o = heat loss in $kcal \cdot h^{-1}$, V = velocity in $m \cdot s^{-1}$, T = environmental temperature in °C, 10.5 = a constant, 33 = normal skin temperature in °C.

Radiation

Radiation is a process of losing or gaining heat by electromagnetic energy waves and the sun is a prime example of this radiation process. Radiation is expressed as:

$$R = \sigma (T_s^4 - T_R^4) A_r \qquad (11.6)$$

Where R = radiation, σ = Stefan–Boltzmann constant = $5.67 \times 10^{-8} \times m^{-2} \times K^{-1}$, T_s = average surface temperature, T_R = average radiant temperature, A_r = effective radiant surface area.

Radiation is dependent not only on the temperature of an object but also on the colour and surface. Therefore to measure radiant temperature, a globe thermometer is used. This is a 15.2 cm diameter globe or sphere painted black with a thermometer suspended inside. This black globe then absorbs all the radiation that falls upon it. Because the human body absorbs most of the radiation that falls on it, the body is often compared to a black globe or a 'black box'. Hence black clothing absorbs more heat than lighter coloured clothing, which reflects more and thereby absorbs less heat. The surface of an object also influences radiation, as a rougher surface will absorb less heat than a smoother one. If the sports of tennis and cricket are considered, clothing tends to be white, and made of synthetic material that is rough to the touch rather than smooth, and loose fitting rather than tight to the body. All these features will help keep an athlete cooler than wearing tight-fitting, dark-coloured and cotton-type clothing.

Work

Work can by definition be both positive and negative because of operating against both internal and external forces. During restful conditions there is production of heat through metabolism but work is considered to be zero. As discussed in previous chapters on energy metabolism, children have the potential for a 10-fold increase in oxygen consumption and therefore a large range for the production of work and transfer of heat.

Heat storage

The final concept to consider is heat storage. If equation 11.1 is rearranged, the heat storage of a human body can be expressed as:

$$S = M - E \pm R \pm K \pm C - W \tag{11.7}$$

Heat storage is calculated by measuring the change in the mean body temperature (comprising both the core and skin temperature) and utilizing a constant value for the body's specific heat capacity. The heat capacity value of the body is assumed to be $3.47 \text{ kJ} \cdot \text{kg}^{-1} \cdot {}^{\circ}\text{C}^{-1}$.

Therefore, all the above factors need to be considered when investigating issues of environmental conditions and exercise in children whether this is indoors or out-doors. It is important not to become too fixated on the ambient temperature alone as humidity, air movement (wind or lack of) and the effect of solar radiation, particularly from surfaces such as snow or artificial pitches, are just as crucial. The acknowledgement of the importance of these other factors, aside from the ambient temperature, has been recognized by environmental physiologists who devised the wet bulb globe thermometer (WBGT). The WBGT was originally designed for use in the military and consists not of one thermometer but three, a dry bulb, a wet bulb and a black bulb measuring air temperature, humidity and radiation, respectively. The equation for WBGT is:

$$\text{WBGT} = 0.7_{wb} + 0.2_g + 0.1_{db} \tag{11.8}$$

The above equation weights more highly the wet bulb or humidity (70%) compared to radiation at 20% ($_g$ or black globe) and 10% for dry bulb ($_{db}$ or the air temperature). The wet bulb component is weighted more heavily because it is the most important environmental factor due to the emphasis upon evaporative processes. When the radiant heat (g) is not considered to be a major factor then the black globe and dry bulb components can be combined to form a new constant of 0.3_{db}.

Stable core temperature

As discussed earlier, the human body maintains a stable core temperature of about 37°C subject to the daily fluctuations already mentioned as well as due to the effects of evaporation, conduction, convection, radiation, work and metabolism. Core temperature is usually measured by rectal thermometry but there are ethical issues concerning the use of this procedure with children. Since the mid-1990s, there has been a shift away from ascertaining the rectal temperature as a surrogate of core temperature to that of measuring the temperature closer to the brain. Wilson et al (1971) stated that the tympanic membrane temperature might be a better representation of core temperature because it is situated closer to the vascular supply of the tympanic membrane to the hypothalamic area. As the tympanic membrane is closer to the centralized specialized neurons responsible for homeostatic temperature control, it may reflect thermoregulatory processes better. The hypothalamus gland is responsible for monitoring core temperature and is perfused by the internal carotid arteries. These arteries also vascularize the tympanic membrane and auditory canal and provide an intimate link for monitoring temperature.

Tympanic temperature is a non-invasive measure and is better suited for temperature studies with children, although it too is not without limitations. The tympanic membrane is sensitive and easily damaged and insertion into the ear must be performed carefully. Most devices used are infrared and measure the temperature of the auditory meatus, approximately 1 cm inside the ear canal. The ear should be insulated as environmental temperatures easily affect it. Shinozaki et al (1988) measured the tympanic membrane from 34 to 39.5°C and concluded that it can accurately measure temperatures in vivo which are reproducible. Infrared devices like these also have the advantage that they are much more rapid in measuring temperature than rectal devices. Rectal thermometry is not thought to be the best measure of core temperature when the temperature is changing rapidly, for example during exercise protocols. The measurement of the tympanic membrane has been correlated well to oesophageal temperature and tracks core changes faster than rectal temperatures. It is also possible to measure oesophageal temperature but this is more likely in a clinical setting with children than a sports and exercise science one. Whichever method is utilized for monitoring core temperature it is important to represent data as a delta value (the difference between baseline and actual reading) rather than establishing absolute values because different tissues have different temperature gradients.

It is also possible to use thermometers to measure skin temperature, which at rest is usually 4°C below core temperature. Skin thermometers can be taped to the skin over a variety of body places such as the chest, thigh, finger and subscapula and have been used to ascertain a mean skin temperature (Klentrou et al 2004). The temperature gradient between the core and the skin is an important determinant of heat transfer in which heat is effectively transferred to or away from the body. The closer the two values are the less heat is lost from the body.

Thermoneutral zone

The thermoneutral zone (TNZ) represents a range of temperatures in which a stable core temperature is maintained. The TNZ is a criterion measure, which uses a naked 70 kg man with temperatures between 27 and 31°C. The lower of the two values is known as the critical temperature. The use of a naked person clearly forsakes the influence of clothing but as this would vary core temperature too much, the TNZ is defined using this standard criterion.

In order to maintain TNZ simple processes such as vasodilation and constriction of peripheral blood vessels are activated. These processes either increase or decrease the amount of blood moving from the core to periphery or skin, thus promoting or inhibiting heat loss. Temperature control is an excellent example of a negative feedback mechanism such that an increase in temperature of the body initiates a decrease in temperature. Cold receptors known as Aδ fibres are present in the peripheral areas of the body such as the skin and are stimulated by low ranges of temperatures. Warm receptors, also known as C fibres, are stimulated by a higher range of temperature and comprise about one tenth the number of cold receptors. Cold and warm receptors are also found centrally in the hypothalamus and the spinal cord. The pre-optic and anterior region of the hypothalamus is considered to be responsible for changes that will result in heat loss whereas the posterior hypothalamus responds to changes that result in heat gain. These changes involve manipulating the levels of hormones such as renin and angiotensin, the activation of the sweat glands as well as innervation of arteriole smooth skin muscle to control constriction and regulate blood flow.

Thermoregulation outside the neutral zone

To a large extent thermoregulation outside of the TNZ will be influenced by behavioural and environmental factors. If we are cold we will generally seek shelter and/or put on more clothing and the reverse with hot climates. If, however, ambient temperature is falling below the TNZ heat losses from the body will increase and core temperature will fall. If this imbalance is not addressed then clearly this represents a danger and normal body temperature must be returned as soon as possible. In the above example of a cold climate, if the physiological responses fail to restore normal heat balance or human behaviour cannot influence the situation, hypothermia will occur. Hypothermia is defined as a core temperature of 35°C or below. Conversely, if ambient temperature is greater than the TNZ and heat gains outweigh heat losses, core temperature will increase. If the behavioural or normal physiological responses fail to reduce core temperature hyperthermia will occur. Hyperthermia is defined as a core temperature of 40°C or more.

A major problem in newborn babies or neonates is retaining heat. Neonates have a TNZ that is higher than that of adults, between 32 and 36°C. Neonates possess a large head in proportion to the rest of their body, which is supplied by an excellent blood flow. Therefore, they have a high surface area to body mass, which creates problems in the retention of heat. They also possess a poorer evaporative cooling mechanism than toddlers and adults and are not able to dissipate heat as easily. This poorer mechanism is due to the fact that the temperature at which sweating is stimulated, and as a consequence evaporated, is higher in neonates. Therefore it is much easier for neonates to overheat. Neonates' autonomic nervous system is not as well developed as children's and adults' and so they do not react as well as older children and adults to small temperature changes. This is not usually a problem as babies can be dressed appropriately, but it is a very serious problem for premature babies because often they cannot be fully clothed because of the need for incubating tubes etc. The use of incubators that are equipped with heating systems is a response to the temperature retention problem of newborn babies. Early heating system incubators encountered problems with an increase in CO_2 levels in the incubator that affected the babies' respiration. However, this has now been resolved by a 'flow through' air system, which has removed the problem of the recirculation systems of the past.

PHYSIOLOGICAL RESPONSES TO HIGH TEMPERATURES

In this section details of the physiological differences during high temperatures between children and adults are highlighted. It would appear that in thermoneutral conditions (27–31°C) children are effective thermoregulators. The majority of the research studies investigating children exercising in the heat have been performed in a warm environment (30–40°C). For ethical reasons there are only a few studies that have required performance in temperatures above 40°C. Although the physiological mechanisms that respond to high temperatures are considered to be the same in children as in adults, there are some significant differences between the two groups. These mechanisms include differences in peripheral blood flow, lower cardiac output and sweat patterns.

One of the first physiological responses to high temperatures is vasodilation. The hypothalamus can directly affect the smooth muscles of metarterioles to control blood flow between vessels that are located deep within the body and those located superficially. Hence, by redirecting warm blood from the deep vessels or core of the body to the surface, heat can be dissipated. The processes of conduction and convection will assist in transferring heat from the deep vessels to other vessels for transportation to the body's surface to the environment via radiation and conduction. Providing the temperature between the blood and the vessels it bypasses is cooler, heat will be transferred away from the vessels via the blood to the body's surface (principle of a positive temperature gradient or ΔT). Furthermore, if this process continues such that the skin temperature is lower than the environmental temperature, heat will be lost. Of course the danger is when the environmental temperature is so high that the skin temperature becomes warmer than the core temperature; in this case these processes will be reversed and core temperature will begin to rise due to increased heat absorption.

One of the consequences of vasodilation is that because an increased blood flow is being diverted to the peripheral tissues such as the skin, there is a compromise in flow to other areas of the body. In an exercising child this will present problems because of the competing nature of blood flow with other metabolically active organs such as the brain, muscles, heart and lungs. Compared to adults, children have a lower cardiac output ($\dot{Q}$) per volume of oxygen uptake ($\dot{V}O_2$). This difference in $\dot{Q}$ will mean that there is a lower capacity for convection to the body's surface. However, it has been reported that children appear to have a higher peripheral blood flow both during exercise and immediately after. Falk et al (1992b) found in 10 prepubertal, 13 midpubertal and 8 late pubertal boys during cycling at 50% $\dot{V}O_2$max that significant differences in forearm blood flow occurred. During three 20-minute cycling bouts at 42°C and 20% RH, prepubertal boys were found to have a forearm blood flow which increased over time and was consistently higher compared to the more mature boys. This finding has been replicated in girls when compared to adult females

(Drinkwater et al 1977). A key assumption in the interpretation of these results is that the increased blood flow is to the skin and not to other areas such as muscle.

The observed increased blood flow and therefore enhanced convective process in children might be advantageous to dissipate heat. However, in combination with a greater surface area to body mass ratio and a lower $\dot{Q}$ these factors might compromise blood flow to other vital organs such as the brain. The greater surface to body mass ratio is an important geometrical difference between children and adults. Because the movement of heat is dependent on the contact area or surface area and the heat transfer between the environment and a child's body it will result in a greater transfer than an adult's relative to each kilogram of body mass. The surface area per body mass ratio is approximately 35–40% greater than in an adult. However, care must be taken with geometrical dimensional theory when extrapolating to biological law, as it does not mean that the surface area to body mass ratio can be used to predict chronological age differences in thermoregulation, due to the impact of maturation.

Another important differentiator in the heat is that children expend more energy per mass than adults whilst exercising. Therefore, if a child and an adult are running at the same treadmill speed a child will generate up to 20% more metabolic heat per kilogram body mass. How comparisons are made between two different groups is very important because if the comparisons are not equitable then any conclusions will lack validity. This lack of equivalence was demonstrated in early studies that examined sexual differences in heat tolerance in adults. As adult men and women were always assigned the same absolute running speed or cycle power output, the women, who were also not as aerobically fit as the male participants, did less well in these studies. The conclusion was that women tolerated exercising in the heat less well than men. Studies that then corrected for these inequalities and used male and female participants of equal cardiovascular fitness found no difference. This indicated that women were just as able to tolerate the heat as their male counterparts. In studies between children and adults or between children in different categories of maturity, it is important that all subjects are exposed to the same heat stress. This includes accounting for fitness, level of acclimatization to the heat and relative intensity of the exercise bout.

Simultaneous to the occurrence of vasodilation is the initiation of the sweat response. It is important to stress that the sweat response is not just about the rate of sweating but also the onset of its initiation, its composition and the population density of heat-activated sweat glands (HASG). It is thought that by age 2 years children have a similar number of sweat glands to adults at approximately 2 million. That averages out to around 120 sweat glands per square centimetre. However, this calculation is not strictly valid as most eccrine sweat glands are not evenly distributed and over 50% of sweat production is located on areas of the chest and back. On average, children have been found to produce about 400–500 mL $\cdot$ m^{-2} $\cdot$ h^{-1} compared to adults' 700–800 mL $\cdot$ m^{-2} $\cdot$ h^{-1}. It not uncommon for adult endurance athletes to sweat over 3 L $\cdot$ h^{-1}. There are clear sex and maturational differences; women sweat more than girls but the difference is not as great as between men and boys. Boys sweat more than girls and postpubertal children sweat more than pre- and midpubertal children. As the evaporation of sweat is one of the key mechanisms to heat loss, children's lower sweating response to central thermal stimuli seriously disadvantages them in warm and hot environments. Children also have a delayed onset of sweating with a greater rise in skin temperature at a given thermal stress, as well as a higher core temperature at which sweating commences compared to adults (Araki et al 1979). It is important to re-emphasize that it is the evaporation of the sweat droplet that initiates heat loss and not its production or even the droplet dropping to the ground.

Consequences of increased sweating are potential shifts in body fluid. As sweat is hypotonic (concentration is lower) to plasma water, the major elements of potassium (K^+), sodium (Na^+) and chloride (Cl^-) are found in lower concentrations. But as sweat production increases the concentration of the electrolytes increases, as more water is lost. Consequently, plasma osmolarity increases. This response in turn increases the secretion of the antidiuretic hormone (ADH) from the pituitary gland. ADH, by acting on the distal tubules of the kidneys, causes a reabsorption of water and the conservation of Na^+. Hence, during exercise in the heat it is as important to replace water as it is electrolytes, because far more of the solvent (water) is lost from the body than solutes (electrolytes). The strategy of adding Na^+ to drinks is as much because it has been found to encourage more drinking of the fluid as it is about replacing lost electrolytes. There have been some cases of adult athletes drinking too much water leading to what has been referred to as 'water intoxication', defined clinically as hyponatraemia (low blood sodium), which at its most extreme can lead to a coma. However, there are no published data for this symptom in children.

Epidemiological evidence on the incidence of heat injuries or illness is difficult to gather on children. Although some authors claim young children are at high risk during times of high climatic stress (Ellis et al 1976), to the best of the author's knowledge there are no peer-reviewed published data to support such a claim. Investigators have recently attempted to monitor heat-related injuries in junior athletes. Bergeron (2002) studied nationally ranked US tennis players aged 13–14 years playing during a tournament (San Antonio, Texas in August) and a different group of similar aged players during tennis training sessions, and found that many were dehydrated at the commencement of competition or training. Core temperatures often approached 39°C and players often lost up to 1–2 $L \cdot h^{-1}$ of fluid through sweating. Bergeron reported that for some adolescents as much as 3 $L \cdot h^{-1}$ was lost, but interestingly Bergeron also noted that these responses were very individual and this fact might negate the use of average values when working with children. It was also reported that fluid-electrolyte deficits worsened as the day progressed, particularly where a second match was played or daily training sessions ensued, suggesting a lack of recovery between matches or training sessions. It was also found that sweat losses of Na^+ and Cl^- were greater than sweat losses of other electrolytes.

Secondary consequences of an elevated body temperature include alterations to ventilation. Increases are usually found in ventilation rate and volume but because little heat is lost by this mechanism, it has minimal effect on temperature regulation. An increased ventilation rate can continue to acerbate the problems found with high body temperature by causing hyperventilation, a decrease in PCO_2 leading to respiratory alkalosis and in severe cases fainting. Table 11.1 shows the symptoms and consequences brought about by high body temperatures. These include heat cramps, syncope, heat exhaustion and heatstroke (hyperthermia).

Therefore, in summary in thermoneutral conditions, children's higher body surface area enables them to dissipate heat more effectively by R, K and C than by evaporative cooling. But in warm and hot conditions evaporative cooling is less than that for adults. However, it should be pointed out that boys have performed most thermoregulatory studies during aerobic exercise, and there are few studies examining sprint type or anaerobic activities. More studies are clearly needed to fully explain the thermoregulatory mechanisms for boys and girls in relation to age, sex and maturational effects (see Table 11.2 for a review of studies).

Table 11.1   Signs, symptoms and remedial action of heat-related illness

Condition	Signs and symptoms	Action
Heat cramps	Tightening of muscles, usually in stomach or legs. Often brought on by exertion and insufficient electrolytes	Stretch the muscle and replace electrolytes with appropriate drinks
Heat syncope (fainting)	Dizziness, headache, increased heart rate, feelings of nausea, possible vomiting, resulting in loss of consciousness	Lie person down or seated, elevate feet slightly, give small amount of fluid. Ensure no injury because of fainting episode. Avoid vigorous activity for several days
Heat exhaustion (volume depletion) Fluid losses from sweating are greater than internal fluid reserves, lack of fluid causes body to vasoconstrict blood vessels especially in the periphery. Core temperature ≤40°C	Intense thirst Rapid, shallow breathing Headache Severe sweating, skin pale in colour and clammy Nausea often accompanied by vomiting Decreased urine volume Core temperature may be normal or slightly elevated Irrational behaviour Whole body weakness, particularly musculoskeletal	Seek immediate emergency help Aim is to get core temperature below 39°C Seek shade or take indoors Loosen or remove as much clothing as practical Lie child down, elevate feet slightly If child conscious and aware and a bath available, place in cool but not cold water or alternatively sponge bathe the child repeatedly If outdoors find some sort of spray device and cool the child
Heatstroke – fluid depleted (slow onset) Lack of fluid has prevented the body's heat loss mechanism from operating functionally, the core temperature rising >41°C, which can lead to death	Severe headache Difficulty in breathing, which is often rapid Hot skin, skin may be wet or dry. This is the key identifier of heatstroke	Move to a cooler spot Remove clothing Pour water on arms and legs and fan the person to create a cooler air circulation system Alternatively cover the legs and arms with cool wet cloths and fan the person

(Continued)

Table 11.1 (Continued)

Condition	Signs and symptoms	Action
	Increased heart rate Muscular weakness Decreased urine volume Confusion and dizziness Pupils dilated and unresponsive to light Child can become comatose, possible seizures	Immerse in water if possible Ensure legs and arms are massaged to help shunt the cooler blood to the core of the body If these measures are successful, the temperature should fall but take care to avoid hypothermia as this may trigger shivering which will create heat Provide fluid, small sips Basic life support and cardiopulmonary resuscitation will be needed if the heatstroke is life-threatening
Heatstroke – fluid intact (fast onset) Heat transfer has overwhelmed the body even though fluid balance adequate	Same as above	Same as above

Table 11.2 Summary of existing thermoregulatory studies in children

Authors	Title	Aims	Methods	Key findings	Conclusions	Evaluation
Drinkwater, Kupprat, Denton et al (1977)	Response of prepubertal girls and college women to work in the heat	Examine the responses to three different environments when matched for aerobic workload	$N = 5$ girls (12.0 (0.9) years) $N = 5$ women (20.6 (0.7) years) 28°C 45% RH 35°C 65% RH 48°C 10% RH 2 × 50 min walks 30% $\dot{V}O_2$max	Women achieved HR stability at 28 and 35°C 4 of the 5 girls removed from 48°C 10% RH session before completion of first 50 min	Low tolerance of girls to heat Circulatory instability – lower total blood volume to surface area increases difficulty to maintain adequate peripheral blood flow Girls had a higher mean skin temp – due to delayed onset/distribution of sweat glands, i.e. on limbs	Small sample of subjects Onset and distribution of sweat activated glands not measured Body composition not determined
Araki, Toda, Matsushita et al (1979)	Age difference in sweating during muscular exercise	(1) Determine age difference in sweating (2) Physical training effects on age-related sweating	All except in 29(1)°C, 60% RH Experiment 1A – manipulation of workload $N = 4$ from each age 7–16 years 15–35 min at three workloads: 110–120, 130–150, 160–170 bts · min^{-1}	(1A) No difference in sweat volume at light load. Increase in sweat volume >13 years	(1) Age difference in sweating evident for high intensity work. Pre-adolescents have a reduced secretory capacity of sweat gland. Increased T_{sk} results	Very complex article with six experiments included Major limitation is lack of use of relative workloads, i.e. fixed resistance of 1 kg load etc.

(Continued)

Table 11.2 (Continued)

Authors	Title	Aims	Methods	Key findings	Conclusions	Evaluation
			Experiment 1B $N = 5$ from 7, 9, 11, 12, 15, 20 years 1.5 kg resistance 110 revs · min⁻¹ for 40 min or 60 min, 20 years	(1B) Increase in T_{re} represented a very significant age difference. No difference in age for sweat volume		Disadvantage of using HR to determine intensity, i.e. CV drift
			Experiment 1C $N = 7$ from 9 and 20 years 2 levels of workloads: light – to induce a slight increase in T_{re} followed by a plateau heavy – linear increase in T_{re} November – cycle at 40 or 60 min, same as experiment B	(1C) At light load no significant difference in pectoral sweat volume, T_{sk} and total sweat volume; heavy – pectoral sweat volume of 20-year-old increased from early stages very rapidly 9 years – much slower		
			Experiment 2A Pre-adolescent 3–11 years Post-adolescent	(2A) Sweat volume of 11-year-old less affected by training than	(2) Pre-adolescents' sweating mechanism less affected by	

Author	Title	Aim	Method	Results	Comments
			>20 years >9 years – 5 min outdoor running 3–4 × week, once a day for 5–7 wk Others – 500 m 2–5 × week, 8–16 weeks Assessment: >9 years 5 min outdoor running Others – 3 min indoor running	20-year-old 11 years and under: less affected in sweat concentration	physical training. In adults heavy workload invokes an increase in T_{re} offset by evaporation, in pre-adolescents offset by increase in T_{sk}
			Experiment 2B Pre-adolescents: 3 male 10 years 2 female 11 years 5 min running, 5 days a week for 7 weeks 60 min at 1 kg	(2B) T_{sk} unaffected and rise in T_{re} became less	
Araki, Tsujita, Matsushita et al (1980)	Thermoregulatory responses of prepubertal boys to heat and cold in relation to physical training	Effect of thermoregulatory responses from physical training adults vs. children	Three experiments (A) $n = 12$ vs. $n = 13$ physical vs. untrained 25 11-year-olds (pre-)	A) HR lower in the trained. No significant difference in T_{re} or T_{sk}	Trained vs. untrained children – differences associated with CV adaptations, i.e. higher cardiac output Study did not examine effect of exercise, i.e. other work has demonstrated that differences in evaporative

(Continued)

Table 11.2   (Continued)

Authors	Title	Aims	Methods	Key findings	Conclusions	Evaluation
			30 min periods of heat and cold alternately. Heat stress – legs dipped in 42°C and 30°C, 70% RH ambient. Cold stress – 20°C, 0% RH 2 h total exposure (B) n = 4 pre-adolescents (11 years) = 3 male adults (20 ± 0.8 years) 60 min heat and cold stress as Experiment A. Training 5–7 km per day for 40 days (C) n = 17 prepubertal boys (11 years) trained and untrained n = 16 male adults (19–21 years)	(B) HR reduced post training. Increase in 4 km performance, therefore training increased performance. Exposure to heat post training: children lower HR, adults lower HR, T_{re}, T_{sk} (C) Age difference evident in T_{sk}, HR. Children had higher HR and T_{sk} with exposure to heat	Previous work showed inferior ability to sweat vs. adults. At given $\dot{V}O_2$ children have a lower Q̇ therefore heat exposure to periphery is lower, T_{sk} will increase	mechanisms become evident for intense work

Study	Topic	Aims	Methods	Results		
Davies (1981)	Thermal responses to exercise in children	To increase information of thermoregulation of exercising children	N = 8 boys 12.9 (0.8) years N = 5 girls 13.8 (0.70 years) N = 8 adults (36.1 (6.7) years) T_A 21°C, RH<50% 60 min at 68% $\dot{V}O_2$max	Sweat rate lower in children vs. adults Children 51% E, 5% stored, 44% R + C Adults ~64% E, 2% stored, 32% R + C	Radiation and convection forced due to less effective sweat mechanism? Evaporation is modulated by T_{sk} – higher in children therefore must be limited mechanism	Maturation development not acknowledged – implications upon development of apoeccrine glands etc. Pre- and post-acclimation would determine whether sweat response would increase
Mackova, Sturmova & Macek (1984)	Prolonged exercise in prepubertal boys in warm and cold	To establish a temperature suitable for school gymnastics	N = 10 (12.3 (0.3) years) 60 min at 50% $\dot{V}O_2$max 25°C vs. 10°C	In warmer environment HR, T_{re}, SR via weight loss were all increased	Increased thermoregulatory demands from the warmer environment	Gymnastics dependent upon force development; therefore increased muscle temperature more favourable? Cycling does not fully meet research aims?
Piekarski, Morfeld, Kampmann et al (1986)	Heat stress reactions of the growing child	(1) Age- or fitness-related change in body temperature, HR, sweat loss during heat stress? (2) Increased heat tolerance from	Longitudinal study N = 4 boys N = 1 girl (10 years) T_A = 25–55°C sitting or walking 3 h exposure	HR and T_{RE} showed decrease with increasing age. SR increased to 13 years then stopped	Increased tolerance. Body temperature and HR show a negative trend Girl had reduced tolerance during	Three research questions unanswered. Limited observations due to small sample

(Continued)

Table 11.2 (Continued)

Authors	Title	Aims	Methods	Key findings	Conclusions	Evaluation
		increased physical fitness? (3) Gender difference			puberty to heat – link to adiposity, i.e. higher specific heat capacity?	
Houmard, Costill, Davis et al (1990)	The influence of exercise intensity on heat acclimation in trained subjects	To determine whether continuous, short-duration, moderate intensity exercise (30–35 min, ~75% $\dot{V}O_2$max) would result in heat acclimation	$N = 9$ trained runners (25.6 (2.2) years) 2 counterbalanced 9-day heat stress protocols Heat tolerance test (HTT) performed on day 1 and 9 = 90 min walking or jogging at 50% $\dot{V}O_2$max Protocol 1 = days 2–8, running at 75% $\dot{V}O_2$max Protocol 2 = walking or jogging	Final HR and T_{re} reduced in HTT2 vs. HTT1; no difference between 2 HA protocols. No changes in sweat rate, lowering of T_{sk} and an expansion of resting PV	Similar degree of heat acclimation using short duration high intensity – implications for sport-specific requirements. Same sweat rate during HTT2 at lower T_{re} infers that sweating did occur earlier during HTT2 enhancing heat dissipation	Does 56–63 days allow complete de-acclimation from each protocol?

		at 50% $\dot{V}O_2$max for 60 min 40°C, 27% RH Protocols separated by 56–63 days		HA reduces metabolic rate whereas endurance training does not; 4% reduction, which would decrease metabolic heat and reduce T_{re}	Comparisons made to adults from a study 15 years ago. Protocol differences likely
Delamarche, Bittel, Lacour et al (1990)	Thermoregulation at rest and during exercise in prepubertal boys	Effects of exercise-induced thermal load in children	$N = 11$ (10–12 years) 45°C, 20% RH 90 min passive 60 min at 60% $\dot{V}O_2$max	Passive test – 2 phase response to sweating. Initial 10 min heat stored due to absence of sweating, second phase began at onset of sweating and resulted in thermal equilibrium

Active test – sweating occurred more rapidly | Comparisons made to adults from work of Bittel (1975) Passive test – children thermoregulate as efficiently as adults but with greater reliance upon convection and radiation During exercise test – dissipation of heat by evaporation smaller vs. adults |

(Continued)

Table 11.2   (Continued)

Authors	Title	Aims	Methods	Key findings	Conclusions	Evaluation
Falk, Bar-Or, Calvert et al (1992a)	Sweat gland response to exercise in the heat among PP, MP and LP boys	Determine the association between the heat-activated sweat gland response to exercise in the heat and the level of physical maturity using a refinement of the macrophotographic technique	PP, $N = 16$ (10.8 (0.2) years) MP, $N = 15$ (13.6 (0.4) years) LP, $N = 5$ (16.2 (0.2) years) 41–43°C, 18–22% RH 2 × 20 min bouts, 10 min interval Cycling at 50% $\dot{V}O_2$max	No significant difference in HR rise, initial and final T_{re} or initial and final T_{sk} SR was higher for PP when expressed per body surface area PD of HASG in PP was significantly higher than MP during bout 1 and significantly higher than MP and LP during bout 2 % A (skin % covered by sweat) not significantly different between groups SR per gland was significantly lower in PP vs. MP and LP	PD decreases while mean area of sweat drops (DA) increases. This is accompanied with a higher whole body SR and a higher calculated SR per gland with increasing maturity Increase in SR from bout 1 to 2 was due to an increase in the SR per gland as opposed to an increase in the number of active glands (Due to increase in DA without a concomitant increase in PD)	Regional differences in PD exist – not accounted for. However, this is thought to be proportional across all three groups Body surface area increase and sweat gland size increase with age, which contributes to an increase in sweat rate per gland No difference in proportion of skin area covered by sweat; therefore difference in evaporative cooling unclear

| Falk, Bar-Or & MacDougall (1992b) | Thermoregulatory responses of pre-, mid-, and late pubertal boys to exercise in dry heat | Thermoregulatory responses to dry heat when matched for metabolic heat load production | PP, $N = 10$
MP, $N = 13$
LP, $N = 8$
41–43°C, 18–22% RH
3×20 min bouts at 50% $\dot{V}O_2$max | PP – 2 stopped
MP – 2 stopped
LP – 6 stopped
Sweat rate lower in PP vs. LP
HS highest in LP | Increase in DA and SR towards end of puberty as no difference in MP and PP found

SR per kg equal. Lower HS due to calculations not accounting for heat adiposity?
PP had increased HASG population density

Is thermoregulation linked to puberty?
Validity of calculations to children |
| Falk, Bar-Or, MacDougall et al (1992c) | Longitudinal analysis of sweat response of pre- mid- and late pubertal boys during exercise in the heat | Effect of growth and maturation on thermoregulation: Sweat rate HASG | PP, $N = 16$
MP, $N = 15$
LP, $N = 5$
3×20 min cycle at 50% $\dot{V}O_2$max
41–43°C | During the 18 month study 4 of PP became MP and 5 of MP became LP

Sweat rate per body surface area and per gland were higher among LP vs. PP

Increased sweat lactate in LP | Physical maturation is characterized by enhanced sweating rate per body surface area and per gland

Increased sweat lactate reflective of increased anaerobic metabolism

Indications of sweat threshold and acceleration at puberty, i.e. increase

Fixed intensity work in the present study, therefore the use of different intensities would help determine whether increases in sweat rate are due to age or metabolic load?
Low transition of children across groups, therefore |

(Continued)

Table 11.2 (Continued)

Authors	Title	Aims	Methods	Key findings	Conclusions	Evaluation
Meyer, Bar-Or, MacDougall et al (1992)	Sweat electrolyte loss during exercise in the heat: effects of gender and maturation	(1) Compare sweat electrolyte concentration and sweat rate of three maturation groups, male and female (2) Compare total amount of sweat electrolyte loss in these different groups	$N = 51$ (25 females, 26 males) PP = 8 female, 10 male P = 9 female, 8 male YA = 8 female, 8 male Exercise in heat trial: 40–42°C, 18–20% RH 2 × 20 min bout, 10 min rest, 50% peak $\dot{V}O_2$	Male YA higher sweat vs. PP and higher [Cl]− than all Sweat [K]+ lower in YA (males and females) vs. children (YA [K]+ vs. P not significant) PP and P lower sweat rate even with surface area accounted for YA lost more [Na]+ and [Cl]− compared with PP and P	from PP which then decreased from MP PP and P lower [Na]+ and [Cl]− and higher [K]+ vs. YA in addition to lower sweat rate. Amount of [Na]+ and [Cl]− lost from sweat (absolute and relative) lower in PP and P. No maturational difference in [K]+ Maturational differences in sweat electrolyte concentration likely to occur in reabsorptive duct rather than acinus as precursor sweat from interstitial fluid has similar electrolyte concentration to that of plasma	low power of statistics Is there any evidence that documents sweat gland response on the lower back reflects the total body response? Maturational differences and gender responses may not have been determined due to lack of sensitivity of sweat glands analysed in one location

Study	Focus	Aim	Subjects	Findings	Comments
				Differences not thought to be due to plasma aldosterone levels but differences in sensitivity of receptors or no. of receptors. Higher sweat rate decreases time for Na$^+$ to be reabsorbed, $r = 0.15$. Higher plasma [K]$^+$ increase in YA vs. young children due to higher shift from contracting muscles since working with greater mass and higher absolute intensity	
Anderson & Mekjavic (1996)	Thermoregulatory responses of circumpubertal children	To analyse the core temperature threshold for sweating and its magnitude of response in prepubescent	N = 9 non-obese young adults 26.6 (5.2) y; N = 9 non-obese circumpubertal children 11.4 (1.2) years	Slope of sweat rate in relation to change in tympanic temperature relationship lower in PP vs. young adult (YA). PP able to maintain core temperature as effectively but different effector mechanisms, i.e. previous	Mechanisms for regulation unclear, greater attention to surface area calculations

(Continued)

Table 11.2 (Continued)

Authors	Title	Aims	Methods	Key findings	Conclusions	Evaluation
		children vs. young adults	1 trial 5 × min pre-exercise data 20 × min submaximal steady-state exercise in 22–24°C 65–70% HRmax Post-exercise immersion in 28°C until $\dot{V}O_2$ doubled	Null zone (absence of sweating/shivering) narrower in PP Sweat thresholds similar in PP and YA	attributions to surface area:body mass not substantiated	

CV, cardiovascular; DA, drop area; HASG, heat-activated sweat glands; HR, heart rate; HS, heat storage; P, pubertal; PD, population density; PP, MP, LP, pre-, mid- and late pubertal; SR, sweat rate; T_{re}, rectal temperature; T_{sk}, skin temperature; YA, young adults; values are mean (standard deviation).

PHYSIOLOGICAL RESPONSES TO LOW TEMPERATURES

There have been fewer studies of children's physiological responses to the cold than to the heat (Table 11.3). However, the few studies that have been conducted provide evidence that children's thermoregulatory responses are as effective as those of adults. If the stored body heat (S) is negative then heat is being lost at a faster rate than it is being produced. Of the components discussed in the thermal balance equation, convection and radiation are the most important processes of heat loss in the cold. For radiation, the temperature gradient between the skin or clothing and the surrounding air is the major factor that will influence heat loss. Convection is also influenced by the temperature gradient between skin or clothing and air but also critically by air velocity.

In water it is not just convection that is the important process but also conduction. Water is 20 times greater a conductor than air. Children face a real danger in cold water temperatures; their large surface area to body mass ratio permits large losses of heat and heat will be conducted away from the body to the surrounding water. This heat is then lost by convection as the warmer water around the body is replaced by colder water, which is why cross-channel swimmers often cover themselves in insulating layers of grease or fat-like substances. The additional layers of fat help to insulate against the cold. Body fat, something younger children have less of than adults, has the highest insulator capacity of any structure or organ in the human body.

The primary physiological response to cold temperatures is thermogenesis due to shivering. This mechanism is initiated by declines in both skin and core temperature. This involuntary action has the resultant effect of an increased heat production that is capable of causing a fivefold increase in metabolic rate. The disadvantage of thermogenesis is that it cannot be sustained for long time periods as it is still an energy-deriving process. Another form of thermogenesis called non-shivering thermogenesis has often been reported. This process, which produces heat by not involving muscular contractions, has been found to increase the metabolic rate by two to three times. However, this mechanism, which is associated with brown adipose tissue, has been largely confined to studies in animals such as rats. Although it is acknowledged that in newborn human babies brown fat does contribute to non-shivering thermogenesis, in adults this mechanism is less clearly understood. Alternatively, increasing heat production by increasing activity such as foot stamping or rubbing of hands and arms can often be seen when it is cold and is an obvious behavioural response.

Whilst thermogenesis is a heat-producing mechanism in the cold, antagonistic to this is peripheral vasoconstriction, a process to reduce heat loss. The usual physiological response to the cold is a decreased blood flow through the peripheral circulation in order to reduce heat loss through convection. By shunting the blood to deeper vessels this effectively works to insulate deeper layers and conserve heat. The rate of heat loss is inversely related to tissue thickness; therefore as blood is shunted away from cooler peripheral tissues, the temperature gradient between the skin and the core increases. The initial response of vasoconstriction does not remain for long as there then occurs a period of vasodilation which results in some heat loss. Thereafter, an alternating period of vasoconstriction and vasodilation ensues. This process is known as the 'hunting reflex' and is thought to prevent tissue damage most notably in the fingers and toes.

Few studies have been conducted in cold conditions with children. The first studies involved swimming and showed that children were at a considerable disadvantage compared to adults (Sloan & Keatinge 1973). Proficient swimmers aged 8–19 years

Table 11.3 Thermoregulatory responses to exercise in the cold

Authors	Title	Aims	Methods	Key findings	Conclusions
Klentrou, Cunliffe, Slack et al (2004)	Temperature regulation during rest and exercise in the cold in premenarcheal (PM) and menarcheal (EM) girls	(1) To determine the thermoregulatory responses in EM and PM (2) To examine the differences during follicular vs. luteal phase	EM, $N = 6$ PM, $N = 7$ (13–18 years) Thermoneutral Cold stress test 5°C, 40% RH 20 min rest 40 min exercise at 30% peak $\dot{V}O_2$	(1) No difference in heat production but higher in PM vs. EM at rest (2) 79% variance in core temperature from body fat	PM – higher metabolic heat production but core temperature not maintained due to ineffective vasoconstriction Thermosensitivity affected by phase, i.e. warmer in luteal phase due to increased progesterone Temperature responses more affected by metabolic responses than morphology

were monitored in water temperatures of 20.3°C whilst swimming at a constant speed. The youngest swimmers had to be taken out after 10 min whilst the adults managed to complete 30 min. Oral temperature, although not the best measure of core temperature, was found to be 2°C lower than in adults. These results can be explained by the significant differences in the surface area to body mass ratio and the differences in skinfold thickness. Both of these explanatory variables disadvantage children in water environments even more so than in similar temperatures in air. The smaller and leaner the child and the colder the water, the greater is their disadvantage in water compared to adolescents and adults.

Several research groups (Araki et al 1980; Matsushita & Araki 1980) have found that children resting with minimal clothing in a cool environment of 16–20°C maintained their core temperature, and their physiological responses to the cool conditions were as effective as those of the adults. However, as conclusions are based on so few studies and mostly male participants, the implications must be viewed with caution. Another limitation to these studies was the short exposure times (<60 min). Indeed Falk et al (1997) showed that for boys at rest and exposed to conditions of 7, 13 and 22°C for 110 min each, rectal core temperature continued to fall even after the boys had been removed from the chamber and were back in thermoneutral conditions. The only study to have investigated maturity and exposure to cold conditions is by Smolander et al (1992). Eight prepubertal and early pubertal boys (11–12 years) were compared to 11 adult men (19–34 years) when resting and cycling (30%$\dot{V}O_2$max) for 40 min at 5°C and 40% RH wearing only shorts, socks and trainers. In agreement with previous studies, thermoregulation was found to be similar to and as effective as that in adults. The boys achieved this by a higher thermogenesis at rest and during exercise, and a greater reduction in skin limb temperature (possibly due to greater peripheral vasoconstriction). This was accomplished despite their disadvantage in surface area to body mass ratio. The main threats emanating from a cold environment are hypothermia, frostbite and bronchoconstriction. Unless appropriate protection is taken to reduce these threats, children will be vulnerable. Epidemiological evidence tends to be retrospective but certain groups of children appear more vulnerable than others. These groups include children with anorexia nervosa, cystic fibrosis, chronic asthma, and those with poor blood supply, particularly to the extremities.

ACCLIMATIZATION AND ACCLIMATION

Acclimatization and acclimation are relevant to the physiological responses of both hot and cold conditions. However, presumably because there are fewer volunteers willing to be subjected to long exposures of cold temperatures there are more details related to acclimatization and acclimation in hot conditions. Therefore, this section will be confined to acclimatization and acclimation in the heat. The process of acclimatization relates to the physiological changes exhibited by a person who is repeatedly exposed to altered natural environmental conditions. It differs from acclimation, where the process is artificially created, usually in an environmental chamber in which such factors as heat, humidity and pressure can be rigorously controlled and monitored.

The key aims of acclimatization and acclimation are to initiate an earlier onset of sweating, produce sweat that is more dilute, increase the rate of sweat at the same absolute temperature, reduce the heart rate and therefore the stress of the exercise for a given exercise intensity, and improve the pacing of effort and perception of environmental conditions.

In adults, these changes typically take about 2 weeks to occur and ideally should occur in the climate where the training or competition is happening. If this is not possible then the use of environmental chambers is effective in initiating acclimation changes. Both acclimatization and acclimation procedures initiate a sweat response earlier following a smaller rise in body temperature. This will allow the acclimatized person to sweat more than an unacclimatized one. Although there will be a greater rate of sweat loss, the loss of sodium in sweat is also reduced due to the hormonal action of aldosterone. Acclimatization also allows a better distribution of blood flow around the body and to the skin. For acclimatization and acclimation purposes in adults it is not enough to passively experience the increased temperature conditions; exercise must be performed to achieve optimal benefits. The intensity of exercise is usually lower at the beginning of the acclimatization and acclimation programme. Passive procedures in adults have been found to be ineffectual as it is thought that the thermal load is too low and therefore limits the thermal and cardiovascular adjustments.

In children, there is limited information on acclimation procedures and the investigators suggest that the rate of acclimation is physiologically slower but perceptually faster in children. The level of acclimation is postulated to be lower and less stringent in children compared to adults and can be achieved through passive strategies. Most studies comparing children and adults have shown decreases in body temperature and heart rate and increases in sweat rates during a 2-week acclimation period. The main difference has been that adult change has occurred earlier, often after two sessions compared to four or five for children. Whilst adults appear to acclimate through large increases in their sweating rate, moderate changes are only shown in children. Although acclimatized children have been shown to sweat at a higher rate than unacclimatized children (Riveria-Brown et al 1999), it appears that children can acclimate to heat whether in thermoneutral conditions or whilst resting in the heat. Therefore, a child's acclimation programme can be very different to that of an adult. For a review of studies see Table 11.4.

STRATEGIES IN THE HEAT

It is difficult to find specific UK guidelines for strategies to safeguard against heat illness or injury because the ambient temperature is rarely threatening. Based on the above research findings, and in conjunction with the American Academy of Pediatrics (2000), the American College of Sports Medicine (Armstrong et al 1996) and the Australian Sports Medicine Federation (1989), the following guidelines for anyone with responsibility for children exercising in the heat are recommended:

1. That the intensity of activities that last 30 min or longer should be reduced whenever relative humidity and air temperature are above critical levels.
2. At the beginning of a strenuous training programme or on arrival in a hot country, the intensity and duration should be lower and gradually increased over a 2-week period.
3. Before prolonged training (>30 min), children (10 to 12 years) should be fully hydrated by consuming 300–400 mL 30 minutes prior to exercise. Periodic drinking of 100–125 mL of fluid should be consumed every 15–20 min for 10-year-olds and under, 200–250 mL for older children.
4. The clothing that children should be wearing whilst exercising should be light coloured and loose fitting to encourage evaporation. The replacement of sweaty

Table 11.4 Summary of studies in acclimatization and children

Authors	Title	Aims	Methods	Key findings	Conclusions	Evaluation
Wagner, Robinson, Tzankoff et al (1972)	Heat tolerance and acclimatization to work in the heat in relation to age	Controversy of young vs. old men acclimatization, i.e. rapidity of process in young men	Study 1 – sedentary 20–29 years vs. 46–69 years 5.6 km · h⁻¹, 50–90 min, 49°C Acclimatization in summer via sports Study 2 – prepubertal (11–14 years) vs. postpubertal (15–16 years) vs. non-athletic young men 8-day acclimatization	Older men – increased mean evaporative rate Increased sweat sensitivity post acclimatization Younger – decreased mean skin temperature, rectal and above post acclimatization Young boys unable to regulate temperature due to limited sweating Acclimatization resulted in reduced rectal temperature. HR and mean skin temperature – not as low in younger subjects	Process more effective in younger men Prepubertal athletes do not have same sweat secretion/sensitivity	Difference in acclimatization process and duration, i.e. intensity of sports and time of exposure 21.2 h – young 16.2 h – old 8-day acclimatization enough exposure as rate of acclimation known to be slower in children vs. adults?

(Continued)

Table 11.4 (Continued)

Authors	Title	Aims	Methods	Key findings	Conclusions	Evaluation
Bar-Or & Inbar (1977)	Relationship between perceptual and physical changes during heat acclimatization in 8–10-year-old boys	Examine RPE changes of acclimatization vs. physical conditioning	Heat and exercise group ($N = 9$) (H + E) Exercise group ($N = 8$) (E) Baseline assessment = 3 × 20 min cycle rides, 90 min total exposure 43°C 21% RH Power = 85% HRmax 5 physical exercise sessions H + E: 43°C, 21% RH E: 23°C, 50% RH	RPE, HR and rectal temperature decreased in both cohorts SR increased 10% in heat and exercise group; not significant	Pre and post subjective ratings decreased by acclimatization and conditioning	Differences in anthropometric values – impact due to minor alterations in surface area:body mass? Impact of humidity? i.e., physical training group worked in more humid environment
Inbar, Bar-Or, Dotan et al (1981)	Conditioning versus exercise in the heat as methods to acclimatize 8–10-year-old boys to dry heat	Physical conditioning vs. heat acclimatization in 10-year-old boys	$N = 18$ (8–10 years) 2 groups: work and work + heat Baseline = 3 × 20 min, 5 sessions in heat 43°C predetermined power 85% HR max w = 23°C, 21% RH w + h = 43°C, 21% RH	w + h = increase in HASG and sweat rate w = increase in O_2 pulse w and w + h = decrease in HR and T_{re}	Only significant difference was HASG Two different time courses of change, i.e. HR decrease evident after 30–35 min in w + h group but from onset in w group	Impact upon performance not determinable from study; i.e. may have been useful to look at higher intensity/ time trial to determine benefits of two different methods

Reference	Aim	Subjects/Methods	Results	Mechanisms	Comments
Inbar, Dotan, Bar-Or et al (1985)	Passive versus active exposures to dry heat as methods of heat acclimatization in young children	To determine the effect of an active and passive protocol in dry heat of 8–10-year-old boys – 43°C	$N = 18$ (8–10 years) 2 groups – passive (PHA) ($n = 8$) and active (AHA) ($n = 9$) Baseline and criterion test 3 × 20 min cycle ~85% HRmax, ~40 W and ~40–45% VO_2max 7–8 min rest between each bout 10-day alternate acclimation	Both procedures resulted in: T_{re}, T_{sk}, HR reductions PHA = reduction in heat storage AHA = increase in sweat sensitivity when reported per degree rise in core T_{re} above 37°C	PHA – due to thermal stress not CV stress or conditioning effect. Result was a reduction in peripheral blood flow thereby reducing radiation and convection processes. Skin has increased thermal conductance and acts as a barrier to penetrating heat gain AHA – due to increased sweating apparatus sensitivity and increased evaporative cooling mechanism. Increase in HASG	No significant difference found between the two different protocols for acclimation benefits. PHA due to favourable geometric morphology of children, i.e. more conducive to heat gain so thermal stress induces physiological change. AHA – combination of thermal and exercise thought to be too high to induce optimal acclimation benefits, i.e. when a function of stored heat each session
Wilk & Bar-Or (1997)	Heat acclimation and sweating pattern in prepubertal boys	Partial acclimation to heat in 9–12-year-olds and associated changes	$N = 12$, 9–12-year-old boys 3 h intermittent 35°C, 50–60% RH 3 × 70 min	Mean sweat rate similar before and after Sweat pattern alterations No difference in per cent skin covered, population density	Minor changes in sweat pattern at rest and exercise	Full study details required

AHA, active heat acclimatization; CV, cardiovascular; HASG, heat-activated sweat glands; HR, heart rate; PHA, passive heat acclimatization; SR, sweat rate; T_{re}, rectal temperature; T_{sk}, skin temperature; YA, young adults.

garments with dry ones should be encouraged to initiate heat loss. Rubberized suits should never be used to produce weight loss and procedures that promote weight loss through dehydration must be discouraged for child athletes.

5. Before departure to a hot country, whilst training at home young athletes should seek out an environment with the highest thermal load available and begin a process of acclimatization or acclimation.

6. If possible, use an environmental chamber and enlist specialist advice.

7. Saunas have limited use and should be discouraged.

8. Young athletes should habituate to a regular and enforced drinking schedule of water and sports drinks during both training and competition.

9. Young athletes' body mass before and after exercise should be monitored as a precursor to the assessment of fluid balance.

FLUID BALANCE

Water forms the largest proportion of the human body. For children aged between 9 and 17 years this can equate to approximately 75% of their fat-free mass. Approximately two thirds of this water is located in the intracellular fluid with the remaining distributed between cells (interstitial fluid) and in the plasma. The fluid balance is achieved by gains in the intake of fluids, food and the production of metabolic water. This is counterbalanced by the losses due to evaporation of water through the lungs/skin, sweat loss, and losses through faeces and urine.

Exercise will naturally disrupt the fluid balance as the body seeks to adjust to the varying circulatory and thermoregulatory demands. These demands include a reduction in blood volume, a diversion of blood away from the muscles, a reduced ability to transfer internal body heat via vasodilation, and a reduction in the capacity of sweat glands to continue to secrete sweat. In adults, as little as a 2% loss of body mass through sweating is found to have a significant impact on performance (Armstrong et al 1996). Little is known about the physiological responses of trained children and the effect on performance but there are subtle differences in sweat composition between children and adults.

In our laboratory with a group of adolescent cyclists who performed cycling for 60 minutes at a moderate to hard intensity, the average sweat loss was 1100 mL; this was despite a mean fluid intake of ~750 mL $\cdot$ h^{-1}. Therefore, a deficit of ~350 mL was observed. Data from the one female cyclist involved in the study showed she was able to remain hydrated with 750 mL of fluid intake with no change in body mass. Table 11.5 shows the average sweat loss per hour, per minute, per body mass and relative to body mass per minute. The same values for the female cyclist were 628 mL $\cdot$ h^{-1}, 6.4 mL $\cdot$ min^{-1}, 9.6 kg^{-1} $\cdot$ h^{-1} and 0.16 mL $\cdot$ kg^{-1} $\cdot$ h^{-1}, respectively.

Sweat contains similar substances to blood plasma but because sweat is more dilute than other body fluids, it is hypotonic compared to blood plasma. This is largely due to the fact that sweat contains only a third of the Na$^+$ and Cl$^-$ content compared to plasma. In Table 11.6 it is shown that although the plasma content of different minerals is similar, the largest differences are between children's and adults' sweat content. Children's sweat Cl$^-$ and Na$^+$ content is less but K$^+$ content higher than adults' sweat. Therefore, children have a more dilute solution because of their lower NaCl content in sweat. Hence children's and adolescents' sweat is more hypotonic than adults' and their salt loss will be lower than that of adults.

In the extracellular fluid, Na$^+$ and Cl$^-$ maintain water content, which is important particularly during exercise when total body water is being redistributed and sweat

Table 11.5 Sweat loss of eight male adolescent cyclists during 60 minutes of cycling

Sweat loss[a]	Mean (SD)
$mL \cdot h^{-1}$	1066 (220)
$mL \cdot min^{-1}$	18 (4)
$mL \cdot kg^{-1} \cdot h^{-1}$	16 (3)
$mL \cdot kg^{-1} \cdot min^{-1}$	0.27 (0.02)

[a]Values representative of 30 min moderate and 30 min hard intensity cycling under neutral environmental conditions, 20–25°C.
Fluid loss calculations do not consider respiratory losses.

Table 11.6 Plasma and sweat composition of children and adults

	Plasma (mEq · L⁻¹)	Sweat (mEq · L⁻¹)
Children[a]		
Sodium	139	20–40
Chloride	105	15–25
Potassium	4.0	12–15
Magnesium	1.2	–
Adults		
Sodium	140	40–60
Chloride	100	30–50
Potassium	4.0	5.5
Magnesium	1.5	1.5–5.0

[a]Figures adapted from Meyer et al (1992).

loss is occurring. This process results in the minerals becoming more concentrated because the loss of body water is greater than the loss of minerals. Therefore, from the structure of the cell there becomes an excess or greater concentration of minerals rather than a loss and it is more important that water content is replaced than minerals.

Although studies on dehydration are more common in adults, there are some studies that have investigated this process in children. Although there are few data it would appear that the processes are similar to those in adults. This process involves initial changes at the beginning of exercise by a decrease in plasma volume accompanied by an efflux of K^+ and other metabolites from the active muscle sites. As exercise continues, plasma volume decreases further due to sweat losses, and in a partial attempt to offset the sweat loss there is a reduced urinary output. Decreasing the renal plasma flow reduces the urinary output and glomerular filtration rates, which is also accompanied by an increase in antidiuretic hormonal activity. It is only when the fluid deficit from the body exceeds 5% of its initial pre-exercise mass that the sweat rate will begin to decrease. In one study investigating athletic acclimatized boys in Puerto Rico, one child lost 4.5% of initial pre-exercise body mass during a triathlon race (Riveria-Brown et al 1999). To support this heat loss and in an attempt to maintain a thermal balance the body gives up trying to defend its fluid balance.

Children are similar to adults in that when offered water ad libitum dehydration is progressive. Why this is the case is unknown but several factors have been implicated. First, there is the possibility that there are thirst perception impairments facilitated by the ingestion of water as its taste does not induce significant volumes to be consumed. It is known that the desirability of the drink is an important determinant of the total volume consumed. Therefore, to be adequately consumed it must taste good. In one adult study (Wilmore et al 1998) the ad libitum intake of water was compared to two carbohydrate-electrolyte drinks (one containing 6% carbohydrate, the other 8% carbohydrate) to determine the relationship between taste preference and total fluid intake during a 90 min run at 60%$\dot{V}O_2$max and during a 90 min recovery period. It was concluded that although there was no difference in the volume of fluid consumed during exercise for the three drinks, subjects consumed >50% more fluid from the sports drinks compared with water during recovery. When the drinks were subdivided into the most liked compared to the least liked drinks, the results showed subjects drank more of the most liked fluid during exercise. Therefore, it was concluded that perceived taste of the drink was an important factor for fluid replacement. Secondly, thirst is considered to be a late indicator of hydration status and therefore to drink only when you become thirsty is too late, as the process of dehydration has usually begun. There are, however, proponents who argue that this mechanism is subtle enough and that we should not ignore our thirst mechanism for fluid replenishment (Noakes 2001). Lastly, the addition of Na^+ is considered important in stimulating consumption of fluids, as it not only acts to stimulate receptors that initiate drinking, but also gives the drink flavour. In one study (Wilk & Bar-Or 1996) fluid intake differed significantly between water, flavoured water and flavoured water containing carbohydrate and Na^+ (Fig. 11.2). Body fluid losses were similar irrespective of the drink and there was a negative body fluid balance observed with the flavoured water and water.

Fluid intake strategies have been found to be incomplete (pre-exercise body mass not restored) up to 2 hours following exercise in adults but these strategies are

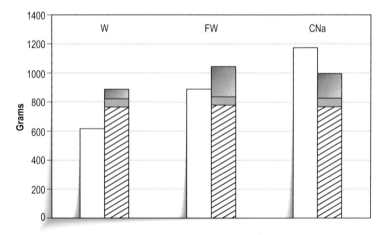

Figure 11.2 Fluid intake and fluid losses through sweat, urine and respiration in water (W), flavoured water (FW) and water containing carbohydrate and sodium (CNa) trials. Open bars, drink; hatched bars, sweat; blue bars, respiration; solid bars, urine. (From Wilk & Bar-Or 1996, used with permission of the American Physiological Society.)

significantly influenced by the content of sodium in the drink. Sodium-containing drinks have been found to rehydrate faster than water. Recently, in children exercising in the heat it was found that the degree of thirst and level of dehydration were positively related. In a study involving Canadian children a preference for grape flavoured drinks over apple, orange and water was reported. Interestingly, as the degree of dehydration progressively increased, the preference for orange, apple and water increased more than the grape flavour. This was explained by a possible ceiling effect on the higher first preference for the grape drink. It is not known if there are cultural or intra-country differences in taste preferences but wide individual variations are likely. Meyer & Bar-Or (1994) also observed that the thirst intensity increased as body mass decreased. This increase in thirst perception with minimal decreases in body mass has been reported in adults exercising in the heat (Hubbard et al 1990). However, the key trigger for thirst is an increasing blood osmolality, which stimulates the hypothalamic and gastrointestinal osmoreceptors, rather than changes in plasma volume and body mass. As these were not measured in children it is difficult to conclude what is triggering the increase in thirst perception. Also important from this study was the finding that children voluntarily overhydrated during recovery from exercise, which contrasts sharply with adult studies.

Ensuring the body is appropriately hydrated is a strategy to ensure that thermoregulation is not impaired when exercising in the heat. Children, like adults, will hypohydrate when exercising in the heat, even when water is offered ad libitum; in past studies this was often referred to as 'voluntary dehydration'. This term has, however, been replaced by 'involuntary dehydration' because of the acknowledgement that some sports, including those with child participants, actively encourage dehydration strategies so as to induce weight loss. Those sports found to employ deliberate dehydration strategies include wrestling, boxing and judo.

Involuntary dehydration appears to be similar to adults, although in children their smaller blood volumes may increase the effects of fluid shift. In addition, the core temperature rises faster than in adults for a given percentage loss in body mass. Bar-Or et al (1980) found that for a 1% loss in body mass in adults there was a 0.15°C increase in core temperature compared to a 0.28°C increase in children. During this study, in which children underwent a rest and exercise protocol for a total of 3 hours at a temperature of 39°C and 45% RH, dehydration was at a rate of 0.2–0.3% body mass $\cdot$ h^{-1}. A later study by Wilk et al (1994), however, found that both a grape flavoured water and grape flavoured sports drink prevented this progressive dehydration. The authors used these findings as evidence that the flavouring was the key factor and prevented dehydration in children. In fact, the body remained euhydrated with only a mild body mass loss of 0.32%. Of course, there are other factors such as palatability, mouth feel, temperature, colour and odour that will affect drinking patterns and there is wide inter-individual variation, but flavouring the drink ameliorated the dehydration.

Practical drinking solutions

1. Drinking recommendations should be focused mainly on fluid losses and less on electrolyte or carbohydrate replacements.
2. As children sweat less than adolescents, they will need less fluid, so if the environment is not too extreme a 0.75–1 L drink should be enough to keep hydrated.
3. Reminding and encouraging children to drink is very important and should be at a minimum able to satisfy their thirst.

4. Experiment with a variety of drinks including but not exclusively, sports drinks, but also diluted fruit-flavoured squash (cordial) drinks and items such as frozen fruit-flavoured icicles.
5. The greater the heat stress and the longer the exercise or match, the more important it is to drink fluids.
6. Avoid drinking large amounts of fluid at any one session, as this increases the feeling of 'fullness' in the stomach and can make it uncomfortable to continue playing. Smaller amounts every 15 min might be more appropriate.
7. Drinking approximately 300–400 mL 45 min before exercise or a match should ensure most children are adequately hydrated.

SUMMARY

It appears that under normal environmental conditions (20–25°C) children are as effective thermoregulators as adults, even though children rely more on convective heat loss. However, even though children have a smaller absolute surface area than adults, their surface area relative to their body mass is considerably greater than that of adults. Children will therefore experience heat transfer, which will become a major factor at the extremes of temperature. A greater stress will be placed on their thermoregulatory system because of their metabolic inefficiency producing more heat per body mass than adults and also having a lower cardiac output. This lower cardiac output will have consequences for the transfer of heat to the periphery. Additional limitations in sweat production further disadvantage children in the heat. The amount of sweat produced per gland is considerably less in children than in adults and is lower in prepubertal compared to circumpubertal and late pubertal children. Results from heat-activated sweat gland studies suggest that physical maturation is characterized by an enhanced sweat rate per body surface area and per gland that may be associated with increased sweat gland anaerobic metabolism. Although a lesser ability to sweat might be thought of as a disadvantage, this function does conserve water and perhaps protects a child from dehydration. This mechanism is also coupled with the fact that children require a greater core temperature to activate sweating.

Although there are fewer data available on the effects of cold temperature on children, the same principles apply. The greater surface area to body mass ratio will result in faster heat loss in children. Although children can compensate for exercising in cool temperatures by an increased peripheral vasoconstriction and higher metabolic heat production, this poses risks for children who are small and lean. In extreme cold, the enhanced peripheral vasoconstriction might result in frostbite.

KEY POINTS

1. The thermoregulatory system is regulated by the contributions of radiation, convection, conduction and evaporation, and the production of metabolic heat through physical activity to the heat balance equation.
2. Technological advances such as the use of infrared aural thermometry and telemetry pills may make studying thermoregulation in children less invasive and more practical. These techniques are as valid as traditional methods using rectal thermometry.
3. Children compared to adolescents and adults are able to sustain exercise in the heat providing temperatures are not extreme.

4. Children produce more heat relative to their body surface area, and have a lower sweating rate but a higher blood flow to the skin compared to adolescents and adults.
5. Children appear to utilize conductive processes more to lose heat over evaporative heat loss but during puberty this process begins to change with evaporative cooling dominating.
6. More studies are needed to conclusively define physiological responses in the heat. These studies should examine sex and maturational differences as well as ensuring the thermal load is equivalent; this is particularly important for studies of child–adult comparisons.
7. In air with temperatures as low as 5°C an increased peripheral vasoconstriction and heat production offsets some of the heat loss. Children, particularly those that are young and lean, are particularly disadvantaged in water because of the faster heat loss compared to air and the child's large surface area to body mass ratio. Hypothermia, frostbite and bronchoconstriction are all serious symptoms of an inability to respond to the cold environment.
8. Acclimation is generally slower compared to adults and it has been found that significant benefits can be attained from passive strategies as well as active ones. Guidelines recommend checking environmental temperatures, humidity and wind chill before exercising in the heat. Training intensity should be reduced and then built up gradually over a 2-week period.
9. Results from voluntary hydration studies in children mirror adult ones. Children often do not drink enough even when encouraged to do so. This situation is worse for children than adults as any degree of hypohydration results in a faster rise in their core temperature.
10. Drinks that have been flavoured appear to maintain euhydration status better than non-flavoured drinks. More studies are needed examining a wider range of exercise protocols, drink composition and environmental conditions.
11. Optimal flavours and content of electrolytes for children are not known at present but it is thought drinks that are more palatable and contain sodium will stimulate drinking. There are no good reasons for a normal healthy child to be ingesting salt tablets when exercising in the heat.

References

American Academy of Pediatrics Committee on Sports Medicine and Fitness 2000 Climatic heat stress and the exercising child and adolescent. Position statement. Pediatrics 106:158–159

Andersen G S, Mekjavic I B 1996 Thermoregulatory responses of circum-pubertal children. European Journal of Applied Physiology 74:404–410

Araki T, Toda Y, Matsushita K et al 1979 Age differences in sweating during muscular exercise. Japanese Journal of Physical Fitness and Sports Medicine 28:239–248

Araki T, Tsujita J, Matsushita K et al 1980 Thermoregulatory responses of prepubertal boys to heat and cold in relation to physical training. Journal of Human Ergonomics 9:69–80

Armstrong L E, Maresh C M, Castellani J W et al 1996 American College of Sports Medicine position stand: heat and cold illnesses during distance running. Medicine and Science in Sports and Exercise 28:i–x

Australian Sports Medicine Federation 1989 Guidelines for safety in children's sport. ASMF, Canberra ACT

Bar-Or O, Inbar O 1977 Relationship between perceptual and physiological changes during heat acclimatization in 8–10 year old boys. In: Lavallée H, Shephard R J (eds) Frontiers of activity and child health: Proceedings of the VIIth International Symposium of Paediatric Work Physiology. Editions du Pelican, Quebec, p 205–214

Bar-Or O, Dotan R, Inbar O et al 1980 Voluntary hypohydration in 10- to 12-yr-old boys. Journal of Applied Physiology 48:104–108

Bergeron M 2002 Playing tennis in the heat: can young players handle it? August 2002 www.acsm.org

Davies C T M 1981 Thermal responses to exercise in children. Ergonomics 24:55–61

Delamarche P, Bittel J, Lacour J R et al 1990 Thermoregulation at rest and during exercise in prepubertal boys. European Journal of Applied Physiology 6:436–440

Drinkwater B L, Kupprat J E, Denton J E et al 1977 Responses of prepubertal girls and college women to work in the heat. Journal of Applied Physiology 43:1046–1053

Ellis F P, Exton-Smith A N, Foster K G et al 1976 Eccrine sweating and mortality during heat waves in very young and very old persons. Israeli Journal of Medicine and Science 12:815–817

Falk B, Bar-Or O, Calvert R et al 1992a Sweat gland response to exercise in the heat among pre-, mid-, and late-pubertal boys. Medicine and Science in Sports and Exercise 24:313–319

Falk B, Bar-Or O, MacDougall J D 1992b Thermoregulatory responses of pre-, mid-, and late-pubertal boys to exercise in dry heat. Medicine and Science in Sports and Exercise 24:688–694

Falk B, Bar-Or O, MacDougall J D et al 1992c Longitudinal analysis of the sweating response or pre-, mid- and late pubertal boys during exercise in the heat. American Journal of Human Biology 4:527–535

Falk B, Bar-Eli M, Dotan R et al 1997 Physiological and cognitive responses to cold exposure in 11–12-year-old boys. American Journal of Human Biology 9:39–49

Houmard J A, Costill D L, Davis J A et al 1990 The influence of exercise intensity on heat acclimation in trained subjects. Medicine and Science in Sports and Exercise 5:615–620

Hubbard R W, Szlyk P C, Armstrong L E 1990 Influence of thirst and fluid palatability on fluid ingestion during exercise. In: Gisolfi C V, Lamb D R (eds) Perspectives on exercise science and sports medicine: Vol 3. Fluid homeostasis during exercise. Benchmark Press, Carmel CA, p 39–96

Inbar O, Bar-Or O, Dotan R et al 1981 Conditioning versus exercise in heat as methods for acclimatizing 8- to 10-yr-old boys to dry heat. Journal of Applied Physiology 50:406–411

Inbar O, Dotan R, Bar-Or O et al 1985 Passive versus active exposures to dry heat as methods of heat acclimatization in young children. In: Binkhorst R A, Kemper H C G, Saris W H M (eds) Children and exercise XI. Human Kinetics, Champaign IL, p 329–340

Klentrou P, Cunliffe M, Slack et al 2004 Temperature regulation during rest and exercise in the cold in premenarcheal and menarcheal girls. Journal of Applied Physiology 96:1393–1398

Mackova J, Sturmova M, Macek A 1984 Prolonged exercise in prepubertal boys in warm and cold environments. In: Ilmarinen J, Valimaki I (eds) Children and sport: paediatric work physiology. Springer, Berlin, p 135–141

Matsushita K, Araki T 1980 The effect of physical training on thermoregulatory responses of preadolescent boys to heat and cold. Journal of Physical Fitness in Japan 29:69–74

Meyer F, Bar-Or O 1994 Fluid and electrolyte loss during exercise: the paediatric angle. Sports Medicine 18:4–9

Meyer F, Bar-Or O, MacDougall J D et al 1992 Sweat electrolyte loss during exercise in the heat: effects of gender and maturation. Medicine and Science in Sports and Exercise 24:776–781

Noakes T 2001 IMMDA advisory statement on guidelines for fluid replacement during marathon running. Online. Available: http://www.aims-association.org/guidelines_for_fluid replacement.htm

Piekarski C, Morfeld P, Kampmann B et al 1986 Heat stress reactions of the growing child. In: Rutenfranz R, Mocellin R, Klimt F (eds) Children and exercise XII. Human Kinetics, Champaign, IL, p 403–412

Riveria-Brown A M, Gutierrez R, Gutierrez J C et al 1999 Drink composition, voluntary drinking, and fluid balance in exercising, trained, heat-acclimatized boys. Journal of Applied Physiology 86:78–84

Shinozaki T, Deane R, Perkins F M 1988 Infrared tympanic thermometer: evaluation of a new clinical thermometer. Critical Care Medicine 16:148–150

Sloan R E G, Keatinge W R 1973 Cooling rates of young people swimming in cold water. Journal of Applied Physiology 35:371–375

Smolander J, Bar-Or O, Korhonen O et al 1992 Thermoregulation during rest and exercise in the cold in pre- and early-pubescent boys and young men. Journal of Applied Physiology 72:1589–1594

Wagner J A, Robinson S, Tzankoff S P et al 1972 Heat tolerance and acclimization in the heat in relation to age. Journal of Applied Physiology 33:616–622

Wilk B, Bar-Or O 1996 Effect of drink flavour and NaCl on voluntary drinking and hydration in boys exercising in the heat. Journal of Applied Physiology 80:1112–1117

Wilk B, Bar-Or O 1997 Heat acclimation and sweating pattern in prepubertal boys. Pediatric Exercise Science 7:2

Wilk B, Meyer F, Bar-Or O 1994 Effect of electrolytes and carbohydrate drink content on voluntary drinking and fluid balance in children (abstract). Medicine and Science in Sports and Exercise 26:S205

Wilmore J H, Morton A R, Gilbey H J et al 1998 Role of taste preference on fluid intake during and after 90 min of running at 60% of $\dot{V}O_2$max in the heat. Medicine and Science in Sports and Exercise 30:587–595

Wilson R D, Knapp C, Traber D L et al 1971 Tympanic thermography: A clinical and research evaluation of a new technique. Southern Medical Journal 64:1452–1455

Further reading

Falk B 2000 Temperature regulation. In: Armstrong N, Van Mechelen W (eds) Paediatric exercise science and medicine. Oxford University Press, Oxford, p 223–239

Noakes T D 2002 Exercise and the cold. In: Reilly T, Greeves J (eds) Advances in sport, leisure and ergonomics. Routledge, London, p 13–31

Chapter **12**

Perceived exertion

Roger G. Eston and Gaynor Parfitt

CHAPTER CONTENTS

LEARNING OBJECTIVES

After studying this chapter you should be able to:

1. understand the basis of ratings of perceived exertion (RPE) and the theoretical interplay of the three effort continua
2. understand the need for the conceptual development of children's scales of perceived exertion
3. understand the difference between active and passive paradigms in the study of perceived exertion and the problems associated with comparing the results from different paradigms
4. understand the effect of intermittent and continuous protocols
5. understand methods of anchoring perceived exertion in children
6. encourage critical evaluation of the various scales of assessing perceived exertion in children
7. recognize the importance of practice in using effort perception in children.

INTRODUCTION

Humans possess a remarkable ability to sense the strain, aches and degree of effort and fatigue resulting from physical work. The pioneer who introduced the concept of perceived exertion together with methods of applying psychophysical principles to enable measurement of overall exertion, breathlessness and localized sensations of fatigue is Gunnar Borg. He described the perception of exertion as a kind of 'gestalt' or configuration of sensations of strain, aches and fatigue from the peripheral muscles and pulmonary system, along with other sensory cues (Borg 1998). Borg highlights that the antecedents of perceived exertion include the memory of exercise or physical work experiences and the emotions associated with them. However, due to the strong relationship with objective measures of exercise intensity such as power, work, speed and physiological factors such as heart rate (HR), ventilation and blood lactate, these antecedents are often forgotten. Therefore, in discussing scale development and utility, it is important for all relevant factors to be considered.

In this regard, Borg's original thesis is that subjective responses to an exercise stimulus involve three main effort continua – perceptual, physiological and perform-ance (Borg 1970). A number of more complex models of perceived exertion have been developed, although in essence these models have used the same three effort continua as the fundamental and underlying basis to explain the perception of physical exertion. For the purposes of this chapter, we will use this model to highlight how these three continua may interact to influence the rating of perceived exertion (RPE) in children (Fig. 12.1) and the degree to which different scales may accommodate specific elements. It is notable that Borg used the 'perceptual continuum' as the initial basis from which to explore the derivations of the ratings of perceived exertion. This is founded on the premise that perception plays a fundamental role in our behaviour and in how we adapt to a situation (Borg 1998). He also stressed that starting the inquiry from the perceptual continuum is fundamental since the meaning of a concept has to start from a person's subjective experience. This is a crucial factor for consideration

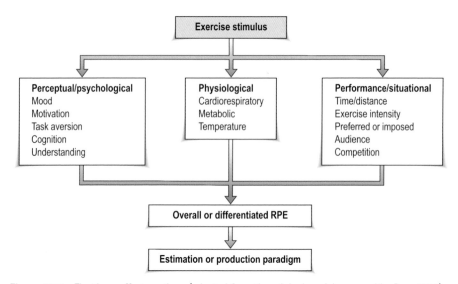

Figure 12.1   The three effort continua (adapted from the original model proposed by Borg 1970).

when attempting to compare, describe or apply the concept of perceived exertion in children.

The physiological continuum includes a wide variety of variables such as HR, blood lactate, oxygen uptake, respiratory frequency and rate of ventilation, among others. These factors are relatively easy to measure and may be characterized by different growth functions to the stimulus of exercise intensity. For example, HR and oxygen uptake are characterized by linear growth to increases in intensity as measured by power output (watts), whereas blood lactate concentration and rate of ventilation are characterized by a non-linear (positively accelerating) growth function.

The effect of the interplay of the perceptual continua and the unique patterns of physiological responses on the rating of perceived exertion will also be influenced by the situational characteristics of the performance. In this regard, one has to take into account the nature of the test and the environment in which it takes place. Maximal physiological testing has many variations, which may involve timed (short or long) incremental stages to exhaustion, the highest exercise intensity a subject can maintain for a specific period of time, the greatest distance one can cover in a given time period or the fastest one can cover a given distance. Submaximal performances may involve monitoring the time to exhaustion at a given exercise intensity, for example at a given percentage of maximal oxygen uptake or at an intensity corresponding to a ventilatory threshold reference point. Alternatively, the individual's preferred level of exercise intensity may be used in a work task, in which case the prior experience of the individual will impact upon the intensity selected. Consideration of the nature of the situation must also include the interaction of the subject with the tester (e.g. the RPE of some boys or 'macho' men may be influenced by the perceived attractiveness of the female experimenter), the expectations of the tester and the perceived expectations of the subject (e.g. the subject may think that the person supervising the test may expect a given response which is based on behavioural cues exhibited by the tester), and the conditions manipulated by the experimenter. These may include the provision of verbal or visual feedback during the experiment, the use of deception (e.g. deceiving the individual over time to end task or total distance completed or to be completed), the influence of audience, positive or negative feedback, or the influence of external distraction factors (e.g. music, noise from equipment, video display, etc.).

ESTIMATION AND PRODUCTION OF EFFORT (PASSIVE AND ACTIVE PARADIGMS)

The rating of perceived exertion can be employed using two different paradigms: passive (estimation) and active (production). These two paradigms place different demands upon the three effort continua (perceptual/psychological, physiological and performance/situational as indicated in Fig. 12.1) with memory of exercise experience particularly relevant in the active paradigm. Following an exercise situation, memory will degrade and this degraded memory will impact upon future active productions. In comparison, the passive paradigm is based upon the interpretation of current stimulation. The estimation paradigm requires the individual to provide a rating of perceived exertion in response to a request from the investigator to indicate how 'hard' the exercise feels at that moment in time. This information may then be used to compare responses between conditions after some form of intervention or to assist in the prescription of exercise intensity. In the active production paradigm, the individual is required to actively produce an intensity based upon his/her interpretation of effort sense and the cognition and understanding of the RPE prescribed.

Eston (1984) first proposed the application of this procedure for use as a complementary means of controlling exercise intensity in the endurance or cardio-vascular health component of secondary school physical education lessons. Although the idea was not empirically tested at the time, he proposed that it may be possible to teach an 'awareness of effort' to children to enhance understanding of the more objective measures of exercise intensity. In this way measures of metabolic demand could be compared at each RPE-derived exercise intensity. With few exceptions most studies on children, using a variety of RPE scales and measures of performance, provide evidence for the feasibility and validity of this procedure (e.g. Eston et al 1994, 2000, 2001, Lamb 1996, Lamb et al 1997, 2004, Robertson et al 2002, Williams et al 1991, 1994, Yelling et al 2002). Further detail on these studies is provided in a later section of this chapter. However, fundamental to the application of RPE in an active paradigm is the ability of the children to understand the scale.

PROBLEMS WITH ASSESSING PERCEIVED EXERTION

The application of an individual's RPE to facilitate the assessment and control of exercise intensity is well established, although the majority of the research in this area has been derived from studies on adults using the 6–20 Rating of Perceived Exertion Scale (Borg 1998). Research on the efficacy of using the RPE scales to assess and control exercise intensity in children is a relatively new area. The pioneering studies of Bar-Or (1977), using multistage cycle ergometry data on 1307 males aged 9–68 years of age attempted to address whether there were differences in the perception of exercise intensity in boys and men. He observed an age-related pattern in the ratio of RPE to percentage maximal HR (RPE/% HRmax), in which the ratio was lower in children than in adolescents, and even lower in comparison to adults. It was therefore con-cluded that exercising at the same physiological strain was perceived to be easier by children than by older individuals. However, more recent studies by Mahon et al (1997) contradict this finding. They observed that the RPE at the ventilatory threshold was no different compared to adults, and more recently that children's RPE was higher at this exercise intensity threshold (Mahon et al 2001). A noticeable finding in the study by Bar-Or (1977) was that the youngest group of 7- to 9-year-old gymnasts had a much higher rating than any other child or adolescent group. It is also worth noting that the correlation between HR and RPE in that group was lower than in the older groups. Bar-Or suggested that this might have been indicative of their inability to provide valid ratings at such a young age. Despite this observation, it is only recently that researchers have realized that adult-derived methods and applications of the RPE are not appro-priate for use with children. This has been the consensus of several critical reviews in the literature (e.g. Eston & Lamb 2000, Lamb & Eston 1997, Robertson 1997). As a consequence, a number of limited numerical-range and pictorial scales have been proposed to expand the age range at which ratings of perceived exertion can be used.

The following sections describe the development of these various scales and highlight their potential utility and limitations before discussing specific methodological issues.

DEVELOPMENT OF CHILD–SPECIFIC RATING SCALES

There have been important advances in the study of effort perception in children in the last 15 years. Despite observations that experience and maturity were important determinants for accurate perception of exercise intensity (Bar-Or 1977) little regard was given to the creation of a more developmentally appropriate scale using meaningful terminology and symbols until 1989. In the first attempt to provide a developmentally appropriate rating of perceived exertion scale, Nystad et al (1989) published an illustrated RPE Scale with all the written descriptors removed. Six stick figures corresponding to ratings of 6–7, 9–10, 11–12, 14–15, 16–17 and 19–20 depicted various stages of effort in a study of 10–12-year-old asthmatic children. Despite their attempts to improve the lucidity of the 6–20 RPE Scale for these children, it was apparent that the children continued to experience difficulty in interpreting the scale accurately. The investigators concluded that children lacked the physical experience and awareness of different exercise intensities, and therefore could not understand the concept of perceived exertion. A similar idea was adopted by Mutrie and colleagues, using caricatures at various stages of animation (see Eston & Lamb (2000) for a more detailed description of these and other scales).

The idea for a simplified perceived exertion scale which was more suitable for use with children emanated from the study by Williams et al (1991) on 40 boys and girls aged 11–14 years. In their study, although the children seemed to accept and under-stand the purpose of Borg's 6–20 RPE Scale, the authors asserted that a children's version of the scale would be more meaningful to this age group and younger age groups, and proposed the idea of a 1–10 scale anchored with more developmentally appropriate expressions of effort. This led to a significant development in the meas-urement of children's effort perception in 1994 with the publication of two papers which proposed and validated an alternative child-specific rating scale – the Children's Effort Rating Table (CERT) (Eston et al 1994, Williams et al 1994). Compared to the Borg Scale, the CERT (Fig. 12.2) has five fewer possible responses, a range of numbers (1–10) more familiar to children than the Borg 6–20 Scale and verbal expressions chosen by children as descriptors of exercise effort. This type of scale would of course facilitate the child's perceptual understanding and therefore the ability to use it in either a passive or active paradigm with greater reliability. The CERT initiative for a simplified scale containing more 'developmentally appropriate' numerical and verbal expressions led to the development of scales that combined numerical and pictorial ratings of perceived exertion scales. All of these scales depict four to five animated figures, portraying increased states of physical exertion. Like the CERT, the scales have embraced a similar, condensed numerical range and words or expressions that are either identical to (P-CERT, Yelling et al 2002), abridged from (CALER, Eston et al 2000, BABE, Eston et al 2001) or similar in context to the CERT (OMNI, Robertson 1997,

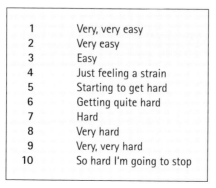

1	Very, very easy
2	Very easy
3	Easy
4	Just feeling a strain
5	Starting to get hard
6	Getting quite hard
7	Hard
8	Very hard
9	Very, very hard
10	So hard I'm going to stop

Figure 12.2 The Children's Effort Rating Table (from Williams et al 1994).

Robertson et al 2000). Due to the importance of the CERT in the advancement of the study of perceived exertion in children, the following section describes the derivation and validation of the CERT in some detail.

Derivation of CERT

The development of the CERT is described in more detail by Williams et al (1994) and is summarized here. The initial phase involved introducing several children aged 4–9 years to walking and running on a treadmill, stepping continuously on and off a 30 cm gymnasium bench, and pedalling a cycle ergometer in a laboratory environment. The children were questioned generally during the exercise about how it felt when the speed, tempo or resistance was varied particularly as it related to their interpretation of the Borg 6–20 Scale. Although the children had a rudimentary idea of the feelings that accompanied 'hard work', the authors noted that the children were generally puzzled by the RPE Scale. The next stage in the development of the CERT involved a field project entitled 'Exercise: how it makes you feel' with 257 children of similar age from two elementary schools in the Merseyside area of England. The children exercised in the playground by walking, running, skipping (jumping rope) at different speeds and time periods. As soon as the children returned to the classroom, they were encouraged to write about and draw pictures to depict their efforts and to discuss how the activities felt with the teachers and research group. A selection of words and expressions that the children used were then placed at each point on the 1–10 scale. The numerical range of the CERT reflects a conceptual model in which RPE and HR in the range of 100 to 200 bts · min^{-1} are assumed to be linearly related by the regression equation:

$$HR = 100 + 10x$$

where x is the CERT value reported at any one time.

The initial validation of the CERT involved estimation and production methods. In the estimation method, 112 children (four groups of 14 boys and 14 girls from age groups ~5, 6–7, 7–8 and 8–9 years) performed four 2 min stages of a step test at 25 steps per minute, with load increases corresponding to 0%, 5%, 10% and 20% of body mass added to a backpack. Perceived exertion was recorded in the final 15 s of each stage. The results for each age group are shown in Figure 12.3. The RPE:HR correlation (r) by grade was 0.73, 0.95, 0.99 and 0.99 for the ~5, 6–7, 7–8 and 8–9 year age groups, respectively. As can be seen from Figure 12.3, the increase in RPE was commensurate with the increase in exercise intensity and HR response, providing evidence of validity of the scale, particularly with regard to the three older age groups. The authors noted that the youngest age group did not respond as consistently and predictably as the older children. This was attributed to their phase of cognitive development. The authors reported that exercise for this group is typically characterized by spontaneous movement of varying levels of activity necessary for play. It was recognized that at this early stage of development, physical activity is perceived as 'go' (perceived as 'easy') or 'stop' (perceived as 'hard').

The production method of validation of the CERT was somewhat limited in the original study by Williams et al (1994). Using the lines of best fit for the HR:RPE in the estimation trial, the authors compared the predicted HR response to the actual HR response elicited at randomized CERT values of 5 and 7 in the three older age groups. Whilst stepping, the child instructed the tester to add weight to the backpack until it

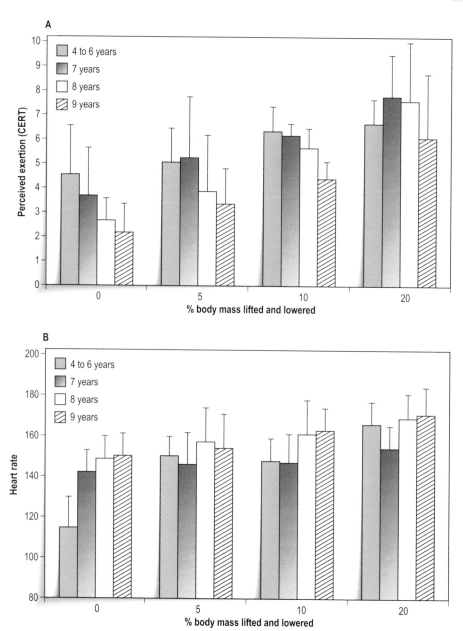

Figure 12.3   Perceived exertion (A) and heart rate (B) for stepping exercise with increased external loading in children aged 5–9 years. Values are mean ± SD.

was felt that the randomized intensity level of 5 or 7 was reached. HR was then recorded at the end of a further minute of stepping at this level. The authors reported no significant association between the predicted HR from the estimation protocol and the HR elicited in the production protocol. The authors reported that the lack of association was a reflection of the children's inability to produce the predicted HR response. As noted by Williams et al (1994), it is important to note the limitations of comparing physiological responses from passive estimation tasks with the responses from effort production (active) tasks. The problems with this procedure have already been highlighted (Eston & Lamb 2000). Caution is recommended when interpreting the results from studies that have adopted an estimation-production paradigm, such as in the study by Williams et al (1994). As indicated earlier, the process of using perceptions of effort to actively self-regulate exercise intensity levels using predetermined RPEs is not the same as that used to passively appraise exercise intensity. Nevertheless, it can be seen from Figure 12.4 that the children in the study of Williams et al (1994) could indeed use the randomized CERT 5 and 7 values to produce correspondingly higher exercise intensities.

Support for a 1–10 scale

Another study explored the notion of using the CERT to control exercise intensity in young children (Eston et al 1994), and is worthy of comment here. In this study, 16 boys and girls aged 9–10 years performed three separate exercise tests on a mechanically braked cycle ergometer. The initial test was a graded exercise test with HR and perceived exertion (CERT) recorded in response to a graded exercise test incremented by 10–25 W over a series of 4 min stages. The children subsequently performed two production tests at randomized CERT values of 5, 7 and 9. The tests were separated by several days.

The results from the study by Eston et al (1994) were encouraging and provided strong supporting evidence for the validity of a simplified perceived exertion scale to regulate the intensity of exercise during structured activity. The correlations (*r*) between HR:CERT and power output:CERT during the estimation test were 0.76 and 0.75, respectively. The exercise intensities and HRs produced by the children at CERT

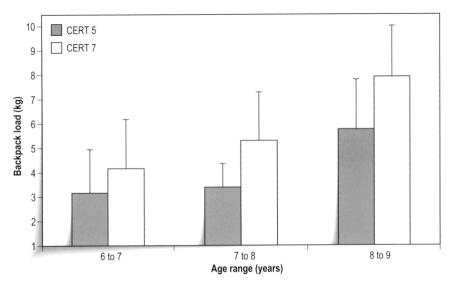

Figure 12.4 Average backpack load (± SD) produced at randomized CERT values of 5 and 7 during a 1 min step test. Data from the study of Williams et al (1994).

levels 5, 7 and 9 correlated well with those estimated for the corresponding CERT levels in the estimation test (stage I) for power output, $r = 0.84$, 0.89 and 0.91; for HR $r = 0.65$, 0.78 and 0.79 for all subjects. However, both power output and HR values were 13–18% lower in stage II compared to the expected values predicted from stage I. The authors attributed this apparent 'underestimation' or rather 'underproduction' of the task to the difference in the psychophysical processes involved: the reproduction of a given exercise effort from memory is not the same as estimating exercise intensity during ongoing exercise. It was also noted that the production of a given effort may be influenced by the sequence of the perceptual regulators of exercise intensity (CERT). Those subjects required (by random selection) to produce levels of effort from low to high may be more successful than other subjects required to produce effort from high to low.

An important observation from this study was the high degree of repeatability of the production task between stages II and III. An intraclass correlation of 0.91 for power output values provided evidence that the CERT could be used to reliably regulate exercise intensity. This is particularly notable as the production tasks were randomized and could not therefore be attributed to expectation or order effects.

The CERT is recognized as a notable advancement in the study of paediatric effort perception (Robertson 1997). Studies that have compared the CERT to the 6–20 RPE during stepping in children aged 5–9 years (Williams et al 1993) and during cycling exercise in children aged 8–11 years (Lamb 1996) and 10–11 years (Leung et al 2002) provided further support for the CERT. The latter study on 69 Chinese children, which assessed the concurrent validity and the reliability of a Chinese-translated (Cantonese) version of the Borg 6–20 RPE and the CERT, observed that the correlations for CERT, power output, HR and oxygen uptake were consistently higher than those for the 6–20 RPE Scale. They also reported higher reliabilities (intraclass correlations, ICCs) for the CERT (0.96 vs. 0.89) derived from two continuous, incremental cycling tests.

PICTORIAL RATINGS OF PERCEIVED EXERTION SCALES

Pictorial versions of the CERT

As indicated earlier, several pictorial versions of the CERT have been developed and tested. The first illustrated version of the scale was piloted in a study to assess whether young children could reliably regulate exercise intensity production after several practice trials, without reference to objective feedback measures (Eston et al 2000). Figure 12.5 presents a child pulling a cart that is loaded progressively with bricks (Cart and Load Effort Rating, CALER, Scale).

The number of bricks in the cart is commensurate with numbers on the scale. The verbal descriptors are selected from the CERT to accompany some of the categories of effort.

In the study by Eston et al (2000), 20 children aged 7–10 years performed four intermittent, incremental effort production tests at CALER 2, 5 and 8 over a 4-week period. To reach the specific CALER level the child instructed the experimenter, in the first 2–3 min, to adjust the cycling resistance by adding or taking away weights, available in units of 0.1, 0.5 and 1.0 kg units. Sight of the cradle was obscured by a copy of the CALER Scale so that the child could not see the loads added or removed from the cradle. On each trial, the child worked at each of the three CALER levels for 3 min, with a 2.5 min rest between each bout. This was repeated on three further

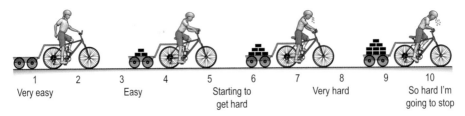

1	2	3	4	5	6	7	8	9	10
Very easy		Easy		Starting to get hard		Very hard			So hard I'm going to stop

Figure 12.5 The Cart and Load Effort Rating Scale. (From Eston R G, Parfitt G, Campbell L et al 2000 Reliability of effort perception for regulating exercise intensity in children using a Cart and Load Effort Rating (CALER) scale. *Pediatric Exercise Science* 12(4), page 390, Figure 1. © 2000 by Human Kinetics Publishers, Inc. Reprinted with permission from Human Kinetics (Champaign, IL).)

occasions in the next 4 weeks. An increase in power output across trials (44, 65 and 79 W at CALER 2, 5 and 8, respectively) confirmed that the children understood the scale. A Bland & Altman (1995) limits of agreement (LoA) analysis and an ICC analysis between trials (T) indicated that reliability improved with practice. Inter-trial comparisons of overall reliability from T1 to T2 and from T3 to T4 ranged from 0.76 to 0.97 and an improvement in the overall bias ±95% limits of agreement from −12 (19) W to 0 (10) W. This study was the first to apply more than two repeated effort production trials in young children and provides strong evidence that practice improves the reliability of effort perception in children of this age. The data also provided preliminary evidence for the validity of the CALER Scale in children aged 7–10 years.

The Bug and Bag Effort (BABE) Scale, introduced at the International Society of Sport Psychology conference in 2001 (Fig. 12.6, Eston et al 2001), depicts a cartoon bug-like character at various stages of exertion stepping up and down on a bench. The character carries a backpack that is progressively loaded with rocks. Like the CALER, the number of coloured rocks in the backpack is commensurate with numbers on the linear scale. The limited verbal descriptors are also the same as those used for the CALER Scale.

Preliminary validity data for the BABE Scale, and the intermodal validity of the CALER, were reported by Eston et al (2001). In their study, three groups of six children (7–10 years) were randomly allocated to one of three groups, CERT, BABE or CALER. They performed three separate intermittent effort production protocols, at least 1 week but no greater than 2 weeks apart, which involved stepping up and down on a bench (0.30 m high) for 2–3 min at a rate of 25 steps per minute. Bouts were separated by 5 min rest. Exercise intensities were adjusted by loading a backpack fitted to the subject. Backpack loads were calculated according to 0, 5, 10, 15, 20 and 25% of body weight. The exercise intensity was adjusted to randomize effort rating levels of 3, 5 and 8. Whilst stepping, the child asked the tester to add weight to the backpack until they reported the target rating. When the child reported that the target rating had been reached, the stepping was continued for a further minute and HR and power output were recorded at the end of this period. Effort production was confirmed in each child within 2–3 min.

An increase in power output across both trials at randomized ratings of 2, 5 and 8 confirmed that the children understood the scale. A limits of agreement (LoA) analysis and an ICC analysis on HR between trials (T) also indicated that reliability improved with practice for the CERT (T1–T2 = 0.78, T2–T3 = 0.81) and BABE (T1–T2 = 0.81, T2–T3 = 0.87). Although the values for the CALER did not show improvement across trials, they were nevertheless very high (T1–T2 = 0.91, T2–T3 = 0.87).

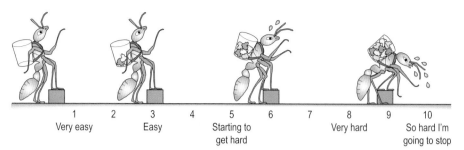

1	2	3	4	5	6	7	8	9	10
Very easy		Easy		Starting to get hard			Very hard		So hard I'm going to stop

Figure 12.6 The Bug and Bag Effort (BABE) Scale. (From Eston & Lamb 2000, Figure 1.9.10 (p. 89), by permission of Oxford University Press.)

More recently, the same group of investigators have evaluated the validity and reliability of the CALER and BABE Scales for intra- and intermodal regulation of effort production in a triple repeated, randomized, intermittent, production paradigm using cycling and stepping protocols (Parfitt et al in press). In this study, 30 boys and girls, aged 7–11 years were randomly allocated into a CALER or BABE group. Each group performed a discontinuous effort production protocol on six occasions, 1 week apart. For both the CALER and BABE groups, the first three trials were on a cycle ergometer. The second three trials consisted of a stepping protocol with and without a loaded backpack. All children were tested individually. Immediately prior to each effort production trial, the child was refamiliarized with either the CALER Scale (group 1) or BABE Scale (group 2) and given standard instructions concerning its use and the purpose of the test.

On each of the six production trials, the child was instructed to regulate exercise intensity on a cycle ergometer to match a range of three randomly presented effort production levels of 3, 5 and 8. For the cycling task, the child instructed the experimenter to adjust the cycling resistance (to add or subtract weights in multiples of 0.1, 0.5 or 1.0 kg units), in accordance with the specified perceived levels. A shield was placed to hide the weights being applied to the basket. For the stepping protocol, the backpack loads were calculated according to 0, 5, 10, 15, 20 and 25% body mass (Eston et al 2001, Williams et al 1993). For both the cycling and stepping protocols, the exercise intensity was adjusted by instruction from the child to the investigator to add or remove weights in the first 2 min until the child was confident that the randomly assigned effort rating level of 3, 5 or 8 was attained. The child then exercised for a further minute. HR was recorded at the end of the third minute. Exercise bouts at RPEs 3, 5 and 8 were interspersed with a 2.5 min rest period.

For both scales, used in both modes of exercise, the increase in power output and HR at RPE levels 3, 5 and 8 confirmed that the children understood the effort rating scales. This is exemplified in Figure 12.7, which shows the average HRs generated at ratings of 3, 5 and 8 in the CALER group whilst cycling. Similar results were observed for stepping, although the average HR produced was significantly lower by about 5 bts · min^{-1}. There were no differences in the HR response between the CALER and BABE groups. Thus, when the children were instructed to exercise at randomized intensities of 3, 5 and 8, the HR response was not influenced by which scale was used. This was true for the cycling and stepping tasks.

The ICC for HR at the three RPE levels (3, 5, 8) for the CALER and BABE groups across trials for cycling and stepping demonstrated good reliability. For cycling, the ICCs between T2 and T3 (0.81–0.90) were higher than between T1 and T2 (0.74–0.84)

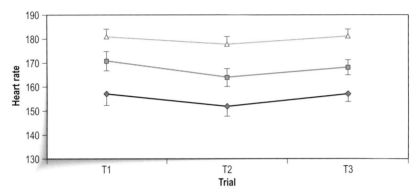

Figure 12.7 Average heart rate generated at ratings of 3, 5 and 8 in the CALER group whilst cycling. Values are mean ± SEM. (From Parfitt et al, in press.)

across the three RPE levels for both groups. The overall ICCs for cycling were highest in the BABE group (0.90). For the stepping task, the ICCs show highly reliable HR production at all RPE levels for both the CALER and BABE groups (>0.84).

Results from the study by Parfitt et al (in press) provide evidence that children aged 7–11 years were able to regulate exercise efforts during intermittent cycling and stepping tasks (with randomized order of levels) by applying their understanding of the CALER or BABE Scale. The general trend of increasing reliability across trials concurs with the results of earlier effort production studies using the CALER Scale (Eston et al 2000), described above. In this study, the authors highlighted the importance of using three or more trials to enhance the reliability of producing exercise efforts in children aged 7–10 years during intermittent cycle ergometry tasks.

This study also indicated that the CALER and BABE Scales, which are pictorially quite different, could be used interchangeably to produce equivalent physiological intensities during cycling and stepping exercise. The results suggest that either of the two scales may be used for these activities in children aged 7–11 years – i.e., they are 'intermodal'. To some extent, these results question the necessity of developing multiple mode-specific pictorial scales, which have appeared in the literature in the last 5 years.

With regard to preference of a particular scale, previous validation work on the BABE and CALER Scale has observed that children preferred the BABE Scale (Eston et al 2001). Most of the children were disappointed not to be assigned to a BABE group. The BABE Scale was developed to appeal to children, particularly as it contained characters that were similar to characters depicted in the Walt Disney film 'A Bug's Life', the central characters of which were familiar to most children at the time of scale development. During informal discussions it was indicated that reasons for their preferred choice were that the scale was 'fun-looking' and 'interesting' due to the use of colours, and the character association with a recent hit movie which all participants were familiar with. This does of course beg the question as to how 'fun-looking' and 'interesting' the scale would be to 7–11-year-old children 5 years on when the character is potentially not as popular.

A further pictorial version of the CERT (P-CERT), initially described by Eston & Lamb (2000), has been validated for both effort estimation and effort production tasks during stepping exercise in adolescents (Fig. 12.8, Yelling et al 2002). The scale depicts a child running up a 45° stepped gradient at five stages of exertion, corresponding to CERT ratings of 2, 4, 6, 8 and 10. All the verbal descriptors from the original CERT are included in the scale.

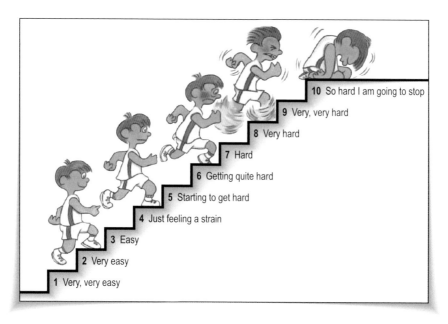

Figure 12.8   The pictorial CERT. (From Eston & Lamb 2000, Figure 1.9.7 (p. 88), by permission of Oxford University Press.)

Yelling first proposed the P-CERT at a perceived exertion symposium in 1999. The scale had immediate appeal and was considered to be a significant improvement on the CERT. To facilitate the development of the P-CERT, Yelling et al (2002) employed a similar strategy to that used in the development of the CERT (Williams et al 1994) by engaging the children (48 boys and girls aged 12–15 years) in a series of play and running activities. Throughout the lessons the children were asked to focus on the exercise sensations of breathlessness, body temperature and muscle aches. Immediately after the lesson, the children were presented with a copy of the CERT in the form of a stepped gradient and five pictorial descriptors and asked to locate the positions which best reflected their own perceptions of effort. The frequency with which the children positioned the visual character at given points along the scale was recorded and the most commonly chosen format was selected, resulting in the pictorial scale above.

The validity of the P-CERT was determined in a separate group of 48 similarly aged boys and girls in two exercise trials separated by 7–10 days (Yelling et al 2002). In trial 1, the children completed five 3 min incremental stepping exercise bouts interspersed with 2 min recovery periods. HR and RPE were recorded in the final 15 s of each bout. They observed that perceived exertion increased as exercise intensity increased. This was also reflected by simultaneous significant increases in HR. In trial 2, the children were asked to regulate their exercise intensity during four intermittent 4 min bouts of stepping to match randomly assigned ratings of perceived exertion at 3, 5, 7 and 9. Bouts were separated by a 2 min recovery period. The desired step height and frequency were determined in the first 2 min of the 4 min exercise bout by verbal feedback from the child. HR and power output were recorded in the last 15 s of each bout. The HR and power output produced at each of the four prescribed effort levels were also significantly different. Yelling et al (2002) concluded that the children could discriminate between the four different exercise intensities and regulate their exercise intensity according to the four prescribed ratings from the P-CERT.

OMNI Scale

In recognition of the advantages of using a comparatively narrow numerical range to assess perceived exertion, such as that used in the CERT, Robertson proposed the idea of using pictorial descriptors along the scale for assessing perceived exertion in children (Robertson 1997). As part of a special symposium on effort perception at the European Pediatric Work Physiology Conference in 1997, he presented the idea for a 1–10 pictorial scale (now 0–10) which would be applicable to variations in race, gender and health status, hence the term Omni Scale (Fig. 12.9). His original idea was to employ 'pictorially interfaced cognitive anchoring procedures, eliminating the need for mode-specific maximal exercise tests to establish congruence between stimulus and response ranges' (Robertson 1997, p. 35). However, since then, a number of different pictorial scales have been validated for various modes of exercise in children, for example cycling (Robertson et al 2000), walking/running (Utter et al 2002) and stepping (Robertson et al 2005). Robertson and colleagues have also proposed 'adult' versions of the OMNI Scale for resistance exercise and cycling, although we are sceptical as to the necessity for developing such pictorial scales given the well-established validity of the Borg 6–20 RPE and Category-ratio scales of perceived exertion. The original idea behind the development of pictorial scales was to accommodate the cognitive ability of children. In other words, it was to simplify the cognitive demands placed on the child. This is not necessary in normal adults.

In the original OMNI validation study described by Robertson et al (2000), four equal groups of 20 healthy African-American and white boys and girls aged 8–12 years performed a continuous, incremental exercise test on a cycle ergometer. Exercise intensities were increased by 25 W every 3 min. Differentiated (chest and legs) and

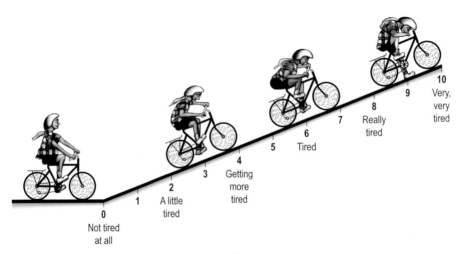

Figure 12.9 The OMNI perceived exertion scale. (From Robertson R J, Goss F L, Boer N F et al 2000 Children's OMNI scale of perceived exertion: mixed gender and race validation. *Medicine and Science in Sports and Exercise* 32(2):452–458, with permission of Lippincott, Williams & Wilkins.)

undifferentiated (whole body) RPE, HR and oxygen uptake were monitored in the final minute of each test stage. The authors reported similarly high positive linear associations between HR, oxygen uptake and RPE for each gender/race cohort of children. The r values for the entire cohort ranged from 0.85 to 0.94 for the relationships between RPE, HR and oxygen uptake. The RPE for the legs was significantly higher than the chest RPE and overall RPE values.

This study formed the basis for a number of subsequent validation studies with various forms of the OMNI (see above), forming a popular publication theme in *Medicine and Science in Sports and Exercise*, particularly. These studies include data on the validity of the children's OMNI Scale to self-regulate exercise intensity during cycling (Robertson et al 2002), which is described later.

Although they were developed independently, there are marked similarities between the P-CERT and the OMNI Scale. With the exception of the '0' starting point on the OMNI Scale, there is the same limited range of numbers, a linear gradient and culturally familiar verbal cues derived from common verbal expressions used by the children in the two respective countries (UK and USA) to describe their feelings of exertion.

With regard to the specificity of the verbal anchors, it is important to note that the original derivation and validation of the CERT was based on children aged 5–9 years of age in the UK, whereas the OMNI was based on children aged 8–12 years of age in the USA. This difference in maturational status and cognitive development, in addition to cultural semantics and socioeconomic status, should be taken into account regarding the differences in terminology that were originally derived for the two scales.

The common cue throughout the OMNI Scale is 'tired', the degree of which is indicated by various adverbs: 0 – not tired at all, 2 – a little tired, 4 – getting more tired, 6 – tired, 8 – really tired, 10 – very, very tired. In the initial validation of the scale, this trunk word appeared 475 times out of a total of 1582 verbal expressions (Robertson et al 2000). Conversely, the verbal cues derived for use in the CERT describe degrees of exertion according to various levels of being 'easy' or 'hard' to the extent that the exercise becomes so hard that the child will stop ('so hard I am going to stop'). The appropriateness of the latter term is supported by frequent observations by the authors that young children will often stop exercising when it becomes too uncomfortable. Sometimes, there is little pre-warning of this occurrence.

The connotations of the wording in the two scales are quite distinct. In this regard, the OMNI Scale assumes a baseline level of 'tiredness' from the starting point of 0. From a purely semantic and literal perspective, feeling 'tired' is a term used to describe a general condition or state of fatigue, weariness or sleepiness rather than effort. It is not an indication of exertion. Anchoring the scale around the central condition of varying states of 'feeling tired' could be perceived as portraying a negative perspective on the feelings experienced during physical activity, such as that experienced in children's play. Indeed, feeling tired is a common psychological barrier to engaging in physical activity. We therefore feel that the use of this term to describe states of physical exertion is somewhat inapt. It is notable that the more recent adult versions of the OMNI Scale, developed initially for resistance exercise and later to be re-illustrated for cycling, utilize the terms 'easy' and 'hard'. The authors did not divulge the rationale for changing the terminology in the adult scales, although we are of the opinion that these terms are much better suited for purpose. These are the terms used in the CERT.

Independent validation of P-CERT and OMNI

In recognition of the dearth of data for the OMNI walking/running scale (Utter et al 2002) and the P-CERT in young children (Yelling et al 2002), Roemmich et al (2006) have recently validated the two scales for submaximal exercise. In their study, 51 boys and girls aged 11–12 years performed a perceptual estimation paradigm, comprising a five-stage incremental treadmill test to elicit about 85% of the HRmax. Increases in the P-CERT and OMNI Scale were correlated with increases in oxygen uptake ($r = 0.90$ and $r = 0.92$) and HR ($r = 0.89$ and $r = 0.92$), respectively. There was no difference in the slopes of the P-CERT and OMNI scores when regressed against HR or oxygen uptake. There was also no difference in the percentage of maximal P-CERT and OMNI at each exercise stage. In effect, the results showed that the two scales could be used with equal validity. This result is not that surprising since the scales utilize basically the same number range. This observation raises the question as to where the child's focus of attention is based. Is it mainly based on the number scale, the figures, or equally combined between the two? If attention is focused primarily on the limited number range, it perhaps questions the need for pictorial scales of perceived exertion for children of this age range.

Other more recent pictorial scales

Curvilinear scale

All the pictorial scales developed so far to assess the relationship between perceived exertion and exercise intensity in children have used either a horizontal line or one that has a linear slope. We are currently exploring the notion of using a pictorial curvilinear scale, which is similar in construction to that shown in Figure 12.10. Our rationale for exploring the use of such a scale is founded on its inherently obvious face validity. As noted previously (Eston & Lamb 2000), it is readily conceivable that a child will recognize from previous learning and experience that the steeper the hill, the harder it is to ascend. This may also be helpful in the process of 'anchoring' effort perceptions

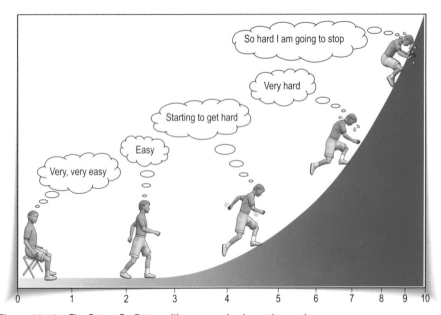

Figure 12.10   The Eston–Parfitt curvilinear perceived exertion scale.

(see later). Further, given the indisputable evidence that ventilation is a physiological mediator for respiratory-metabolic signals of exertion during endurance exercise, and given that this variable rises in a curvilinear fashion with equal increments in work rate, we propose that a curvilinear gradient may be more ecologically valid.

For the initial development of this scale, 20 children aged 8–11 years were requested to place a sitting figure and four ambulatory figures on a progressively increasing gradient. The figures were stylized to represent different stages of exertion and the children located them according to where they perceived they should be on the gradient. The area under the gradient is also filled by progressively darker shades of red. We believe that the face validity of this scale is self-evident. Preliminary studies in our laboratory have shown that children can use the scale to self-regulate exercise intensities at RPE levels of 2, 5 and 8. On six separate occasions, separated by at least 1 and no more than 2 weeks, the children were requested to bench step for 3 min at an exercise intensity corresponding to RPEs of 2, 5 and 8, in that order, without reference to objective feedback measures. The protocol was continuous. Intraclass correlations of HRs collected in the last 15 s of each 3 min bout revealed good potential for the reliability of repeat effort productions across the six trials with values of 0.71, 0.75 and 0.76 for RPEs of 2, 5 and 8, respectively. Research to explore the acceptability and validity of variations of this scale with children is recommended.

Dalhousie Leg Fatigue Scale

In recognition of the difficulties in interpreting the Borg 6–20 RPE Scale, Pianosi & colleagues (personal communication) have recently explored the utility of a 'leg fatigue scale' in both adults and children (Fig. 12.11). This novel scale depicts seven figures in various states of exertion. In each figure the legs are highlighted in an attempt to portray how the legs feel. For example, the illustrations utilize the analogies of the legs feeling like wood, lead and spaghetti at the higher exertion levels to depict the various perceptions of localized fatigue. At the present time, there are no validity data on this scale, although the authors report that it appears to be preferred in comparison to the Borg 6–20 Scale in children aged 11–14 years.

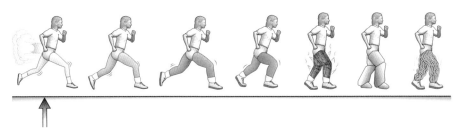

Figure 12.11   The Dalhousie Leg Fatigue Scale. Note the analogies of the legs feeling like wood, lead and spaghetti at the higher levels of exertion to depict the various perceptions of localized fatigue. (Reproduced with permission of Paul Pianosi and Pat McGrath.)

METHODOLOGICAL CONSIDERATIONS

Anchoring effort perceptions

Whatever scale is used, it is important to provide the child with an understanding of the range of sensations that correspond to categories of effort within the scale. This is known as 'anchoring'. There are three ways by which perceptual anchoring may be accomplished – from memory, by definition or from actual physical experience. The memory method requires the child to remember the easiest and hardest experiences of exercise and use these as the anchor values on the scale. The 'definition' method involves the experimenter defining the anchors with terms such as 'the lowest effort imaginable' for the low anchor or the 'greatest effort imaginable' as the high anchor. The third method (experience) allows the child to physically experience a range of perceptual anchors. Eston & Lamb (2000) stated that the experiential method is the best of the three methods. They recommended that the child should be exposed to a range of intensities that can be used to set the perceptual anchor points at 'low' and 'high' levels. This can be achieved during habituation to the test or exercise procedures. They recommended that, following a warm-up, the child should be allowed to experience exercise that is perceived as being 'hard' or 'very hard'. To avoid fatigue, a period of time should be allowed to regain full recovery.

However, a recent study by Lamb et al (2004) has questioned this assertion. In their study, 41 boys and girls aged 11–13 years, randomly assigned to either an experiential anchor group or a non-anchor group, undertook two identical production-only trials (three 3 min cycle ergometer bouts at randomized CERT levels 3, 6 and 8). Before each trial, the anchor group received an experiential exercise trial to provide a frame of reference for their perceived exertions, at levels 2, 1 and 9, in that order. The authors reported slightly better test–retest reproducibility (ICC) for HR and power output in the non-anchor group, with values ranging from 0.86 to 0.93 and 0.81 to 0.95, respectively. A 95% limits of agreement analysis indicated no marked differences between the two groups in the amount of bias and within-subject error. The implementation of an experiential anchoring protocol therefore had no positive effect on the reproducibility of the children's ability to self-regulate exercise using prescribed CERT levels.

Comparing different experimental paradigms

An underlying problem concerning the interpretation of data from studies on perceived exertion in children is the wide variation in methodology and procedures used. Problems associated with comparing data from estimation, production, continuous and intermittent procedures have been discussed previously (Eston & Lamb 2000, Robertson et al 2002). Most investigations have studied perceived exertion in children using a passive estimation process (perceptual estimation paradigm). In these studies the RPEs are typically compared against such measures as HR, power output or oxygen uptake. Most studies have also used a continuous testing protocol in preference to intermittent testing protocols. For example, the CERT was validated using a single continuous perceptual estimation paradigm in which the work rates were incremented by 10–25 W, depending on age, every 4 min to CERT 9 or 10 (Eston et al 1994). The OMNI was validated using a similar procedure (Robertson et al 2000).

If the relationship between perceived exertion and exercise intensity in children is robust, it should be possible to utilize the RPE to control exercise intensity. However, relatively few studies have applied effort production procedures in which young children are requested to self-regulate exercise intensity to match prescribed effort ratings. One of the problems with studies that have examined the ability of children to self-regulate exercise intensity is the use of various methodologies. These include estimation-production paradigms and repeat-production paradigms.

In the estimation-production paradigm, expected or derived values of objective intensity measures derived from a previous estimation trial are compared to values produced during a subsequent exercise trial(s) in which the child actively self-regulates exercise intensity levels using predetermined RPEs (e.g. Eston et al 1994, Robertson et al 2002). With the exception of the latter study, most studies have observed that children ranging in age from 8 to 14 years are not very good at self-regulating exercise intensity to produce prescribed target RPEs, when these are based on passive estimation tests. In other words, there is a lack of 'prescription congruence' (Robertson et al 2002). In the two studies by Eston et al (1994) and Robertson et al (2002), the perceptual production mode was performed on two occasions to assess the reliability of effort production. A direct comparison of the two studies is difficult, as the paradigms employed different exercise formats (continuous vs. intermittent) and perceived exertion scales (CERT vs. OMNI). As indicated earlier, Eston et al (1994) reported that power output and HR were lower in the production trial than those predicted from the estimation trial (at CERT RPEs 5, 7 and 9), whereas Robertson et al (2002) reported no differences (at OMNI 2 and 6). However, in terms of the ability to reproduce a given exercise intensity from two production trials, the results from the two studies provide limited evidence that children could reliably produce a given effort (HR) when requested to exercise at a given RPE. Further research is required in this area.

The assessment of perceived exertion using a repeat-production paradigm examines a child's ability to discern between different target RPEs while self-regulating exercise intensity on more than one occasion (e.g. Eston et al 2000, 2001, Lamb 1996, Lamb et al 1997). Studies by Eston & colleagues (2000, 2001) are the only ones to apply three or more repeated effort production trials in young children (7–10 years). The increase in ICCs between paired comparisons of the successive production trials in both studies support the importance of practice. For example, in the 2000 study, the ICCs improved from 0.76 to 0.97 and the overall bias ±95% limits of agreement from –12 (19) W to 0 (10) W. These data provide the strongest evidence available to date to demonstrate that practice improves the reliability of effort perception in children of this age.

Lamb et al (1997) used a production-only paradigm to assess the influence of a continuous and intermittent exercise protocol on the relationship between perceived exertion (CERT) in children aged 9–10 years. Common to both groups was the requirement to regulate exercise intensity to match a range of four randomly presented effort rating levels (3, 5, 7 and 9). The children were allowed 2 min to settle on the appropriate resistance before cycling for a further 1 min at the prescribed RPE. For subjects allocated to the discontinuous group, each bout was separated by a 3 min rest period. The provision of 3 min recovery periods between exercise bouts produced higher relationships between CERT and HR ($r = 0.66$ and $r = 0.46$, for the intermittent and continuous protocol, respectively). HRs tended to be lower in the discontinuous protocol. These results indicate that children may be more able to use effort ratings to control exercise intensity when the exercise is intermittent, rather than continuous in nature.

A study to compare the effects of an intermittent versus continuous incremental exercise protocol on perceived exertion using a passive estimation paradigm on the same group of children has yet to be conducted. However, we have limited data to suggest that an intermittent protocol may be preferred.

Figure 12.12 shows the HR and RPEs during a graded exercise test to exhaustion in an 8-year-old boy. The first three data points are the responses to a continuous protocol in which the treadmill speed and gradient were 8 km · h⁻¹ and 0% at 4 min, 8 km · h⁻¹ and 2% at 7 min, and 8 km · h⁻¹ and 4% at 10 min, respectively. At the point of increasing the gradient at the end of the 10th minute, the boy expressed a wish to stop the test. He'd had enough! After a brief period (1–2 min) of rest and reassurance, the protocol was modified to 2 min bouts with 2 min recovery, starting at 8 km · h⁻¹ at 2%, and increasing by 2% gradient for each bout. The intermittent nature of the protocol is shown by the HR response in Figure 12.12. Although these data are limited, they show a clearly different perceived exertion response to the continuous and discontinuous protocols. The perceived exertion response was higher at a given HR during the continuous protocol. For this boy, the intermittent protocol was preferable. This is perhaps to be expected as this type of protocol reflects the intermittent activity pattern that characterizes children's play activity.

On the basis of the limited data available on perceived exertion in young children, further research is recommended. As exemplified above, it would appear that there

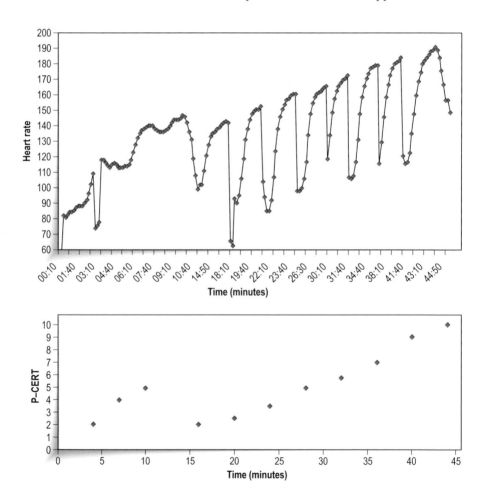

Figure 12.12   A comparison of perceived exertion (P-CERT) and heart rate during a continuous and intermittent graded exercise test to exhaustion in an 8-year-old clinically normal boy.

are some problems with comparing perceived exertion data from studies that have used passive, continuous, estimation trials with studies that have employed active, intermittent, production trials. Furthermore, most of the studies that have used intermittent protocols have been incremental in nature. Most of our understanding of children's effort perceptions has evolved from measuring responses to a situation in which they realize that the exercise is getting progressively harder. Few studies have randomized the order of exercise intensities. Future investigations into children's effort perception should consider these factors.

SUMMARY

Given the importance of encouraging physical activity in children, studies on the accuracy and reliability of effort perception in this population are essential. Most recent studies now take into account the respective cognitive abilities of each age group and attempt to use appropriate scales and methods of assessing the relationships between effort perception and objective markers of effort. Time will tell which scales are the most sensible and valid. Whatever scale is used, consideration should also be given to the type of perceptual paradigm, the temporal nature of the exercise protocol and the influence of learning and practice as each may affect, and be differentially affected by, the three effort continua.

KEY POINTS

1. Exercise stimuli impact upon three effort continua – perceptual/psychological, physiological and performance/situational – that collectively influence the rating of perceived exertion.
2. Young children's ability to utilize traditional rating scales is affected by their numerical and verbal understanding. Pictorial scales with a narrower numerical range and fewer verbal references simplify the conceptual demands of the user.
3. An active paradigm places greater demands upon memory of exercise experience in order to generate a specific intensity in comparison to the passive paradigm that requires an instant response to the current exercise stimulation. Following an exercise situation, memory will degrade and be affected by a combination of factors associated with the three effort continua. This will impact upon future active productions.
4. The perceived effort response varies according to whether the exercise protocol is intermittent or continuous. The perceived exertion response appears to be higher in a continuous protocol. The intermittent protocols are preferred with young children.
5. There are three methods of anchoring: from memory, by definition or from actual experience.
6. There are now various scales for assessing RPE in children. These include a focus upon different modes of exercise, the use of different verbal anchors and a linear versus curvilinear conceptualization of the perceived exertion–exercise intensity relationship. Each scale has strengths and weaknesses.
7. The accuracy of children's effort perception increases significantly with practice.

References

Bar-Or O 1977 Age-related changes in exercise perception. In: Borg G (ed) Physical work and effort. Pergamon Press, Oxford, p 255–266

Bland J M, Altman D G 1995 Comparing two methods of clinical measurement: a personal history. International Journal of Epidemiology 24:S7–S14

Borg G 1970 Perceived exertion as an indicator of somatic stress. Journal of Rehabilitation Medicine 2:92–98

Borg G 1998 Borg's perceived exertion and pain scales. Human Kinetics, Champaign, IL

Eston R G 1984 A discussion of the concepts: exercise intensity and perceived exertion with reference to the secondary school. Physical Education Review 7:19–25

Eston R G, Lamb K L 2000 Effort perception. In: Armstrong N, Van-Mechelen W (eds) Paediatric exercise science and medicine. Oxford University Press, Oxford, p 85–91

Eston R G, Lamb K L, Bain A et al 1994 Validity of a perceived exertion scale for children: a pilot study. Perceptual and Motor Skills 78:691–697

Eston R G, Parfitt G, Campbell L et al 2000 Reliability of effort perception for regulating exercise intensity in children using a Cart and Load Effort Rating (CALER) Scale. Pediatric Exercise Science 12:388–397

Eston R G, Parfitt G, Shepherd P 2001 Effort perception in children: implications for validity and reliability. In: Papaionnou A, Goudas M, Theodorakis Y (eds) Proceedings of 10th World Congress of Sport Psychology, Skiathos, Greece, Volume 5, p 104–106

Lamb K L 1996 Exercise regulation during cycle ergometry using the CERT and RPE scales. Pediatric Exercise Science 8:337–350

Lamb K L, Eston R G 1997 Effort perception in children. Sports Medicine 23:139–148

Lamb K L, Trask S, Eston R G 1997 Effort perception in children. A focus on testing methodology. In: Armstrong N, Kirby B J, Welsman J R (eds) Children and exercise XIX – promoting health and well-being. E F & N Spon, London, p 258–266

Lamb K L, Eaves S J, Hartsorn J E 2004 The effect of experiential anchoring on the reproducibility of exercise regulation in adolescent children. Journal of Sports Sciences 22:159–165

Leung M L, Cheung P K, Leung R W 2002 An assessment of the validity and reliability of two perceived exertion rating scales among Hong Kong children. Perceptual and Motor Skills 95:1047–1062

Mahon A D, Duncan G E, Howe C A et al 1997 Blood lactate and perceived exertion relative to ventilatory threshold: boys versus men. Medicine and Science in Sports and Exercise 29:1332–1337

Mahon A D, Stolen K Q, Gay J A 2001 Differentiated perceived exertion during submaximal exercise in children and adults. Pediatric Exercise Science 13:145–153

Nystad W, Oseid S, Mellbye E B 1989 Physical education for asthmatic children: the relationship between changes in heart rate, perceived exertion, and motivation for participation. In: Oseid S, Carlsen K (eds) Children and exercise XIII. Human Kinetics, Champaign, IL, p 369–377

Parfitt G, Shepherd P, Eston R G (in press) Control of exercise intensity using the children's CALER and BABE perceived exertion scales. Journal of Exercise Science and Fitness

Robertson R J 1997 Perceived exertion in young people: future directions of enquiry. In: Welsman J, Armstrong N, Kirby B (eds) Children and exercise XIX, volume II. Washington Singer Press, Exeter, p 33–39

Robertson R J, Goss F L, Boer N F et al 2000 Children's OMNI scale of perceived exertion: mixed gender and race validation. Medicine and Science in Sports and Exercise 32:452–458

Robertson R J, Goss J L Bell F A et al 2002 Self-regulated cycling using the children's OMNI scale of perceived exertion. Medicine and Science in Sports and Exercise 34:1168–1175

Robertson R J, Goss J L, Andreacci J L et al 2005 Validation of the children's OMNI RPE scale for stepping exercise. Medicine and Science in Sports and Exercise 37:290–298

Roemmich J N, Barkley J E, Epstein L H et al 2006 Validity of the PCERT and OMNI-walk/run ratings of perceived exertion scales. Medicine and Science in Sports and Exercise 38:1014–1019

Utter A C, Robertson R J, Nieman D C et al 2002 Children's OMNI scale of perceived exertion: walking/running evaluation. Medicine and Science in Sports and Exercise 34:139–144

Williams J G, Eston R G, Stretch C 1991 Use of rating of perceived exertion to control exercise intensity in children. Pediatric Exercise Science 3:21–27

Williams J G, Furlong B, MacKintosh C et al 1993 Rating and regulation of exercise intensity in young children. Medicine and Science in Sports and Exercise 25(Suppl):S8 (Abstract)

Williams J G, Eston R G, Furlong B 1994 CERT: a perceived exertion scale for young children. Perceptual and Motor Skills 79:1451–1458

Yelling M, Lamb K, Swaine I L 2002 Validity of a pictorial perceived exertion scale for effort estimation and effort production during stepping exercise in adolescent children. European Physical Education Review 8:157–175

Further reading

Bar-Or O, Rowland T W 2004 Pediatric exercise medicine. Human Kinetics, Champaign, IL, p 40–44, 359–362

Eston R G, Williams J G 2001 Control of exercise intensity using heart rate, perceived exertion and other non-invasive procedures. In: Eston R G, Reilly T (eds) Kinanthropometry and exercise physiology laboratory manual: tests, procedures and data. Volume 2: Exercise physiology, 2nd edn. Routledge, London, p 213–234

Lamb K L, Eston R G 1997 Measurement of effort perception: time for a new approach. In: Welsman J, Armstrong N, Kirby B (eds) Children and exercise XIX, volume II. Washington Singer Press, Exeter, p 11–23

Noble B J, Robertson R J 1996 Perceived exertion. Human Kinetics, Champaign, IL

Robertson R J, Noble, B J 1997 Perception of physical exertion: methods, mediators and applications. Exercise and Sports Sciences Reviews 25:407–452

Chapter **13**

The young athlete
Adam D. G. Baxter-Jones and Clark A. Mundt

LEARNING OBJECTIVES

After studying this chapter you should be able to:
1. define what is meant by an elite young athlete
2. describe the statural, body composition, physique and physiological characteristics of young athletes
3. discuss the possible influence of training on stature, body composition, physique and physiological characteristics of young athletes
4. discuss the possible influence of training on maturation of the young athlete
5. evaluate how age, growth and maturation may influence an individual's inclusion or exclusion into sport
6. define and discuss the components of the female triad
7. define the prevalence of common injuries in a variety of sports.

INTRODUCTION

In recent years there have been an increasing number of children participating in sports at an elite level, at ever decreasing ages; with systematic training starting as young as 5 or 6 years of age. Children and adolescents taking part in high-level elite competition are likely to have undergone several years of intensive training prior to the event, highlighting the 'catch them young philosophy', the widespread belief that in order to achieve success at senior level it is necessary to start intensive training before puberty. In addition to long hours of systematic, repetitive training, and dietary regulation, in some sports special schooling and separation from family may also be characteristic of elite youth athletes. The participation of talented individuals in intensive training and competition at young ages gives rise to a number of questions and concerns: What are the effects of high intensity training on growth and maturation of the child athlete? When are children ready for intense training? Are elite young athletes somehow unique and differentiated from others by their response to training? Do the factors that make a young female athlete successful differ from those that make a young male athlete successful? Do young males and females respond differently to training? Perhaps the underlying question to all of the above is: are successful young athletes born or made, i.e. is their success a result of nature or nurture? The following chapter cannot definitively answer all of the preceding questions because an enormous amount of research has yet to be performed. What the chapter will do is summarize some of the existing literature on young athletes and the known effects of training during childhood and adolescence.

THE YOUNG ATHLETE

The first step when discussing the young athlete is to appropriately define what, or who, constitutes a young athlete. Many communities provide some form of agency-sponsored athletic competition for boys and girls, often starting in the preschool years. Many children participating in sports programmes do so for a year or two and then drop out, as their interests change. In this text, when talking about a young athlete we are specifically discussing children who are successful in local, national and or international age-grouped competition. Often researchers talk about elite young athletes; however, there is some debate as to whether or not youth athletes can be considered 'elite'. It has been argued that within a particular sport only the top ten are the true elite. There are a multitude of sports that children can be engaged in, with varying natures, levels of competitiveness, and frequency of involvement. The status of elite youth athletes is usually defined based on their success in: (1) school or club teams, (2) chronological age competitions and (3) regional, national or international competition. Thus definitions of young 'elite' athletes are often vague and include a variety of chronological age groups, skills and competitive levels.

It is also important to consider the distributions of athletes within a population. The young athlete population has been described as having a pyramid shape. Many young people participate in sports at the novice level. As the skill, competition and demands of the sport increase, young people progressively drop out, or are selected out, resulting in fewer participants at the highly competitive and elite levels at the peak of the pyramid. Thus the definition of the young athlete depends on which level of the pyramid they are on (Malina et al 2004).

TRAINING

A term often accompanying the word athlete, regardless of age or elitism, is training. Training is not the same as regular physical activity. Physical activity refers to the complex set of behaviours that encompass body movement produced by skeletal muscle which result in energy expenditure above resting levels. Training could perhaps be considered a special category of physical activity, above and beyond normal levels. It refers to systematic, specialized practice for a specific sport or sport discipline, for most of the year, or to specific short-term training programmes. Training is ordinarily quite specific (e.g. endurance running, strength training, sport skill training, etc.) but it can vary in type, intensity and frequency depending on the sport that an athlete is involved in.

The numerous factors that can vary in a training programme make it very difficult to make a statement on the general effects of training in any population, let alone youth (see Chapter 10 for further details). Also, within and across studies problems arise in measuring, specifying and quantifying training. Many studies classify training as mild, moderate or severe without clear definitions. For comparisons to be made both within and between studies the duration, intensity and type of training needs to be clearly identified. Studying the effects of training in children and adolescents is further complicated by the fact that in many cases the training is designed to induce changes in the same direction as normal growth and maturation. Therefore, the major hurdle when studying young athletes is that the effects of growth and maturation may mask or be greater than the effects of training. In order to identify more clearly the independent effects of growth, maturation and training, physical and physiological changes in the same individuals must be measured repeatedly over a period of time (longitudinal studies). However, much of the existing data on youth athletes to date have been derived from cross-sectional studies.

GROWTH

Stature

There has long been an interest in the effects of intensive training at an early age on a child's growth and maturation. At the beginning of the century it was suggested that exercise was a direct stimulus of growth. More recent publications suggest that intensive training has little, if any, effect on a child's growth (Malina 1994b).

Growth status (size attained at a given age) and progress (rate of growth) are usually monitored by making comparisons with reference percentiles where the 50th percentile represents the average size at any given chronological age. These reference centiles, sometimes called reference standards, are based on cross-sectional data derived from large representative samples of children from infancy to young adulthood. Such charts are useful for comparison or assessment of growth status of a child, or a sample of children, at a given age. However, since growth rates are not linear during childhood and adolescence, the interpretation of these comparisons or assessments may be difficult, particularly during adolescence when there is a marked acceleration in statural growth (peak height velocity (PHV)).

Young female athletes have, on average, statures that equal or exceed the 50th percentile from childhood through to adolescence. Female tennis, volleyball and basketball players, and swimmers have presented mean statures, from 10 years of age and onwards, that are above the average stature of the country-specific general population. The same finding has been observed in other sports such as elite female rowing. In contrast, gymnasts, figure skaters and ballet dancers tend to have shorter statures than average (Malina 1994b).

Young male athletes are generally taller and heavier than their non-athletic peers. The data, however, are not entirely consistent across and within sports. An example of statural development in a sample of elite age-grouped British male gymnasts, swimmers, soccer and tennis players is shown in Figure 13.1A. When compared to reference centiles, male gymnasts were below average for height for most of their growth, apart from the start and end points. In contrast, male swimmers and tennis players were all tall for their age, with average heights well above the 50th centile. Soccer players' heights were, however, above and below the 50th centile (Baxter-Jones et al 1995). The important point to note in this graph is that the figure demonstrates more than simply the positioning on height centiles of possible early and late maturers. It also tells us something about the control of human growth. After the deviations brought about by their adolescent growth spurts, approaching adulthood the gymnasts returned to the same centile position seen in early childhood. When looking at individual growth patterns it is true to say that all children, when in an environment that does not constrain growth, exhibit a pattern of growth that is more or less parallel to a particular centile. This type of growth pattern is known as canalization.

It is not yet known whether physical training is a strong enough stimulus to constrain growth patterns. Although early studies suggested that training increased the

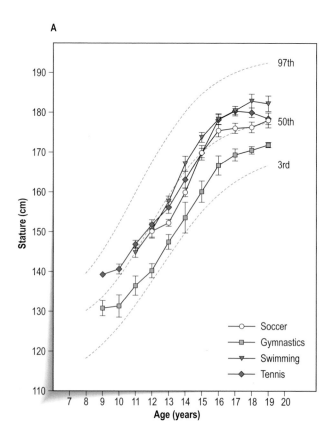

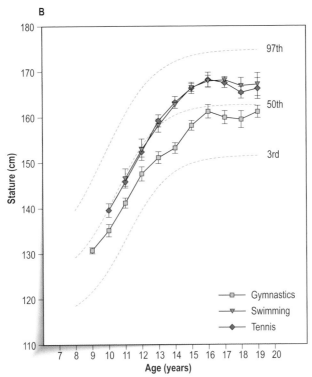

Figure 13.1   The development of stature in (A) male athletes from four sports and (B) female athletes from three sports compared with standard growth centiles (interrupted lines). Means and standard errors are shown at each age.

rate of growth, particularly the height of males, the interpretation of such results is problematic. The apparent acceleration of height, observed in some studies, is likely a reflection of the earlier biological maturation of the males studied, rather than an effect of the intensity of the training programme. However, since biological maturation was not adequately controlled for in these studies, the interpretations cannot be confirmed or refuted.

A major area of study has been the statural growth of elite female gymnasts, who frequently present with shorter heights than average. Theintz and colleagues (1993) suggested that heavy gymnastic training prior to puberty could stunt the adolescent growth spurt, specifically the growth in leg length, thus affecting final adult stature. However, this statement was based on a longitudinal study of only 2 years and assumed that final height had been reached. Since the girls in their study were all late maturers this seems highly unlikely. Long-term longitudinal data suggest that gymnasts in general are shorter than average even before training begins. Furthermore, other studies have found that athletes who drop out of gymnastics early are taller than those who persist in the sport. This suggests that final adult stature is unlikely to be compromised by regular training for sport and that the short stature displayed by some young athletes is a reflection of selection into specific sports (Baxter-Jones et al 2003, Caine et al 2003).

Body mass and composition

Body mass has three components: bone mass, lean mass and fat mass. Total body mass of young athletes presents a similar pattern to that seen for stature. By and large, young athletes have a body mass for their height that equals or exceeds the reference average. Data on young female athletes, from a number of sports, reveal they tend to be heavier than reference populations. In contrast, female gymnasts and figure skaters tend to have appropriate mass-for-height, while ballet dancers have a low mass-for-height. A similar trend of low mass-for-height is indicative of female distance runners. Young male athletes present a similar general trend. For example, in a sample of British male gymnasts, swimmers, soccer and tennis players, body masses of gymnasts were below average up until 16 years of age. However, between 16 and 19 years of age their average body mass approximated the 50th centile. Male swimmers, tennis players and soccer players were close to average for body mass, up until 15 years of age, but between 15 and 19 years of age their body mass increased to well above the 50th centile. In contrast to stature, body mass of young athletes appears to be influenced by regular training for sport. Depending on the sport and age of the athletes, training can either decrease or increase body mass, and it does so via alterations of body composition.

The data on bone mass of young athletes has largely focused on female gymnasts, swimmers, figure skaters, ballet dancers and runners. Findings suggest that athletes participating in these sports have increased bone mass during childhood and early adulthood when compared to their non-athletic peers. Sport-specific effects have also been observed, especially between weight- and non-weight-bearing activities. Weight-bearing sports are those in which an athlete encounters gravitational mechanical loading, such as running. Weight-bearing sports such as weightlifting and gymnastics have been shown numerous times to have a positive effect on bone mass development. The reasons often cited for these improvements are the immense ground reaction forces of up to five times the person's body weight that can occur with these types of activity. Non-weight-bearing exercise results in non-gravitational mechanical loading, for example swimming and cycling. Even though there is no ground reaction or high impact forces on the skeletal system in these sports, the bone is still being loaded by the contractions of the muscular system. These active loading sports generally do not have any significant benefits for increasing bone mass as this type of activity does not apply enough force on the bones to overload them. Again, most data come from adult athletes as the effects of training in children are often masked by the effect of bone mass accrual associated with normal growth and maturation. The most compelling evidence to support a training effect is shown in studies of sports where there is a dominant side. It has been found that youth tennis players have 20% greater bone mineral density (BMD) in their dominant arm. This effect is also observed in the general population, where there is usually an approximately 5% difference in BMD between the dominant and non-dominant arms.

Very few data are available that have assessed the lean mass of young athletes compared to their non-athlete counterparts. This is in part due to methodological problems in assessing lean mass. Findings suggest that young athletes do not have significantly greater lean mass than non-athletes of the same age unless they are more advanced in maturation and/or genetically predisposed to have greater lean mass. It is feasible that once young athletes are close to the fully mature state they may have greater lean mass than non-athletes, but at this point this is mere speculation. Again the training effect on lean mass is particularly difficult to assess given the significant increase in lean mass that occurs naturally with growth. Some studies have associated training with an increase in fat-free mass (lean and bone mass), especially in boys, but these data largely consist of participants who are at the older end of their age-group and therefore probably more advanced in maturity. There are not adequate data available to confidently state that training will influence the lean mass of young athletes, but the low levels of testosterone at younger ages suggest that any increase that might occur would be quite limited (Rowland 2005).

Data on the percent body fat, or relative fatness, of distance runners, middle distance runners, gymnasts, swimmers, jumpers and sprinters reveal some useful body composition comparisons (Malina et al 2004). In general, athletes have less relative fatness than non-athletes of the same age and sex. Young athletes also tend to have thinner skinfolds, an index of subcutaneous fat, than reference samples. During adolescence both non-athletic and athletic males show a decline in relative fatness, as a consequence of normal growth and development. However, at most ages through adolescence athletic males have less relative fatness than non-athletic males. Female athletes also show less relative fatness than non-athletes throughout adolescence. Non-athletic females' relative fatness increases as a result of normal growth and development during adolescence, whereas athletic females' relative fatness appears to remain fairly stable with increasing age. Thus, training appears to affect fat mass development in both genders. Evidence for a training influence on fat mass is further emphasized in studies of young athletes whose continued participation in training (or caloric restriction) is used to maintain their lower fat mass levels. When training is reduced, or terminated, fat mass increases and when training resumes again fat mass declines, suggesting a direct relationship with or influence on body composition.

Physique

The conceptual approach of William Sheldon and colleagues, sometimes called somatotyping, is the most commonly used method of assessing physique (Sheldon 1954). The approach focuses on external dimensions and characteristics of the body and is based on the premise that continuous variation occurs in the distribution of physiques. This variation is related to differential contributions of three specific components that characterize the configuration of the body – endomorphy, mesomorphy and ectomorphy. Endomorphy is characterized by the roundness of contours or fatness, throughout the body. Mesomorphy is characterized by the dominance of muscular and skeletal development, resulting in a sharp definition. Ectomorphy is characterized by linearity of build and limited muscular development. The contributions of the three components define an individual's somatotype, or physique.

Physique is a significant contributor to success in many sports and may be of particular importance in aesthetic sports. Performance scores in subjectively evaluated sports, such as gymnastics, figure skating and diving, may be influenced by the athlete's physique as perceived by the judges. It has been found that young athletes in a given sport tend to have very similar somatotypes and also have similar somatotypes to their elite adult counterparts. This tendency suggests that athletes may be selected or excluded for certain sports based on their physique. Similar to adult athletes, there is typically less somatotype variation among young athletes, compared to the general population. In most youth sports mesomorphy is well developed, endomorphy is low and there is a large variability in ectomorphy. The exceptions seem to be in throwing events in athletics (track and field), and the higher weight categories in weightlifting. Compared to adult athletes, younger athletes tend to be less endomorphic (particularly females), less mesomorphic, and more ectomorphic. The latter component reflects the role of growth in the transition from late adolescence into young adulthood. The fact that mesomorphy is positively associated with skilled performance, that young successful athletes have similar physique to older successful athletes in the same sport, and that outstanding athletes in a specific sport usually have a limited distribution in somatotype is not sufficient evidence to convincingly state that training affects a young athlete's physique. It is conceivable that training could increase a young athlete's mesomorphic score, by increasing muscle mass, and decrease their endomorphic scores by decreasing fat mass. However, as yet there is little existing evidence to substantiate these claims.

Biological maturation

Particular concern has been expressed about the effects of prolonged intensive training and the stress of competition on the maturation of young athletes who specialize in sport at an early age. It has been suggested that high intensity training can alter the maturation process. During childhood and adolescence individuals of the same chronological age can differ dramatically in their degree of biological maturity. The process of maturing has two components, timing and tempo. The former refers to when specific maturational events occur (e.g. age when menarche is attained, age at the beginning of breast development, the age at the appearance of pubic hair, or the age at maximum growth during the adolescent growth spurt (PHV)). Tempo refers to the rate at which maturation progresses (i.e. how quickly or slowly an individual passes from initial stages of sexual maturation to the mature state).

The majority of data investigating biological maturity in young athletes have concentrated on the age of attainment of menarche in female sports such as gymnastics, figure skaters and swimming (Fig. 13.2). Maturity differences among young

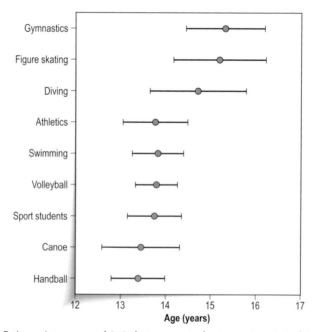

Figure 13.2   Estimated mean ages (circles) at menarche (± standard deviation) in female adolescent athletes from several sports. (Data from Marker 1981.)

female athletes are most apparent during the transition from childhood to adolescence, particularly around the time of attainment of PHV. In general, female youth athletes tend to mature later than non-athletes, with the possible exception of young swimmers. In contrast, young female swimmers appear to be average, or slightly advanced in maturity status. During early childhood (6 to 8 years of age) gymnasts demonstrate average maturity for their chronological age (measured through skeletal age assessment). However, during the adolescent years gymnasts are usually classified as average, or late maturing with very few early maturing individuals seen. During late adolescence female gymnasts are almost exclusively late maturing (Malina 1994b). Therefore, it appears that early and average maturing girls are participating less in elite gymnastics as girls pass from childhood through adolescence. Data on female ballet dancers and distance runners show similar patterns of biological maturity during adolescence.

Late menarche, therefore late maturity, is a common occurrence in some elite female athlete groups. Figure 13.2 shows the mean age of attainment of menarche in several sports; the average age of menarche is 12.8 years in the non-athletic population. Since so many sports demonstrate late attainment of menarche, training has been implicated as a possible delaying factor. However, much of the data on menarche is from small samples of post-menarcheal athletes and does not specify training loads. Furthermore, most studies of athletes do not consider other confounding factors known to affect menarche. For example, mothers of athletes in sports such as gymnastics, on average, attain menarche later than mothers of non-gymnasts, and sisters of elite swimmers and university athletes, on average, attain menarche later than average. These results suggest a familial tendency for later maturation. Training has been implicated for causing a delay in menarche in athletes who began training before menarche, as their menarche is observed to occur later than in athletes who begin training after its occurrence. However, this observation does not imply a cause–effect relationship. The older a girl is when menarche is attained the more likely she would have begun her training prior to menarche. Conversely the younger the girl is when menarche is attained the more likely she would have began training after menarche; she will also have had a shorter period of training prior to menarche. Considering the large number of factors that are believed to influence menarche is it very hard to implicate sport training per se as the causative factor.

Two explanations that have been offered to explain the apparent association between physical training and late menarcheal age are the critical weight–critical fat hypothesis (Frisch & Revelle 1970) and the genetic predisposition theory (or two-part biocultural hypothesis) (Malina 1983). The critical weight–critical fat hypothesis states that a minimum body fatness is necessary for the onset of menstruation. Frisch and colleagues suggested that physical training and/or dietary restriction causes a reduction in body weight and percent body fat, which in turn delays menarche. This hypothesis has been the subject of considerable criticism, particularly concerning the equations and assumptions used to estimate fatness. The genetic predisposition theory suggests that menarche is not delayed by strenuous training, but is simply later in some girls than in others. Girls who tend to have a late menarche also tend to be girls who excel in athletic endeavours. Thus late maturation is a contributing factor in the young girl's decision to take up a sport rather than the training causing the lateness. The characteristics that are generally associated with high skill levels in many sports (slim hips, low percent body fat, longer legs) are also associated with girls who achieve menarche at older ages. Likewise, the characteristics that could be detrimental to performance (gain in body fat, breast development and widening of the hips) are associated with early menarche.

There are limited data on sexual maturation, outside of age at menarche, of girls who are regularly active or training for sport. Available evidence on the sexual development of girls active in sport suggests that training has no effect on timing and progress of breast or pubic hair development. The average length of time it takes to move from one stage to another, or across two stages of secondary sex characteristic development, is similar for active and non-active youth. Furthermore, the time elapsed between ages at PHV and menarche is similar between active and non-active girls. Most researchers agree that training does not effect somatic maturity indicators, such as the age at PHV or the growth rate of height during the adolescent growth spurt (Malina 1994b). All of this evidence suggests that active girls, on average, demonstrate a normal progression of sexual development.

Unlike females, males do not have an easily observable sexual maturational milestone such as menarche, which has limited the study of young male athletes. The evidence available suggests that young male athletes are generally early maturers (as shown through skeletal and sexual maturation). Work in the United States has shown that elite baseball and American football players tend to have advanced biological maturity. This is probably a reflection of the physical advantages associated with advanced maturity (e.g. body size and muscle strength) in these two sports. American football is clearly a sport where a large body size is an advantage and in which many youngsters are selected for a position based on their body size. However, at the senior high school ages, biological maturity status did not consistently differ between elite youth American footballers and non-athletes, probably reflecting the catch-up of late maturers.

Although male youth athletes, on average, have advanced biological maturity, there has been surprisingly little work investigating whether this is the result of sports training. Figure 13.3 shows the mean ages of attainment of PHV in various athlete groups. The average age of attainment for non-athletes is 14 years; the figure clearly shows that there is great variation within and between sports in its attainment. It has been suggested that an increase in muscle mass through regular resistance and strength training during the adolescent years could accelerate pubertal development in boys. However, the limited studies indicate no effects of regular training for sport on the timing and tempo of sexual maturity. Serial observations of the skeletal maturation of the hand and wrist have demonstrated that biological maturity is not affected by regular physical training. Furthermore, age at PHV and magnitude of growth at PHV have repeatedly been shown not to be affected by regular physical activity or training (Malina 1994b).

In summary, although young athletes in several sports demonstrate 'delayed' or 'advanced' biological maturity when compared to non-athletes, the data do not suggest that training alters the biological maturity of the growing athlete. The majority of studies suggesting that physical training alters maturity are cross-sectional in design and thus these results should not be considered causal. Only when a child is repeatedly measured from childhood through adolescence can the independent effects of training be separated from those of normal growth. Results from the few longitudinal studies suggest that young athletes, on average, grow and mature in a similar manner to non-athletes. There is, however, variation in size, physique, body composition and maturity status associated with different sports. Part of the variation in size, physique and body composition is due to variation in maturity status. It may be that late maturation is a contributing factor in the young person's decision to take up a sport, rather than the training causing the lateness. Likewise, the size advantage of the early maturing youngster may be a factor directing him or her towards certain sports.

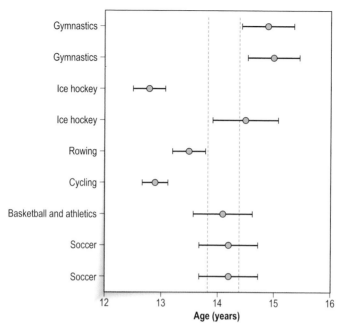

Figure 13.3 Estimated mean ages (circles) at peak height velocity (± standard deviation) in European male adolescent athletes from several sports. Dotted line represents the average range of mean ages at peak height velocity for non-athletes. (Data from Malina et al 2004.)

PHYSICAL PERFORMANCE

Aerobic energy system

Although the effects of training on various physiological systems of adults and adolescents are well documented, extrapolation of physiological variables from adults or adolescents to children should be done with caution due to the differences in body size and the immaturity of the children's developing systems. In other words, children should not be considered to function identically to adults or adolescents nor should they be considered physiologically similar. There is also a need to understand the differences between boys and girls in the development of these physiological systems, particularly given the differences observed in body composition following pubertal development. Specifically, during adolescence females experience an increase in adiposity with a resultant relative decrease in lean body mass whilst males experience an increase in lean body mass with a resultant relative decrease in fat mass.

Aerobic fitness (peak $\dot{V}O_2$) is considered to be the primary definition of physical fitness in children and therefore the aerobic energy system has received the majority of focus in terms of energy systems development in young athletes. When assessing the effects of training on peak $\dot{V}O_2$ in children it is important to determine whether changes are a result of training or growth, or both, as body size directly affects peak $\dot{V}O_2$ (see Chapter 2 for further details). To adequately control for the confounding effects of growth, children ideally should be assessed longitudinally. However, to date the majority of aerobic power development studies in young athletes have been cross-sectional in design. Although conflicting findings exist in the literature, the consensus is that young athletes, even prepubertal athletes, in general have superior cardiovascular function and higher peak $\dot{V}O_2$ values than their untrained peers (Rowland 1990). Although this suggests that children are capable of improving endurance capacity with an adequate training stimulus, it is also possible that genetic determination plays a prominent role in children's endurance capabilities and response to training. In fact, some experts have questioned the effect of endurance training on youngsters at certain developmental ages, suggesting that the effects of training are minimal (see Chapter 10 for further details).

At present there are few studies documenting the young athlete's physiological response to athletic training; therefore, the effect of training on the development of peak $\dot{V}O_2$ during childhood and adolescence is still a contentious issue. Although in adults, regular training has been shown to produce up to a 25% improvement in peak $\dot{V}O_2$, there are conflicting results as to whether aerobic training in children, particularly during the prepubescent years, can cause improvement in peak $\dot{V}O_2$ (Rowland 1990). In studies that have shown no improvement it is suggested that children have greater levels of habitual physical activity which maintains them closer to their maximal oxygen intake potential. Two popular hypotheses have been presented to explain the contentious relationship between a child's biological maturation and aerobic fitness. It has been hypothesized that a maturational threshold exists whereby prepubescent children are unable to elicit physiological changes in response to training. The second hypothesis states that adolescence is a critical period during which children are particularly susceptible to aerobic training. For example, training initiated 1 year prior to the period of rapid growth during puberty has been shown to induce remarkable increases in peak $\dot{V}O_2$. Superior cardiovascular function and higher peak $\dot{V}O_2$ have been observed in a longitudinal study of elite pubescent athletes (Baxter-Jones et al 1993). This study of systematic training in young athletes (gymnasts, swimmers, soccer and tennis players) suggested that when the confounders of growth and maturation were controlled there were age and gender differences present between sports. In addition, in males it was found that pubertal status was a significant independent predictor of peak $\dot{V}O_2$. In summary, although some disagreement remains as to whether aerobic training in prepubescent children causes an improvement in peak $\dot{V}O_2$, most studies conclude that such an effect does exist. If the training stimulus is adequate, the general consensus is that children and adolescents are physiologically more apt to endurance exercise training than adults. However, three main areas of contention still remain: (a) is endurance training limited by a ceiling effect in maximal arteriovenous oxygen difference? (b) do genetics promote a high level of functionality? and (c) does trainability vary with developmental status?

Anaerobic energy system

The anaerobic energy system of young athletes has received relatively little attention compared to the aerobic energy system. It appears that the anaerobic system of young athletes is capable of producing more power than that of young non-athletes. Though some research has assessed the effects of training on the anaerobic energy system of children, the common weakness of such studies is that the training programmes employed were not specifically targeting the performance of the anaerobic energy system. In many cases evaluation of the anaerobic energy system took place after participation in an aerobic training programme. Nonetheless, the results of such studies suggest that the power of the anaerobic system in children and adolescents can increase with training. Though increments observed to date have been small, they may increase with participation in a programme specifically directed at improving the anaerobic system. Post-training metabolic changes have also been reported, such as increases in lactate and phosphofructokinase. However, the ability of the muscle to utilize lactate produced does not seem to improve with training. This area of research in young athletes is a relatively recent development and therefore while it appears training improves performance in short-burst activities it is too early to specify the mechanisms which make this possible (see Chapter 10 for further details).

Muscle strength

Muscle strength development in children is a much debated issue. Resistance training is now recommended by the American Academy of Pediatrics as a safe and effective method of developing strength in children and adolescents, providing the activity is performed in a supervised environment with proper techniques and safety precautions (Washington et al 2001). Although early studies suggested that resistance training in children did not lead to adaptations, the majority of the recent literature would suggest that muscle strength is trainable. Two years of twice-weekly resistance training has been shown to significantly increase muscle strength in boys as young as 9 years of age. The general lack of testosterone in youth may mean that the improvements in strength are mediated by a neural effect rather than a hypertrophic increase in muscle size but an increase in strength seems to occur with training nonetheless. The impact of strength training at a young age on strength development in adulthood is not yet known. Also the impact of strength training in young females has received little attention (see Chapter 10 for further details).

SELECTION INTO SPORTS

Alluded to in the proceeding section but not yet fully discussed is the underlying idea that selection into sport confounds many of the growth and development issues in the young athlete. Athletes, especially elite athletes, competing internationally, are a select group of extremely talented individuals. However, is talent the only factor that separates a young athlete from a non-athlete? Numerous factors, less prominent than talent but possibly interrelated, can influence selection or exclusion into a sport.

The prediction of successful achievement in sporting activities presents a major challenge. The selection and development of talent has intrigued coaches in many different countries for many years. Much time and effort has been spent trying to identify the particular physical and psychological characteristics that contribute to elite performance. Debate has surrounded the relative contributions of genetic, social and environmental factors. Yet, despite the arguments about nature or nurture, most agree that talent has to be identified before potential can be reached. Baxter-Jones & Maffulli (2003) observed, in a sample of young British athletes, that involvement in high-level sport was heavily dependent on the athletes and their parents, with sports clubs and coaches playing an important later role. They concluded that many talented youngsters with less motivated parents were unlikely to undertake sport.

In many sports, however, size and physique can also play an important role in the selection of athletes. For example, a large body size can be advantageous in sports such as basketball and swimming and a small body size can be advantageous in sports such as figure skating, ballet and gymnastics. Malina (1994a) measured the growth and development of young female volleyball players and concluded that body size was likely genotypic, probably reflecting selection at a relatively young age for the size demands of the sport. Available longitudinal data have also indicated that generally the stature of a youth is maintained relative to reference values over the chronological years of growth. This suggests that stature is not influenced by regular training for sport, and is more likely due to the selection practice of specific sports. For example, the smaller size of elite gymnasts is evident before systematic training is started and may contribute to an athlete's success in the sport as well as his/her continued involvement. Furthermore, when parental data were used to predict adult target height in a group of male gymnasts, swimmers, soccer and tennis players, it was found that gymnasts had significantly lower target heights than athletes in the other two sports (Baxter-Jones et al 1995). This indicates again that selection into some sports can be largely dependent on size.

Size and physique are related not only to genetics, but also to biological maturation. Early maturing individuals are generally large for their age, while late maturing individuals are generally small for their age. Therefore, in some sports, biological maturity could play an important role in the selection of youth athletes. For example, coaches of female gymnasts and figure skaters could be concerned with the physical changes that occur during the transition into puberty (increased fat deposits, widening of the hips etc.) as these changes could be detrimental to performance. Therefore youth gymnasts and figure skaters may be selected based on late maturity and, conversely, excluded based on early maturity. The reverse may be true for sports where size and strength are considered an advantage.

In addition to advanced biological maturity, chronological age also plays an important role in talent identification. Numerous studies have demonstrated that many chronological age structured sports are likely to have more participants whose birthdays are early in the selection year than late in the selection year. Such sports include tennis, swimming, cricket, soccer, baseball, American football and ice hockey. The difference in chronological age between individuals in the age group is referred to as the relative age. For example, in a group of 14-year-olds competing in a sport, the youngest player could be 14.0 years and the oldest 14.99 years. The consequence of the relative age is known as the relative age effect (RAE) (Musch & Grondin 2001).

Climate influences have been offered as a cause of RAE. For example, if warm weather during important phases of motor learning and outdoor activities promotes critical sport-related skills, children born in certain months of the year could profit from the fact that their critical sensitive phases occur during summer months rather than winter months. Seasonal influences, however, have frequently been refuted as a cause of RAE in sports. International comparisons reveal that the birth months that appear to give advantage vary to reflect different selection years, as demonstrated in Figure 13.4. The figure shows the birth date distributions of professional soccer players from several countries (Musch & Hay 1999). The players are grouped into the four quarters of the selection year (January–December) and compared to the birth date distributions of the general population. One would expect an even distribution of birthdays throughout the four quarters of the selection year, as shown in the general population data. However, the majority of professional players were born in the first two quarters of the selection year. This bias occurs regardless of the cut-off date for the season. Furthermore, for some sports such as ice hockey, the selection year starts in January and ends in December. January and December are similar climatically but are at opposing ends of the selection year. This suggests that the cut-off date rather than some seasonal influence is related to the RAE.

A 1–2 year chronological age difference can cause a big variation in the stature and body mass of young children in youth sports programmes. Due to this, it is likely that RAE observed in many sports is due to the physical advantages of the relatively older

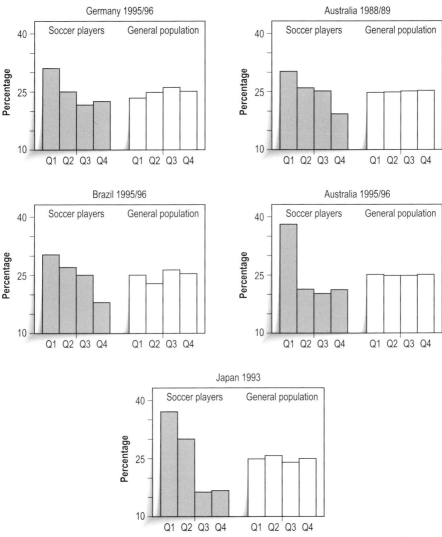

Figure 13.4   Birth date distribution of professional players in the highest national soccer league and the general population. Months included in each quartile differ according to the application cut-off date: 1 August for Germany and Brazil, 1 April for Japan, 1 January for Australia 1998–1989, and 1 August for Australia 1995–1996. (From J Musch and R Hay, 1999, The relative age effect in soccer: cross-cultural evidence for a systematic discrimination against children born late in the competition year. *Sociology of Sport Journal* 16(1):59, Figure 1. © 1999 by Human Kinetics Publisher, Inc. Reprinted with permission from Human Kinetics (Champaign, IL).)

players. These developmental advantages could have a direct impact on perceived athletic potential and predicted sporting success. Researchers have shown that players identified as being talented in sports where size is advantageous not only have birthdays early in the selection year but are also likely to be taller and heavier than average, suggesting above average physical maturity for their chronological age.

Although more evidence is needed, research suggests that these biases have the greatest effect in childhood during times of talent identification. This may be a cause of an over-representation of relatively older boys among those observed to succeed in many youth sports. In light of the maturity and biological age biases that have been observed in youth sports, the appropriateness of using chronological age to index youth sporting talent has been questioned. Two approximate chronological age periods merit special attention; first about 9 through 14 years of age, when maturity-associated variation in size is especially marked, and second, about 15 through 17 years of age, when the catch-up of the late-maturing individuals reduces maturity-associated variation in size and performance (Malina et al 2004).

Along with appropriate skill, physical endowment, maturity levels and timing of their birthday in the selection year, a young athlete's selection or exclusion into a chosen sport can also be dependent on a number of other factors. These include genetics, social and environmental (familial) circumstances, socioeconomic status and psychological constitution. Certainly, elite youth athletes are a highly select group who are not representative of the general population of youth and an abundance of factors contributing to their success are outside their own control. Caution is therefore warranted when making inferences about the effects of training between athletic and non-athletic children.

FEMALE ATHLETE TRIAD

Females' participation in sports has greatly expanded over the past 25 years. With this has come an increased awareness of new conditions and pathologies unique to this population. In 1992, the term female athlete triad was coined to describe three distinct, but frequently interrelated, disorders found in the female athletic population: disordered eating, amenorrhoea and osteoporosis. Individually each of these entities can cause significant morbidity and together their effects appear synergistically detrimental. It has been stated that all female athletes from elite to recreational, in any sport, are at risk of developing the triad. However, athletes competing in sports in which leanness and/or a low body weight is aesthetically pleasing may be at increased risk (e.g. ballet dancers, gymnasts, figure skaters) (Torstveit & Sundgot-Borgen 2005). Though the triad is not well understood it is thought that it may occur in a gradual progression beginning with intentional or unintentional disordered eating patterns, progressing to menstrual disorders, and finally to decreased bone density and osteoporosis. The major concern is whether it has its antecedents in the young athlete.

Disordered eating

The prevalence of disordered eating in young female athletes has been reported to be 15–62%, compared to up to 3% in non-athlete peers (particularly in sports emphasizing leanness) (Torstveit & Sundgot-Borgen 2005). The disordered eating component of the triad is typically initiated by an athlete's desire to lose weight by dieting. To some extent all athletes are concerned with diet and body image, but in susceptible individuals, this preoccupation can become pathological. Disordered eating refers to a wide spectrum of harmful and often ineffective eating behaviours used in an attempt to lose weight or achieve a lean appearance. The spectrum of behaviours ranges in severity from restricting food intake to clinically diagnosed eating disorders. Preoccupation with body weight leading to dieting has become commonplace in childhood and adolescent populations, even amongst those who are of normal weight or underweight. It has been seen in children as young as 9 years of age. The two eating disorders that receive the most media coverage are anorexia nervosa and bulimia nervosa. Anorexia nervosa involves severe self-imposed weight loss, altered body image, an intense fear of being fat and amenorrhoea. Bulimia nervosa involves binge eating followed by inappropriate compensatory behaviours to prevent weight gain such as self-induced vomiting, use of laxatives or diuretics, fasting or exercising vigorously; and great concern about body shape and weight.

The number of individuals who meet the clinical criteria to be diagnosed with an eating disorder is relatively low but there are many more individuals who display subclinical behaviours such as preoccupation with body weight, crash dieting, fasting, binge eating and purging behaviours. In the general population eating disorders can arise as a result of a culture idealizing thinness, families with poor conflict resolution, obsessive-compulsive personality disorders, and being teased about body size. An athlete's predisposition for disordered eating is further increased by pressure to perform, which can sometimes mean meeting unrealistic weight or body fat goals from demanding coaches and parents. Common personality traits of perfectionism, compulsiveness, determination and high achievement expectations among athletes can further influence them to disordered eating (Lebrun & Rumball 2002). Young athletes may also inadvertently engage in disordered eating by simply not consuming an adequate number of calories to compensate for the amount of energy they expend during sport and training.

Amenorrhoea

There are four varieties of amenorrhoea clinically designated as primary, secondary, oligomenorrhoea and luteal deficiency. Oligomenorrhoea refers to menstrual periods that occur at intervals longer than every 35 days. Luteal phase deficiency occurs when the total length of menstruation is normal, yet progesterone levels are low and this can result in decreased fertility (Lebrun & Rumball 2002). The categories of amenorrhoea most commonly referred to are primary and secondary amenorrhoea. Primary amenorrhoea is also known as delayed menarche, and is the absence of menstruation by age 16 years in a girl with secondary sex characteristics. Secondary amenorrhoea is the absence of three or more consecutive cycles after menarche and outside of pregnancy. A study of Norwegian female athletes (13–39 years of age) from a variety of sports revealed a higher prevalence of primary and secondary amenorrhoea in the athletes compared to the controls (Torstveit & Sundgot-Borgen 2005). The highest occurrence was found among athletes competing in aesthetic sports (21.9%), endurance sports (10.6%) and power sports (10.0%). The estimated prevalence of secondary amenorrhoea has further been reported to range from 3 to 66% in athletes compared with 2 to 5% in the general population (Otis et al 1998). The wide range in incidence of secondary amenorrhoea in athletes could be due to a number of methodological factors that vary, such as: (1) definition of menstrual dysfunction, (2) competition level of the athletes and (3) the intensity, duration and frequency of the training. Further studies in this realm should focus on addressing these inconsistencies so that the true prevalence of amenorrhoea amongst young athletes can be ascertained.

Although menstrual dysfunction is relatively common in chronically active post-menarcheal girls and women, no single aetiology has been found. It is known to be mediated by an alteration in function of the hypothalamic-pituitary-ovarian (HPO) axis, with a loss of normal secretion of leuteinizing hormone and subsequent lack of oestrogen production. Figure 13.5 displays some of the factors apparently associated in the pathophysiology of exercise-associated amenorrhoea. Factors involved in the process include dietary changes leading to poor nutrition, hormonal effects of acute bouts of exercise performed chronically, alterations in steroid hormone metabolism, weight loss and/or altered body composition, and the psychological and physical stress of the exercise itself. The fact that the prevalence of amenorrhoea is increased in female athletes involved in sports where a smaller, leaner physique is advantageous has led to the common misconception that the training has caused the amenorrhoea and is a normal outcome. Before drawing such a conclusion it should be remembered that in many of the sports where leanness is advantageous female athletes have also been found to be later maturers (Baxter-Jones et al 1994). Training therefore may not be causing the amenorrhoea, but the delayed menarche may be beneficial to the athlete by allowing maintenance of the favourable physique. Amenorrhoea should never be considered the expected outcome of training but, considering the number of factors involved, it should be considered the symptom of a larger medical problem and treated as such.

Osteoporosis

Athletes with amenorrhoea and/or disordered eating patterns have yet another major concern: osteoporosis. Osteoporosis is a disease characterized by low bone density and microarchitectural deterioration of bone tissue leading to enhanced skeletal fragility and increased risk of fracture. Normal bone mineralization is a bone mineral density (BMD) that is no more than 1 standard deviation (SD) below the mean of young adults. Osteopenia occurs when BMD falls between 1 and 2.5 SD below the mean of young adults. Osteoporosis is defined as a BMD more than 2.5 SD below the mean of young adults, and severe osteoporosis is a BMD more than 2.5 SD below the mean plus one or more fragility fractures (Otis et al 1998).

Amenorrhoea results in low concentrations of ovarian hormones, particularly oestrogen, thereby exerting a negative effect on bone. Oestrogen is needed for calcium

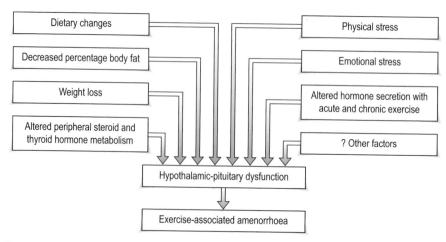

Figure 13.5   Some factors apparently involved in the pathophysiology of exercise-associated amenorrhoea. (From Rebar 1984, with the permission of Elsevier Ltd.)

absorption into bone and therefore with low oestrogen levels bone health is compromised. Amenorrhoea is of particular concern in the young female because most bone mass is gained during the adolescent years. By 18 years of age most women have reached 95% of their peak bone mass and once the peak is attained women lose approximately 1% per year until the onset of menopause, at which point there is a 10-fold increase in the rate of bone loss. The importance of maximizing bone mineral accumulation during adolescence cannot be emphasized enough, and the possible impact of amenorrhoea during the period of peak bone mineral accumulation may have implications on bone strength throughout the remainder of a young female's life. When a young athlete presents with amenorrhoea she may be currently losing bone mineral that has already accumulated, or she may have failed to lay down adequate amounts of bone mineral during critical years. The longer the duration of amenorrhoea, the greater extent of bone mineral loss, and the greater the risk of 'young athletes being left with old bones'. Twenty-year-old women with anorexia have been known to present with a skeletal structure similar to that of a 50- to 60-year-old woman. Not only does low bone mineral density increase one's chance of incurring osteoporotic fractures later in life, it also increases the female athlete's present chances of fracture.

Although numerous studies have shown a positive effect of impact loading on bone mineral density, there is a fear that the effect of loading may not be enough to offset the deleterious effect of amenorrhoea, poor nutritional behaviours or genetic predisposition towards lower-than-average bone density. Among young female athletes, especially those who mature later, this apprehension is heightened as high volumes of strenuous training may be contributing to both amenorrhoea and poor nutrition, therefore exaggerating the negative effects on bone mineral content. These concerns have not yet been substantiated in the literature, however, and further research needs to be performed.

SPORTS INJURIES

Since intensive training and elite competition can start from a very early age in young athletes, there is concern that these young people are at risk for a sporting injury. Sports injury is a collective name for all types of damage to the body that is caused directly, or indirectly, from participation in sporting activity. The specific definition, however, varies considerably between studies and causes problems when comparing results from different investigations. Furthermore, the definition of sports injury incidence and sports participation can also vary between studies. In most studies injury rates, or incidences, are presented as an estimate of risk (i.e. the number of new sports injuries during a particular period, divided by the total number of sports persons at the start of that period). Results presented in this way give an insight into the extent of sports injuries in a specific athletic population. Furthermore, to obtain a true picture of the sports injuries associated with a specific sport one must consider the number of hours of active play during which the athlete actually runs the risk of being injured (i.e. the exposure to injury risk). The severity of sports injury can be determined through data on (a) the duration and nature of treatment, (b) sports time lost, (c) working or school time lost and/or (d) permanent damage. The type of sports injury can further be described, very generally, in terms of medical diagnosis: sprain (of joint capsule and ligaments), strain (of muscle or tendon), contusion (bruising), dislocation or subluxation, fracture (of bone).

The majority of injuries in young athletes can be divided into two categories. The first and more common type of injuries are categorized as acute macrotrauma. They are often impact or twisting derived injuries and are the result of application of a major force to a specific area of the body. The second and perhaps lesser recognized type of injury are those classified as repetitive microtrauma. This type of injury is the product of repetitive stress to an area of the body over a prolonged period of time, and it is typically seen in a strenuous training regimen. Another more common term for this variety of injury is an overuse injury. Concern has been expressed in the past regarding how either type of injury may impact on later growth but the overuse type of injury is of further concern because its occurrence likely indicates overtraining of the young athlete.

Overuse injuries amongst young athletes, at least in developed countries, are more frequently being diagnosed and four main reasons can be suggested for this: (1) more children are participating in organized sport than at any previous time in history; (2) though more children are participating in organized sport, children in general are less active than children of previous generations when outside of sport and are therefore less protected from overuse injuries; (3) there is currently a tendency for young athletes to specialize in one or two sports at a fairly young age; (4) the age at which children in individual and/or team sports become involved in more strenuous and complex training is becoming younger and younger. The overuse injuries most commonly occurring in young athletes are the result of repetitive foot impact of running or jumping, as well as repetitive forces of throwing. The details of all the risk factors that make any given young athlete susceptible to overuse injury are not well understood but research is ongoing and knowledge is slowly accumulating. It is known that overuse injuries can occur in a variety of tissues including articular cartilage, bone, muscle-tendon units, and fascia. Regardless of the tissue involved, the injury consistently has a history of cyclic low level application of forces or repetitive movement, and commonly the affected athlete has associated anatomical or physiological susceptibilities.

Within the literature on sporting injuries there is a lack of randomized prospective or intervention studies, with most information coming from case studies. Although interesting, case studies provide little information about risk factors and influence of prevention of injury. There is a paucity of data on injury rates in children; hence many of the assumptions about prevalence of sporting injuries in specific sports are extrapolated from adult studies. When compared to adult athletes, child athletes tend to be at low risk for sporting injuries (Maffulli et al 2005). Despite this low risk, sports injuries are more prevalent in certain sports. The following discusses the aetiology of sport-specific injuries in contact and non-contact sports, and provides some basic preventive strategies. A list of intrinsic and extrinsic factors that are likely to increase the chance of injury in contact and non-contact sports is shown in Table 13.1. The discussion of injuries in non-contact sports centres around dancing, gymnastics and swimming and in contact sports around American football, soccer and ice hockey.

Injuries in non–contact sports

Injuries tend to be less prevalent in non-contact sports than in contact sports and are more frequently attributed to overuse/overtraining. The following is a discussion of the common injuries observed in ballet, gymnastics and swimming. These sports have been chosen because they are popular activities among the young and often require intensive training from a young age.

The most frequent injuries observed in ballet are attributed to overuse and are most often sprains and strains. Stress fractures have been observed in ballet dancers and are

Table 13.1   Intrinsic and extrinsic risk factors for injury

Sport	Intrinsic risk factors	Extrinsic risk factors
American football	Leg deficiencies Body dimensions Previous injuries	Player's position Lack of well-rounded, full year conditioning Cleats, playing surface, equipment
Boxing	Boxing skills	Sparring Exposure
Soccer	Age Previous Injury Gender	Exposure Player's position Playing surface
Martial arts	Physical characteristics Skill level Technique	Exposure Equipment Opponent
Ice hockey	Physical characteristics	Aggressive play Equipment
Wrestling	Body weight Fatigue Psychosocial characteristics	Exposure Environment Protective equipment
Cycling	Age Gender Pronation Cycling technique	Protective equipment Exposure Training quality Types of roads, intersections, cycle tracks Bicycle fit
Dance	Previous injury Low body mass index (nutrition) Irregular menstrual cycles	
Gymnastics	Larger body size Early maturation (high body fat) Rapid growth High lumbar curvature Previous injury	Competitive level Event

Adapted from Verhagen et al (2000) and Mahler (2000).

most common in girls that have menstrual absence or irregularities. Some dancers may be at increased risk of bone injuries because of restricted diets and heavy training loads. This has been covered in more detail in the discussion of the female triad. Furthermore, dancing 'en pointe' has been proposed to cause lower back stress. To prevent injuries in ballet dancers, injuries needed to be properly treated and adequate rest prescribed. Furthermore, in some circumstances there may be a need for nutritional counselling, monitoring of menstrual irregularities and continual re-evaluation of training intensity and volume.

The incidence of injury in youth gymnasts has received much attention primarily because of the concerns with the high training volume of many young athletes. For example, elite gymnasts have been documented to participate in 40 hours or more of training a week. This can cause significant loads to both the upper and lower extremities which could potentially result in injury. An initial look at injury rates suggests that injuries are much more frequent in training than in competition. However, when one takes into account the length of time (exposure) in both training and competition, it appears that incidence of injury rates is in fact three times higher in competition than in training. This could imply competition pressure as one cause of injuries in gymnasts. It appears that most injuries are of sudden onset (acute injury) and are more likely to occur in the upper extremities. However, this conclusion could be bias as acute injuries could be a reflection of a predisposing overuse injury.

A few factors have been put forward as causes of injuries in gymnastics. Certainly the repetitive nature of the sport, combined with high impact loads and extreme biomechanics, could contribute to both accidental and overuse injuries. Some studies have also suggested biological maturity and anthropometric characteristics as possible contributors. In fact some studies have confirmed that a smaller size, low body weight and decreased biological maturation are associated with reduced injury rates. However, when interpreting these results it is important to consider that small size, low body weight and reduced biological maturation are also characteristic of a younger athlete, who has probably participated in fewer years of intensive training. A reduced exposure to intensive training might therefore confound some of the associations previously found. Other identified risk factors for injury appear to be previous injury, high lumbar curvature, competitive level and exposure. Type of gymnastic event has also been correlated with risk of injury, with floor exercises most commonly associated with injuries in both girls and boys. Gymnastic injuries in the young could be reduced by educating coaches and players about injury prevention and treatment, nutrition and sport specific preparation (both physical and psychological). Ensuring quality training, alternating training loads and providing medical support can also aid in the prevention and treatment of injuries.

There are few data available on the prevalence of sports injuries in youth swimmers. The data available suggest that swimming is a safe sport. The majority of injuries seen in youth swimmers are overuse injuries of the shoulder and arm. This is somewhat to be expected considering the high training loads concentrated on the upper body; thus most authors agree that volume of training is the main source of injury in youth swimmers. Injury incidence has also been correlated with performance/success, with medal winners showing a higher incidence of injury. Furthermore, injury is more frequently seen in free-style, back-stroke and butterfly swimming, and knee injuries are more common in breast stroke. To prevent injuries in youth swimming there is a need to teach correct stroke mechanics and emphasize the importance of a good warm-up and stretching before and after training and competition.

Injuries in contact sports

As previously mentioned, sports injuries tend to be more common in contact, than non-contact sports. The following is a discussion of the common injuries observed in American football, soccer and ice hockey.

American football is a violent collision and contact sport. Thus, as expected, most football injuries are acute, as opposed to overuse or gradual onset injuries. The three most commonly occurring types of injury in football are sprains, strains and contusions. About 50% of all reported injuries occur to the lower extremities and about 30% to the upper extremities. The head is also susceptible to injury with cerebral concussions as the most frequently occurring type of head injury. Leg deficiencies (e.g. lower body strength imbalances), size (i.e. late maturers), previous injury and player position (i.e. defensive and offensive line players) are just a few examples of factors associated with increased injury risk in football. The use of protective equipment and stricter enforcement of rules during training and practice might go a long way towards prevention of injuries. Furthermore, a year-round mandatory football-specific conditioning and training programme aimed at improving muscular and ligament imbalances and weaknesses, as well as coordination, flexibility, mobility and agility, has the potential to reduce injury.

The large number of youths participating in soccer and the increased intensity of participation of youth players results in a high exposure for injury risk in young soccer players. Similar injury rates have been observed in both indoor and outdoor soccer. Relatively low-grade injuries such as strains and sprains are the most common injuries, while more serious injuries, such as fractures and meniscal injuries, are less frequent. Traumatic injuries are most commonly seen in the lower extremity. As in other contact sports, most injuries in soccer result from direct contact with other players. Furthermore, the quick directional changes, sharp turns off a planted foot, and intense contact with the ball and other players make soccer players specifically vulnerable to lower extremity injury. Females playing outdoor soccer have the highest incidence of injury and this has been attributed to the females' lack of experience and inferior technical skills when compared with males of the same age. Age (i.e. younger/less mature players), previous injury, training (i.e. low practice to game ratio), player position (i.e. goalkeeper and defenders) and playing surface (i.e. natural surfaces) are other factors that have been linked to higher rates of injury. As in the other contact sports discussed, youth-specific conditioning and training programmes and tight referee control of games will likely reduce the incidence of injuries. Since females seem to be at a higher risk of injury, possible adjustments to the game, such as ball size, closeness of refereeing, and physical conditioning, need to be explored.

Ice hockey is a collision sport with intentional high energy body contact and thus has a high potential for injury. In general, contusions are the most frequent type of injury in youth ice hockey, followed by concussions, strains and sprains, and lacerations and fractures. The head and neck appear to be the most frequently injured body part. Large proportions of these injuries are localized to the face and are predominantly lacerations caused by the opponent's stick. The types of head injuries that may occur in ice hockey encompass the entire range, from a mild concussion to a progressive neurosurgical emergency such as an epidural trauma. Injuries to the lower extremity include groin muscle strain, contusions of the thigh and knee injuries. Aggressive play and lack of protective equipment have been linked to a higher incidence of injuries. Highlighting the seriousness of dangerous play, such as checking from behind, strict refereeing (i.e. calling penalties), the mandatory use of visors and stretching programmes to reduce muscle strains have the potential to reduce injury among young ice hockey players.

SUMMARY

Young athletes grow in a manner similar to non-athletes. However, athletes tend to demonstrate different body size, physique and biological maturity than non-athletes of the same chronological age. This is probably due to selection into or exclusion from the sport. Participating in regular physical training and competition at a relatively young age does not appear to accelerate or decelerate growth in height or biological maturity. It is likely that the height, physique and maturity characteristics of a young athlete are familial. Regular systematic training can, however, influence body composition and physiological capabilities (e.g. aerobic and anaerobic power, strength) of young athletes. However, more research is needed to elucidate specific relationships. If an athlete (particularly a female athlete) participates in excessive training accompanied by a restricted diet, the growth (specifically in body mass and bone mass) and biological maturity (specifically menarche or the menstrual cycle) can be affected. The term female athlete triad was coined to describe the three interrelated disorders found in the female athletic population: disordered eating, amenorrhoea and osteoporosis. The major concern is that these disorders have their antecedents in childhood and adolescence and that athletes competing in sports in which leanness and/or a low body weight is aesthetically pleasing may be at increased risk (e.g. ballet dancers, gymnastics, figure skaters). Youth sport injures are more prevalent in contact sports than non-contact sports, and are more likely due to impact or collision, whereas in non-contact sports injuries are more likely due to overuse. Intrinsic and extrinsic factors that heighten the risk for sports injury have been identified for specific sports. Strategies such as sufficient training, adequate equipment, stringent refereeing, coaching correct skills/mechanics and promoting 'safe play' can all aid in preventing sport injuries in the young.

KEY POINTS

1. The 'catch them young' philosophy regarding athletes is reflected in the increasing numbers of young elite athletes that have already undergone several years of intensive training prior to puberty.

2. A young athlete's status is determined by their frequency of involvement in a sport, competitiveness and success at increasing chronological age levels; from local clubs and schools, to national and international competitions.

3. Training is a special category of physical activity that refers to systematic, specialized and specific practice for a particular sport or discipline, but it can vary widely in type, intensity and frequency.

4. Training effectiveness in children and adolescents is difficult to elucidate as often it is designed to induce changes in the same direction as normal growth and maturation. However, longitudinal studies provide an appropriate means of studying young athletes' data, to distinguish the independent effects of growth, maturation and training.

5. Although athletes in some sports have been found to be shorter or taller compared to their non-athletic peers there is no evidence to substantiate the claim that training or sport positively or negatively affect stature.

6. Although no substantial evidence is available to justify the claim that sports or sports training alters or influences the timing or tempo of sexual maturation of young male or female athletes, the debate continues.

7. Once maturation and body size are appropriately accounted for, training and sport can influence body mass and body composition via an increase in bone density, an increase in lean muscle mass (in some older 'young athlete' populations), and a decrease in fat mass.

8. Though training may influence the physical performance of young athletes in a positive manner, it should be noted that children and adolescents are not miniature adults and though the mechanisms of improving performance (strength, aerobic and anaerobic) in youth are not well understood they do not appear to mirror the mechanisms of improvement in adults.

9. Numerous factors apart from talent can influence the inclusion or exclusion of a young athlete into any given sport.

10. The three interrelated dynamics of the female athlete triad are disordered eating, amenorrhoea and osteoporosis.
11. The prevalence and nature of the majority of injuries in contact and non-contact sports differ. In contact sports, injuries often relate to the contact and/or lack of proper protective equipment. In non-contact sports, injuries most often relate to training/overtraining; although such injuries occur in contact sports as well and precautions should be taken to avoid overtraining in the young athlete population, which may be more susceptible to such injuries than their adult athlete counterparts.
12. Many areas of study pertaining to child and adolescent athletes remain to be adequately researched.

References

Baxter-Jones A D G, Maffulli N 2003 Parental influence on sport participation in elite young athletes. Journal of Sports Medicine and Physical Fitness 43:250–255

Baxter-Jones A, Goldstein H, Helms P 1993 The development of aerobic power in young athletes. Journal of Applied Physiology 75:1160–1167

Baxter-Jones A D G, Helms P, Baines Preece J et al 1994 Menarche in intensively trained gymnasts, swimmers and tennis players. Annals of Human Biology 21:407–415

Baxter-Jones A D G, Helms P, Maffulli N et al 1995 Growth and development of male gymnasts, swimmers, soccer and tennis players: a longitudinal study. Annals of Human Biology 22:381–394

Baxter-Jones A D G, Maffulli N, Mirwald R L 2003 Does elite competition inhibit growth and delay maturation in some gymnasts? Probably not. Pediatric Exercise Science 15:373–382

Caine D, Bass S L, Daly R 2003 Does elite competition inhibit growth and delay maturation in some gymnasts? Quite possibly. Pediatric Exercise Science 15:360–372

Frisch R E, Revelle R 1970 Height and weight at menarche and a hypothesis of critical body weights and adolescent events. Science 169:397–399

Lebrun C M, Rumball J S 2002 Female athlete triad. Sports Medicine and Arthroscopy Review 10:23–32

Maffulli N, Baxter-Jones A D G, Grieve A 2005 Long term sport involvement and sport injury rate in elite young athletes. Archives of Disease in Childhood 90:525–527

Mahler P 2000 Aetiology and prevention of injuries in youth competition non-contact sports. In: Armstrong N, Van Mechelen W (eds) Paediatric exercise science and medicine. Oxford University Press, Oxford, p 405–416

Malina R M 1983 Menarche in athletes: a synthesis and hypothesis. Annals of Human Biology 10:1–24

Malina R M 1994a Attained size and growth rate of female volleyball players between 9 and 13 years of age. Pediatric Exercise Science 6:257–266

Malina R M 1994b Physical growth and biological maturation of young athletes. Exercise and Sport Sciences Reviews 22:389–434

Malina R M, Bouchard C, Bar-Or O 2004 Growth, maturation and physical activity. Human Kinetics, Champaign, IL

Marker K 1981 Influences of athletic training on the maturity process of girls. Medicine and Sport 15:117–126

Musch J, Grondin S 2001 Unequal competition as an impediment to personal development: a review of the relative age effect in sport. Developmental Review 21:147–167

Musch J, Hay R 1999 The relative age effect in soccer: cross-cultural evidence for a systematic discrimination against children born late in the competition year. Sociology of Sport 16:54–64

Otis C L, Drinkwater B L, Johnson M et al 1998 The female athlete triad. Medicine and Science in Sports and Exercise 29:i–ix

Rebar R W 1984 Effect of exercise on reproductive function in females. In: Givens J R (ed) The hypothalamus in health and disease. Year Book, Chicago, p 245

Rowland T W 1990 Developmental aspects of physiological functions relating to aerobic power in children. Sports Medicine 10:255–266

Rowland T W 2005 Children's exercise physiology, 2nd edn. Human Kinetics, Champaign, IL

Sheldon W 1954 Atlas of men; a guide for somatotyping the adult male at all ages, 1st edn. Harper & Brothers Publishers, New York

Theintz G E, Howald H, Weiss U, Sizonenko P C 1993 Evidence for a reduction of growth potential in adolescent female gymnasts. Journal of Pediatrics 122:306–313

Torstveit M K, Sundgot-Borgen J 2005 The female athlete triad: are elite athletes at increased risk? Medicine and Science in Sports and Exercise 37:184–193

Verhagen E A L M, Van Mechelen W, Baxter-Jones A D G et al 2000. Aetiology and prevention of injuries in youth competition contact sports. In: Armstrong N, Van Mechelen W (eds) Paediatric exercise science and medicine. Oxford University Press, Oxford, p 291–403

Washington R L, Bernhardt D T, Gomez J et al 2001 Strength training by children and adolescents. Pediatrics 107:1470–1472

Further reading

Armstrong N, Van Mechelen W 2000 Paediatric exercise science and medicine. Oxford University Press, Oxford

Bar-Or O 1996 The child and adolescent athlete. Blackwell Science, Oxford

Malina R M 1988 Young athletes: biological psychological and educational perspectives. Human Kinetics Books, Champaign, IL

Tanner J M 1964 The physique of the Olympic athlete. George Allen and Unwin, London

Chapter **14**

Physical activity and health
Jos W. R. Twisk

LEARNING OBJECTIVES

After studying this chapter the student should be able to:
1. describe the three pathways in which physical activity during youth can influence health status at adult age
2. describe the 'historic' development of physical activity guidelines for children and adolescents
3. describe what kind of studies and what kind of results of studies are necessary to obtain guidelines for physical activity
4. evaluate the mechanisms of the assumed relationship between physical activity and traditional cardiovascular disease risk factors
5. evaluate the mechanisms of the assumed relationship between physical activity and 'new' cardiovascular disease risk factors
6. evaluate the mechanisms of the assumed relationship between physical activity and osteoporosis
7. evaluate the mechanisms of the assumed relationship between physical activity and mental health
8. evaluate the scientific evidence from which physical activity guidelines should be derived

9. discuss the possible reasons for the lack of evidence regarding the relationship between physical activity during youth and adult health status
10. describe the concept of 'tracking'.

INTRODUCTION

Habitual physical activity is recognized as an important component of a 'healthy' lifestyle. In adults, it has been shown that physical inactivity is related not only to many chronic physical diseases like coronary heart disease, diabetes mellitus, certain types of cancer, osteoporosis and lung disease, but also to chronic mental diseases. The importance of physical activity is reflected not only in the relative risk of physical inactivity for these chronic diseases but also in the high prevalence of physical inactivity in Western society. The population attributable risks (PAR, i.e. a risk estimate in which both the prevalence of the risk factor (i.e. physical inactivity) and the relative risk for the risk factor for a certain health outcome are combined) of physical inactivity for different chronic diseases are very high; for instance, the PAR for physical inactivity for mortality from coronary heart disease is estimated to be around 35% for coronary heart disease, 35% for diabetes mellitus and 32% for colon cancer. This means that about 35% of the deaths caused by coronary heart disease, 35% of the deaths caused by diabetes mellitus and 32% of the deaths caused by colon cancer could have been theoretically prevented if everyone was (vigorously) active.

Even though the clinical symptoms do not become apparent until much later in life, it is known that the origin of many chronic diseases lies in early childhood. It is therefore often argued that prevention of chronic diseases has to start as early in life as possible. With regard to physical activity, the adolescent period seems to be especially important. It is known that in the Western world the amount of habitual physical activity is decreasing dramatically in this age period. The evidence of this is mostly based on cross-sectional studies. However, the few longitudinal studies investigating the natural course of habitual physical activity during adolescence also show comparable results.

Children and adolescents are, therefore, especially interesting as a target population for preventive strategies aimed at an improvement in physical activity. Because of this, expert committees from all over the world have put much effort into the development of physical activity guidelines for children and adolescents. This has become even more important in light of the 'obesity epidemic' among youngsters that started in the late 1990s, and which is thought to be due to a general decrease in physical activity. However, because the data are ambiguous, the field is seen as confused and controversial.

PHYSICAL ACTIVITY GUIDELINES FOR CHILDREN AND ADOLESCENTS

In 1988, the American College of Sports Medicine developed an opinion statement on the amount of physical activity needed for optimal functional capacity and health. They proposed that children and adolescents should obtain 20–30 min of vigorous exercise each day. In the beginning of the 1990s this recommendation was refined by the International Consensus Conference on Physical Activity Guidelines for Adolescents (Sallis & Patrick 1994), in which new physical activity guidelines for adolescents were developed. The expert committee, with researchers from the USA,

Canada, Europe and Australia, decided not to develop guidelines for children's physical activity, because of a lack of scientific evidence in the younger age groups. The guidelines for adolescent physical activity were twofold: (1) all adolescents should be physically active daily or nearly every day as part of their lifestyle; (2) adolescents should engage in three or more sessions per week of activities that last 20 min or more and that require moderate to vigorous levels of exertion. In 1998, the Health Education Authority symposium 'Young and Active' proposed different recommendations for the physical activity of young people (Biddle et al 1998). Their primary recommendation was that all young people should participate in physical activity of at least moderate intensity for 1 hour per day and that young people who currently do little activity should participate in physical activity of at least moderate intensity for at least half an hour per day. Their secondary recommendation was that at least twice a week, some of these activities should help to enhance and maintain muscular strength and flexibility, and bone health. Nowadays, this recommendation is still believed to be valid. Besides these international-based guidelines there are several national-based guidelines for physical activity in youth. In the USA, for instance, Healthy People 2010 proposed to increase the proportion of adolescents who engage in vigorous physical activity that promotes cardiorespiratory fitness 3 or more days per week for 20 or more minutes per occasion (Office of Disease Prevention and Health Promotion 2003).

PREVALENCE OF PHYSICAL INACTIVITY

One of the problems in assessing the prevalence of physical inactivity (and therefore the estimation of the PAR) is that it is difficult to define physical inactivity. Most of the time, physical inactivity is defined as 'not reaching the guidelines for healthy physical activity'. In the following paragraphs, it will be shown that this definition is rather tricky, because there is no real evidence to support these guidelines for children and adolescents.

However in the beginning of the 1990s, Cale & Almond (1992) reviewed 15 studies conducted on British children and reported that children seldom participate in activity at a level that would have a cardiovascular training effect or a health benefit. On the other hand, in the same period, Sallis examined nine studies and concluded that the average child is sufficiently active to meet the adult recommendations for conditioning activities, with the exception of the average girl in mid to late adolescence (Sallis 1993). It has further been noted that young children are highly and spontaneously active and that children are generally fitter and more active than adults and most of them are active enough to receive important health benefits from their activity. In the United Kingdom, around 70% of boys and 61% of girls, aged between 2 and 15 years, meet the recommended level of 1 hour of physical activity each day (including sport and organized exercise, active play, walking, gardening or housework). For girls, however, participation in physical activity declines after about 11 years of age, so that by age 15 years, only 50% undertake an hour of physical activity each day (Department of Health 2003). On the other hand, from longitudinal studies there is also evidence that for both boys and girls during especially the adolescent period, there is a (huge) decrease in physical activity levels, which continues into the adult period.

Another way of looking at the prevalence of physical inactivity is to look at the prevalence of sedentary behaviours such as television viewing, computer use or video game playing. Survey data from the USA, for instance, show that up to a quarter of American children aged between 8 and 16 years watch more than 4 hours of television each day (American Academy of Pediatrics 2003). However, the amount of time spent watching television and playing video games is not inversely correlated to the amount of time spent in physical activity. They are basically two different phenomena (Biddle et al 2004).

There is some evidence that the level of physical activity of children and adolescents is lower than that of similarly aged children a few years ago. This is mainly based on the finding that the caloric intake today is lower than the caloric intake in previous generations, and yet the previous generations were less fat. This can only be caused by a decrease in physical activity. This secular trend observed for physical activity levels of children and adolescents suggests the importance of this age period for interventions aimed at an improvement (or maintenance) of physical activity levels.

RATIONALE FOR PHYSICAL ACTIVITY GUIDELINES

The expert committees who developed guidelines for physical activity in children and adolescents based these guidelines on the available scientific evidence. This means that there has to be evidence of a relationship between physical activity during youth and health status during youth or more ideally between physical activity during youth and health status at adult age. This also means that there has to be evidence that the relationship has a certain shape on which the guidelines are based. So the first question to address is: is there a relationship between physical activity during childhood and adolescence on the one hand and adult health on the other? Basically the answer to that question can be addressed in three ways:

1. Physical activity during youth is related to health status during youth. This can be important because it is known from the literature that health status during youth is an important predictor of adult health status.
2. Physical activity during youth is related to physical activity at adult age. This can be important because there is extensive evidence that physical activity during adulthood is related to adult health status.
3. Physical activity during youth is directly related to adult health status.

Figure 14.1, which was derived from Blair et al (1989), illustrates the three possible pathways in which physical activity during youth can be related to adult health status.

After answering the question whether or not there exists a relationship between physical activity levels during youth and health status, and before guidelines can be developed, the shape of the possible relationship must be considered. The development of guidelines assumes a certain underlying function to describe the relationship between physical activity and health outcomes. If a linear dose–response relationship (Fig. 14.2A) is assumed, every increase in physical activity will have similar health consequences; in other words there is no threshold value to distinguish, which makes it rather tricky to provide guidelines.

If another shape of the relationship is assumed, threshold values can be distinguished, but the magnitude of the threshold depends greatly on the shape of the curve. Assuming a parabolic function (Fig. 14.2B), health benefits can be gained only in the lowest part of the physical activity scale; consequently, a small increase in physical activity in inactive persons will have beneficial effects, while an increase in physical activity in active persons will not lead to health benefits. Assuming a hyperbolic function, on the other hand (Fig. 14.2C), health benefits can only be gained in the upper part of the physical activity scale, which indicates that the amount of physical activity

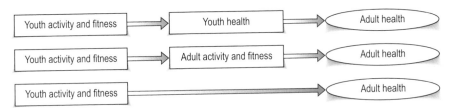

Figure 14.1 Possible relationships between physical activity during childhood and adolescence and adult health (Adapted from Blair et al 1989.)

needed to have health benefits is high. When a so-called S-shaped curve is assumed (Fig. 14.2D), this indicates that there is a threshold value somewhere in between on the scale of physical activity, indicating a more moderate threshold value. In other words, when an S-shaped curve is found for the relationship between physical activity and health outcomes, moderate intensity physical activity guidelines should be given. In fact, both the hyperbolic and the parabolic functions are extreme forms of the S-shaped curve. In a recommendation by the American College of Sports Medicine and the Centers for Disease Control and Prevention, it was suggested that for adults a parabolic function is the best estimate to describe the relationship between habitual physical activity and health benefits. The lower the baseline physical activity level, the greater will be the health benefits associated with a given increase in physical activity (Pate et al 1995). It is also important to distinguish what is on the X axis of these figures. It can be the intensity of physical activity, it can be the frequency of physical activities, or it can be a combination of the two. Besides this, it can also be the case that an increase in physical activity leads to health benefits, but at a certain (high) level of physical activity, the health benefits decrease, or in other words, the risk of physical activity (such as injuries) outweighs the potential health benefits (Fig. 14.2E).

Studies investigating the direct relationship between physical activity during youth and adult health status provide the best information on which the rationale for physical activity guidelines should be based. However, such a study is difficult to obtain. The ideal study to answer the question of whether high levels of physical activity during childhood and adolescence lower the risk of developing chronic diseases later in life is a randomized controlled trial with a lifetime follow-up in which a large group of children and adolescents are assigned to either a sedentary or an active lifestyle, a study that will probably never take place. One classic study investigating the relationship between physical activity in relatively young people and the occurrence of cardiovascular disease at a later age is the Harvard Alumni Study, performed by Paffenbarger et al (1986). In one part of this extensive observational study, physical activity levels during the student period (gathered from university archives) were related to the occurrence of cardiovascular disease later in life. Regarding their former physical activity levels, the students were divided into three groups: (1) athletes, (2) intramural sports players for >5 hours per week, and (3) intramural sports players for <5 (usually none at all) hours per week. The three groups did not differ regarding the occurrence of cardiovascular disease later in life. Student athletes who discontinued their activity levels after college encountered a cardiovascular disease incidence similar to the risk of alumni classmates who had never been athletes. In fact, individuals who became physically active later in life had the same health benefits as individuals who were active throughout the observation period (Fig. 14.3). Therefore, this study provided no evidence for a direct relationship between physical activity during youth and health status in adulthood.

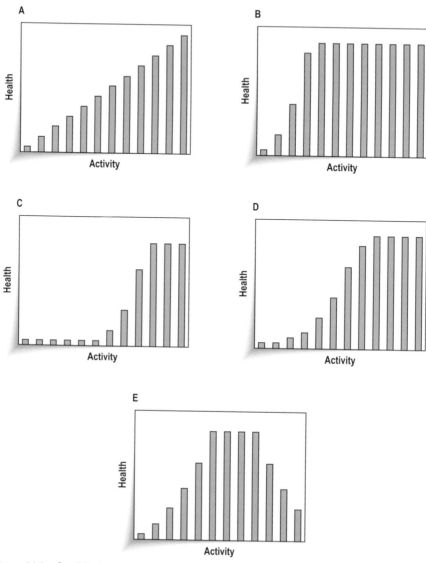

Figure 14.2 Possible dose–response relationships between physical activity and health: (A) a linear relationship, (B) parabolic relationship, (C) hyperbolic relationship, (D) an S-shaped relationship, (E) relationship where at a certain high level of activity, the health risks outweigh the health benefits.

One of the few longitudinal studies in which physical activity during youth can be related to health status at adult age is the Amsterdam Growth and Health Longitudinal Study (AGAHLS). This ongoing study started in 1976 with a cohort of about 600 children with an initial age of about 13 years. Over the last 30 years, this cohort has been measured nine times. Four annual measurements during the adolescent period; four measurements during the young adult period (at 21, 27, 29 and 32 years of age) and up to now, the last measurement was performed at the age of 36 years. In this study physical activity (measured with a detailed structured

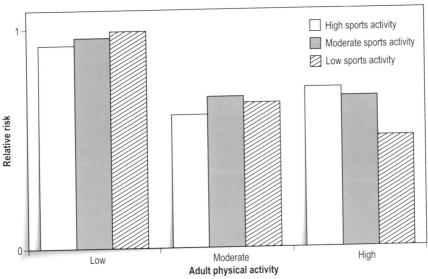

Figure 14.3   Relationship between sports activity during adolescence, physical activity during adulthood and all-cause mortality. Data are expressed as relative risks for all-cause mortality for different subgroups (Data from Paffenbarger et al 1986.)

interview) and several health parameters were repeatedly and extensively measured. Therefore, the AGAHLS provides a unique opportunity to investigate not only the relationship between physical activity during adolescence and health status during adolescence, but also the relationship between physical activity during adolescence and health status at adult age. In the following paragraphs, many examples will be taken from this study.

RELATIONSHIP BETWEEN PHYSICAL ACTIVITY AND HEALTH

Risk factors for cardiovascular disease

Risk factors for cardiovascular disease (CVD) can be divided in the more 'traditional' CVD risk factors, such as lipoprotein levels and blood pressure, and the 'new' CVD risk factors, such as endothelial function of the arteries and the thickness of the artery wall. Both are used as (intermediate) outcomes in the relationship with physical activity during youth.

Lipoproteins

It is known that lipoprotein levels are directly related to the process of atherosclerosis and therefore to the occurrence of CVD. Although total serum cholesterol has been found to be related to CVD, its atherogenic effect depends on the structure of the cholesterol or, in other words, on the ratio between low-density lipoprotein cholesterol (LDL) and high-density lipoprotein cholesterol (HDL). It is assumed that LDL may act directly or indirectly to cause endothelial damage, with subsequent proliferation of arterial smooth muscle cells resulting in an accumulation of lipids and a progression to atherosclerotic plaque formation. HDL, on the other hand, is assumed to be protective against CVD; HDL seems to be responsible for carrying cholesterol from peripheral tissue, including the arterial walls, back to the liver where it is metabolized and excreted. Besides HDL and LDL, very low-density lipoprotein cholesterol (VLDL) and plasma triglycerides (TG) also need to be considered. Although the atherogenic effects of VLDL and TG are not firmly established, both are assumed to be risk factors for CVD. It is further assumed that during exercise, fatty acids are freed from their storage sites to be burned for energy production. Several studies suggest that human growth hormone may be responsible for this increased fatty acid mobilization. Growth hormone levels increase sharply with exercise and remain elevated for up to several hours in the recovery period. Other research has suggested that, with exercise, the adipose tissue is more sensitive to either the sympathetic nervous system or to rises in circulating catecholamines. Either situation would increase lipid mobilization.

From epidemiological studies among adults there is some evidence that physical activity is associated with favourable lipid profiles. However, for children and adolescents there is not much evidence that physical activity has beneficial effects on lipids. The strongest evidence has been found for a positive relationship between physical activity and HDL levels. However, in a recent analysis based on data from the AGAHLS, it was surprisingly shown that high physical activity during adolescence was inversely related to HDL values at adult age. Looking more carefully at the data it was found that this relation was caused by the fact that children who were very active during adolescence show the largest decrease in physical activity between adolescence and adulthood. This unfavourable change in physical activity was found to be related to unfavourable HDL values at adult age. This finding, although preliminary, suggests that it is important to maintain high levels of physical activity throughout life.

Blood pressure

In adults it is known that endurance training can reduce both systolic and diastolic blood pressure by approximately 10 mmHg in individuals with moderate essential hypertension, but exercise does not seem to have an effect on subjects with severe hypertension. However, the mechanisms responsible for the decrease in blood pressure with physical activity have yet to be determined. A reduced cardiac output is mentioned as a reason for the fact that activity lowers blood pressure, although this cardiac output reducing effect of physical activity is not found in all studies. If there is no influence on cardiac output, then the blood pressure decreasing effect may be caused by a reduction in peripheral vascular resistance, which may be due to a reduction of sympathetic nervous system activity. In addition, the relation between physical activity and blood pressure can be caused by the anxiety-reducing effect of physical activity. It is questionable, however, if this mechanism is also present in children and adolescents.

It appears that essential hypertension may begin early in life and that detection and treatment of possible blood pressure abnormalities at young ages is important. There is, however, no direct evidence that elevated blood pressure in children is related to CVD later in life. There is also not much evidence that physical activity has beneficial effects on blood pressure in children and adolescents. There are many cross-sectional studies investigating this relationship, but again the best evidence comes from longitudinal studies and well-controlled intervention studies. In the AGAHLS, for instance, daily physical activity during adolescence was not significantly associated with either systolic or diastolic blood pressure at (young) adult age, nor was the longitudinal development of physical activity related to either systolic or diastolic blood pressure. The latter was also reported in the Cardiovascular Risk in Young Finns Study (Raitakari et al 1994). In the CATCH study, a 30-month multidisciplinary intervention in order to improve physical activity among more than 4000 children and adolescents did not have any effect on blood pressure (Webber et al 1996). It is argued that, as in adults, the possible lowering effect of physical activity on blood pressure only holds for children and adolescents with hypertension and not for young people with normal blood pressure values. This implies that this effect is difficult to observe in population studies in children with low incidence of hypertension. It should also be kept in mind that the effect of reducing blood pressure in hypertensive children and adolescents is probably only true for high intensity aerobic type physical activity and not for normal (or habitual) physical activity.

'New' CVD risk factors

Until the end of the 1990s, research regarding the relationship between physical activity in children and adolescents and CVD later in life had been limited to the analysis of the associations between physical activity and the more 'traditional' biological CVD risk factors. However, in the late 1990s alternative ways became available with which it was possible to 'assess' the degree of atherosclerosis before clinical symptoms occur. With non-invasive ultrasonographic methods it is possible to measure in vivo artery wall thickness, which provides a direct measure of the degree of atherosclerosis. The relative simplicity of these new methods makes it possible to use them not only in small clinical trials, but also in large epidemiological studies. Another new innovation is the assessment of endothelial dysfunction. With high resolution ultrasound the diameter of certain arteries can be measured under different conditions, from which endothelial dysfunction can be determined. Endothelial dysfunction can be seen as an important CVD risk factor. With these new techniques it is therefore possible to analyse the relationship between physical activity during childhood and adolescence and the actual degree of atherosclerosis before clinical symptoms occur.

It has been proposed that the possible effects of physical activity on both the acute and the chronic changes in large arteries are due to the adaptation of the vessel to shear stress. During exercise blood flow increases (especially in arteries supplying the exercise musculature) leading to higher intraluminal shear forces, which stimulates the endothelium to release relaxing factors (e.g. nitric oxide) resulting in arterial vasodilation. In the long term, these repetitive increases in blood flow will result in arterial remodelling (i.e. larger vessel diameters), which occurs in order to restore basal shear stress. Other mechanisms may also play a role, such as a decrease in vascular smooth muscle tone as a consequence not only of an improved local and basal production of nitric oxide, but also of an exercise-induced reduction in sympathetic tone and/or renin–angiotensin system activity. A reduced resting heart rate, which is known as an adaptation to endurance training, may also allow a more complete restoration of the arterial lumen diameter during the diastolic phase of the heart cycle, which results in an increased buffering capacity.

Although there is not much research performed in this area, in a recent study based on data from the AGAHLS, it was found that physical activity during adolescence was not related to arterial properties in adulthood. This was found for intima media thickness as well as for compliance and distensibility of the carotid artery and for compliance and distensibility of the femoral artery.

Body fatness and body composition

The increase in the number of overweight and obese children and adolescents is currently a major health problem. The 'obesity' epidemic started at the beginning of the 1990s and is still increasing. It is assumed that a decrease in the amount of physical activity among children and adolescents is the biggest cause of this epidemic. It has been suggested that adolescence is a sensitive period for the development of a central pattern of body fat. However, the aetiology of childhood obesity is very complex. Besides heredity, which is regarded as the major contributing factor in the development of childhood obesity, neuroendocrine and metabolic disturbances contribute significantly to one's propensity for fatness. Environmental factors, such as cultural background, socioeconomic status, nutrition and physical activity, have also been recognized as causes of childhood obesity.

In light of energy balance, it is obvious that the relationships between physical activity and body fatness and body fat distribution cannot be separated from the influence of food (i.e. energy) intake. There is a theory which states that a certain minimum level of physical activity is necessary for the body to precisely regulate energy intake to balance energy expenditure. A sedentary lifestyle may reduce this regulatory ability, resulting in a positive energy balance and an increase in body fatness. Another theory states that exercise is a mild appetite suppressant; this is based on research in which the total number of calories consumed did not change after a training programme was started, although there was an increase in energy expenditure because of the training programme. It is also suggested that resting metabolic rate is increased because of physical activity and/or aerobic training; some studies have supported this, while others have not.

From studies investigating the relationship between physical activity and body fatness and body fat distribution in children and adolescents, it can be concluded that there is evidence for a relationship between physical activity and body fatness in children and adolescents and that there is some evidence that the amount of physical activity during childhood and adolescence is inversely related to body fatness at adult age. In the AGAHLS, for instance, it was found that 'long-term exposure' to daily physical activity during adolescence was inversely related to body fatness (i.e. expressed as the sum of four skinfolds) at adult age. In another analysis with data from this study, it was shown that the longitudinal pattern (from 13 to 27 years of age) of daily physical activity was strongly related to trends in the sum of four skinfolds.

The evidence for a positive effect of physical activity on body fat distribution is, in contrast to the results for body fatness, weak and the results are ambiguous. In the AGAHLS, it was found that the amount of daily physical activity during adolescence was positively related to the waist to hip ratio (WHR) at adult age. This relation was found for females and not for males. This finding is difficult to explain; firstly because WHR is found to be primarily under genetic control and secondly, if there is a relationship between physical activity and WHR, this relationship is assumed to be inverse. An explanation for this paradoxical finding in the AGAHLS could be that in females inactivity leads to a greater accumulation of fat in the thighs, which would give a lower WHR. In another study with data from the AGAHLS, however, a longitudinal relationship between physical activity and body fat distribution (expressed as the ratio between the thickness of the triceps skinfold and the subscapular skinfold and not as the WHR) was not found. One should realize that it is extremely difficult to measure body fat distribution. In earlier days, body fat distribution was mostly expressed as the WHR, but later waist circumference was shown to be a better indicator. Besides this, different ratios between skinfold thicknesses are also used as indicators of body fat distribution.

A major problem in the investigation of the relationship between physical activity and body fatness or obesity is that it is difficult to distinguish between cause and effect. Physical activity and body fatness are associated with one and another and this cluster of factors is assumed to be a risk factor for CVD. It is difficult to investigate what comes first.

Another problem in the investigation of the relationship between activity and body fatness is the measurement and interpretation of body fatness. In large epidemiological studies, most commonly body fatness is expressed as body mass index (BMI). BMI is easy to measure and therefore widely used as an indicator of body fatness. Another option is using the sum of two or more skinfold thicknesses to indicate body fatness. Although both techniques are used as indicators for the same parameter, they are not the same and analyses with the two techniques can lead to different results, especially when one is interested in the relationship between physical activity and body fatness. This difference in results was shown in a paper by Twisk et al (1998). Based on data from the AGAHLS, daily physical activity was found to be inversely related to the sum of four skinfolds, but not to BMI. One of the reasons for these different results is the fact that BMI is an indicator not only of body fatness, but also of lean body mass (or muscle mass). Subjects with high muscle mass and moderate fat mass will have high values of BMI, but only moderate values for the sum of four skinfolds. When BMI is used as an indicator of body fatness, the inverse relationship between physical activity and body fatness can be more or less counterbalanced by the positive relationship between physical activity and muscle mass. This indicates that results obtained with BMI as an indicator of body fatness should be interpreted cautiously; especially in children and adolescents, because in this particular population the variables concerned are also influenced by natural growth and biological development.

Diabetes

Diabetes mellitus is a disorder of the carbohydrate metabolism characterized by high blood sugar levels. It is known to be an important CVD risk factor and it is often accompanied by overweight or obesity. Diabetes mellitus develops when there is inadequate production of insulin by the pancreas, or inadequate utilization of insulin by the cells. Clinically, two major forms are distinguished: type 1 diabetes, also known as juvenile onset diabetes, and type 2 diabetes, also known as adult onset diabetes. Although about 90% of all diabetes patients suffer from type 2 diabetes, type 1 diabetes is more common among children and adolescents and presents an important health problem in youth. However, the prevalence of type-2 diabetes among youngsters has increased enormously over the last 10 years. This increase has been mainly linked to the 'obesity epidemic' among youngsters.

In adults physical activity has many desirable effects for people with diabetes, particularly those with type 2 diabetes. Glycaemic control is improved, possibly due to the insulin like effect of muscle contractions on translocating glucose from the plasma into the cell. Exercise leads to an increase in muscle mass and therefore to lower blood glucose levels, assisting in better glycaemic and blood sugar control. The latter can reduce insulin resistance. Some researchers believe that physical activity can have an effect on glycaemic control in children with both type-1 and type-2 diabetes, but in other studies this has not been confirmed.

The outcome variables most commonly used in studies relating physical activity to insulin metabolism disorders are glucose and insulin concentrations of blood serum. When reviewing the literature there are not many studies investigating the relationship between physical activity and glucose and insulin concentrations in children and adolescents. Regarding insulin levels the results are quite ambiguous. In the Cardiovascular Risk in Young Finns Study, for instance, for males an inverse relationship was observed between physical activity and insulin levels, while for females this relationship was not found (Raitakari et al 1994). Regarding blood glucose, the few studies carried out have not shown any influence of physical activity in children and adolescents. More consistent results are found in the more limited number of studies on obese children and adolescents. In these studies, a positive (i.e. healthy) effect of physical activity was found on parameters related to insulin metabolism.

Metabolic syndrome

It is known that biological CVD risk factors tend to occur together more frequently than expected by chance. The clustering of risk factors has been shown not only in adults, but also in children and adolescents. Clustered biological CVD risk factors give a higher risk for the development of CVD than just the sum of the risks of the separate biological risk factors. The clustering of dyslipidaemia, hypertension, hyperinsulinaemia and obesity, for instance, has been recognized in children and adolescents and has been termed as 'syndrome X', or 'the deadly quartet'. More generally, the clustering of biological CVD risk factors is known as the 'metabolic syndrome'. Although it seems to be important to investigate clustered CVD risk factors in addition to the study of single risk factors, the relationship between physical activity and this clustering of CVD risk factors has only been investigated in a few studies. In the AGAHLS, clustering concerned the TC: HDL ratio, mean arterial blood pressure, the sum of four skinfolds and aerobic fitness (i.e. $\dot{V}O_2max$). Daily physical activity was found to be strongly inversely related to this cluster of CVD risk factors. In contrast, in the Northern Ireland Young Hearts Project in 12- and 15-year-old boys and girls, no relationship was observed between daily physical activity and a cluster score based on the TC:HDL ratio, diastolic blood pressure, sum of four skinfolds and cardiopulmonary fitness (i.e. the number of laps on a shuttle run test (Twisk et al 1999). In the Cardiovascular Risk in Young Finns Study clustering concerned total serum cholesterol, HDL cholesterol and diastolic blood pressure (Raitakari et al 1994). A large cohort with an initial age between 3 and 18 years of age was followed for a period of 6 years. At the initial measurement, as well as at the follow-up measurement, a 'high risk cluster' was defined as the subjects who belong to the high risk (age and gender specific) tertiles of all three risk factors. A shift from not belonging to this 'high risk cluster' at the initial measurement to belonging to this 'high risk cluster' at the follow-up measurement was associated with a decrease in physical activity.

In another study with data from the AGAHLS, the long-term development of physical activity from adolescence into young adulthood was compared for people with and people without the metabolic syndrome at adult age (Ferreira et al 2005). The metabolic syndrome was defined as having three or more of the following CVD risk factors: (1) systolic blood pressure ≥130 mmHg and/or diastolic blood pressure ≥85 mmHg; (2) triglyceride concentration ≥1.7 mmol $\cdot$ L^{-1}; (3) HDL cholesterol levels <1.03 mmol $\cdot$ L^{-1} for males or <1.29 mmol $\cdot$ L^{-1} for females; (4) HbA1c concentration >6.1% (HbA1c was used instead of plasma glucose levels, because plasma glucose was not measured in the AGAHLS); (5) waist circumference >94 cm for males or >80 cm for females. The prevalence of the metabolic syndrome in this population was relatively low (i.e. about 11%, which corresponds to 35 subjects), so the results of this preliminary analysis should be interpreted with caution. However, from Figure 14.4 it can be seen that there is no difference in the amount of physical activity during adolescence and the prevalence of the metabolic syndrome at adult age. However, if vigorous physical activity is analysed a different picture emerges (Fig. 14.5). First of all, it can be seen that

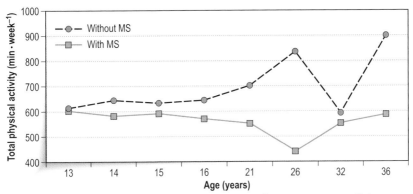

Figure 14.4   Longitudinal pattern of total physical activity (in minutes per week) from 13 to 36 years of age for subjects diagnosed with and without the metabolic syndrome (MS) at the age of 36 years.

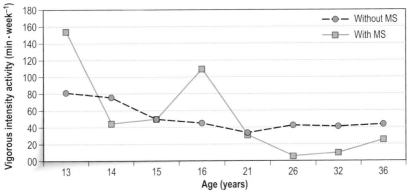

Figure 14.5   Longitudinal pattern of vigorous physical activity (in minutes per week) from 13 to 36 years of age for subjects diagnosed with and without the metabolic syndrome (MS) at the age of 36 years.

especially in young adult age, vigorous activity seems to be quite important in preventing the metabolic syndrome later in life. Secondly, however, it seems to be that children with the highest amount of vigorous activity at 13 years of age are prone to develop the metabolic syndrome at adult age. This is not due to the high amount of vigorous physical activity per se, but more to the dramatic decrease during the adolescent period, a finding that is consistent with the relationship mentioned earlier between physical activity during adolescence and HDL levels at adult age.

Osteoporosis

Osteoporosis is a major public health problem in developed countries and its importance is increasing rapidly because of the increase in average age of developed populations. Peak bone mass, which is achieved in the majority of the population in the third decade of life, appears to be highly under genetic control. However, lifestyle factors also seem to play a role in the development of peak bone mass. Especially dietary intake (i.e. calcium and protein intake) and physical activity appear to be important. It is assumed that the relationship between physical activity and osteoporosis can be twofold. First of all, high levels of physical activity later in life can prevent the natural decline in bone mineral density, which is mostly used as an indicator for bone health. The result will be that the onset of osteoporosis will be postponed. Secondly, it is suggested that high levels of physical activity during youth will increase the peak bone mineral density, also resulting in the onset of osteoporosis being postponed (Fig. 14.6).

Regarding the relationship between physical activity and bone health, a distinction should be made between the energetic (or metabolic) part of physical activity (i.e. energy expenditure) and the mechanical part of physical activity (i.e. weight-bearing activities). With regard to the effects of the energetic part of physical activity on bone density, there seems to be hardly any evidence of long-term effects of physical activity on bone health. However, in adults, there are indications that particularly vigorous physical activity is preventive for osteoporosis and the latest evidence has demonstrated that this is probably also the case in children and adolescents. Results regarding the mechanical part of physical activity show a different picture. It was suggested by animal research that mechanical loading achieved by activities such as jumping will have different effects on bone health than energetic loading from activities such as swimming or cycling. It was argued that small increases in physical activity, which include jumping, will have beneficial effects on bone health, while further increases in physical activity will not be any more beneficial. In other words, the shape of the relationship between the mechanical part of physical activity and bone health seems to be parabolic, while the shape of the relationship between the energetic part of physical activity and bone health can be better described by a hyperbolic function. However, the evidence is preliminary and further research is necessary to establish these findings.

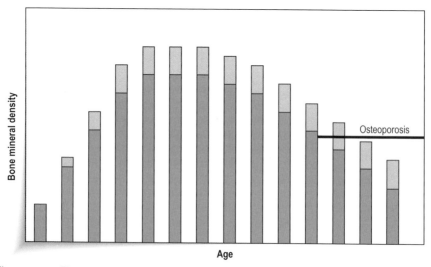

Figure 14.6 The possible influence of physical activity during youth on the natural course of bone mineral density in order to prevent osteoporosis. The blue sections show the possible influence of physical activity during youth on the natural course of bone mineral density in order to prevent osteoporosis.

The fact that physical activity can have an influence on bone health has partly to do with the local mechanical forces of physical activity. First of all, the mechanical forces cause a strain on the bone and calcium accumulation on the concave side of the bending bone (i.e. during flexion of the bone, calcium accumulation takes place at the negative loaded side). Secondly, the mechanical forces cause microtraumas that are removed by osteoclasts and repaired by osteoblasts. Furthermore, osteocytes stimulate the osteoclasts in removing the damaged structures and at the same time they stimulate the osteoblasts to repair the structure of the bone matrix. When the mechanical load falls below the fracture intensity, remodelling activities are stimulated and result in bone hypertrophy. This remodelling process of the bone after a change in mechanical load by weight-bearing activities has been proven in many animal studies.

Mental health

Studies investigating the relationship between physical activity and mental health are mostly limited to adults. In adults, physical activity has been shown to have a short-term mood-enhancing effect. Moderate levels of intensity and duration of physical activity have been shown to have a stress-reducing effect, but an additional increase of either the duration or the intensity will not have further beneficial effects. For children and adolescents, it is assumed that physical activity is associated with good mental health, especially in relation to self-esteem, self-efficacy, greater perceived physical competence, greater perceived health and well-being, but there is almost no evidence that the amount of physical activity is related to better social and moral development or to psychological variables such as body image, academic functioning, social skills, anxiety, hostility and aggression. However, the evidence is only moderate and there is no indication of a certain threshold value or a dose–response relationship between physical activity and mental health.

An important issue that must be considered with regard to the relationship between physical activity and mental health is that it is difficult to distinguish between cause and effect. Physical activity can have a positive effect on self-esteem or perceived physical competence, but on the other hand, children with higher self-esteem and/or perceived physical competence will be more likely to participate in sports activities.

For young children, not much research is performed regarding the relationship between physical activity and mental health. However, the few studies performed also show for this age group that self-esteem is increased by an increase in physical activity. Again, no real dose–response relationship or threshold value could be determined. Surprisingly, in contrast to elderly individuals in whom relatively high levels of physical activity can postpone the natural cognitive decline, in children and adolescents, physical activity does not seem to be related to cognitive (or academic) performance.

Physical activity and physical fitness

Probably the most important health-related benefit from high levels of physical activity is the improvement of physical fitness (i.e. aerobic fitness or peak $\dot{V}O_2$). In fact, aerobic fitness or peak $\dot{V}O_2$ is often used as a proxy measure for physical activity. However, that is a general misunderstanding, because physical activity and aerobic fitness are two related, but different concepts. There is strong evidence for a relationship between physical activity and aerobic fitness, but most of the evidence comes from training studies. In these training studies, in general, high intensity physical activity has been shown to be associated with an increase in aerobic fitness (see Chapter 10).

If a comparison is made between the relationship with health outcomes for physical activity and physical fitness, it is obvious that physical fitness is, in general, more strongly associated than physical activity. However, this mainly holds for CVD risk factors and not for other health outcomes. Table 14.1 presents an overview of the evidence on childhood and adolescence relationships between physical activity and aerobic fitness on the one hand and CVD risk factors on the other.

PHYSICAL ACTIVITY AND OTHER LIFESTYLES

Although physical (in)activity is more or less independently related to some health outcomes, physical inactivity is also often found to be associated with unhealthy lifestyle behaviours such as smoking, alcohol consumption and unhealthy dietary habits. This clustering of unhealthy lifestyles may introduce a health risk that is greater than one would expect from individual unhealthy lifestyles. It is unlikely that these unhealthy lifestyles are related to each other in a causal chain. It is more likely that there is one or more underlying mechanism (caused by genetic predisposition, psychosocial variables, socioeconomic class, environmental factors, etc.) which is cause-related to the construct of 'unhealthy behaviour'. In the Cardiovascular Risk in Young Finns Study, physical inactivity was found to be associated to smoking behaviour, alcohol consumption and having a diet with an excess of fat. This finding was not confirmed in the AGAHLS where physical inactivity was not found to be related to any of these unhealthy lifestyles.

Because of the assumed correlations between unhealthy behaviours it has been argued that a multidimensional view should be used in the prevention of chronic diseases in childhood. As a consequence, there is nowadays the belief that prevention should not only focus on a particular lifestyle, but that multidisciplinary, healthy behaviour oriented preventive programmes should be developed in order to obtain positive health effects.

It is rather surprising that guidelines for physical activity in children and adolescents are not accompanied by recommendations regarding dietary intake. Physical

Table 14.1 Overview of the scientific evidence for the relationship between physical activity and physical fitness on the one hand and CVD risk factors on the other in youth

	Physical activity	Physical fitness
Lipids	+/–	+
Blood pressure	0	0
Body fatness	+	+
Body fat distribution	+/–	+
Arterial properties	0	+
Risk factor clustering	+/–	+
Physical fitness	+	

0 = no evidence for a relationship; +/– = inconsistent evidence for a relationship; + = (strong) evidence for a relationship.

activity and dietary intake are highly linked to each other, particularly if one realizes that body fatness is one of the only health outcomes found to be related to physical activity in this particular age group. A decrease in body fatness is only achieved when an increase in physical activity is accompanied by a decrease in energy intake. In fact, there is some evidence that it is much easier to lose body mass by decreasing energy intake than by increasing physical activity levels. For the relationship between physical activity and bone health, dietary factors (e.g. calcium intake) also play an important role. An adequate amount of calcium is necessary to develop bone and, therefore, to increase bone mineral density by means of physical activity. However, combining physical activity and dietary intake guidelines is very problematic. The rationale behind dietary intake guidelines (better known as daily allowances) is even more doubtful than the rationale behind guidelines for physical activity.

TRACKING OF PHYSICAL ACTIVITY AND INACTIVITY

The predictability of a certain variable measured at a young age for the value of the same variable later in life is known as tracking. For several CVD risk factors tracking is rather high, especially for the lipoproteins and body fatness, indicating that high values of these CVD risk factors during childhood and adolescence are related to high values of these risk factors at adult age. For blood pressure, on the other hand, tracking is rather low. The degree of tracking for a certain variable is mostly expressed in two ways. Firstly, by estimating the correlation coefficient between two measurements of the same variable over time and, secondly, by the percentage of subjects who maintain their position in a certain 'high risk' group over time.

In adults, physical activity is found to be related to a lower prevalence of many chronic diseases. Thus if physical activity during childhood and adolescence is found to be related to physical activity during adulthood, it implies that improvement in physical activity during youth will have beneficial effects for adult health (Fig. 14.2).

The research question to be answered in studies investigating tracking of physical activity is whether or not individuals who are active in their youth (relative to their counterparts) are also more active as adults. There are only a few studies which investigate tracking of physical activity from childhood into adulthood. From several reviews, it can be concluded that tracking of physical activity is low to moderate. It has also been suggested that tracking of physical inactivity is higher than the tracking of activity. In the AGAHLS, however, this was not confirmed.

Therefore, in conclusion, there is only marginal evidence that physical activity/inactivity during childhood and adolescence is related to physical activity/inactivity during adulthood. If a person is very active during youth, it does not imply that he or she will be very active during adulthood as well. The same is probably true for a person who is inactive during youth.

The interpretation of tracking results in the literature can be confusing. First of all, many authors judge the magnitude of the tracking coefficient by looking at the significance level. They suggest that when a tracking coefficient is significant, the tracking (i.e. predictability) is high. However, a significant tracking coefficient does not mean that the predictive value of measurements during childhood and adolescence for values later in life is high. Suppose that tracking is calculated for subjects in a particular risk quartile in a longitudinal study with two measurements in time, and that 50% of the initial 'high risk quartile' maintain their position at the follow-up measurement. In this situation the initial measurement had a predictive value of 50% and a highly significant odds ratio (OR) of 5.0 would be found (an OR of 5.0 calculated for 'risk quartiles' translates to a predictive value of the initial measurement of 50%). So, a highly significant but rather low tracking coefficient. The same problem arises when a large study population is used to estimate tracking coefficients. The larger the population, the lower the tracking coefficient has to be to become significant. The second problem with tracking coefficients is that they reflect the relative position of a certain individual within a group of subjects over a period of time. When tracking for a certain variable over time is high, it does not necessarily mean that the absolute level of that variable does not change over time. Especially for physical activity, it is known that the amount of physical activity in the total population is decreasing from childhood into adolescence and from adolescence into adulthood. So when all subjects are becoming inactive to the same degree, tracking of physical activity will be high, while from a health perspective this is an undesirable situation. Thirdly, one must also take into account that the magnitude of the tracking coefficient is highly influenced by measurement error. Because it is very difficult to measure physical activity, the measurement error is probably high, which results in a low reproducibility of the measurement of physical activity. Consequently, the maximum magnitude of a tracking coefficient for physical activity that can be found in a population is the test–retest reproducibility of the assessment method.

The relative low to moderate tracking for daily physical activity can also be interpreted in another way. In preventive medicine, a lot of attention is given to an improvement of physical activity at an early age (for instance leading to the development of physical activity guidelines for children and adolescents). However, the results of the tracking analyses reveal that the amount of physical activity during adolescence is hardly predictive for the amount of physical activity in adulthood. It is therefore questionable whether possible improvements in physical activity due to intervention programmes during youth endure over time. This suggests that total populations must be considered as target populations for physical activity interventions and that physical activity intervention programmes should not be limited to children and adolescents.

REASONS FOR LACK OF EVIDENCE REGARDING THE RELATIONSHIP BETWEEN PHYSICAL ACTIVITY AND HEALTH

In analysing the effect of physical activity in childhood and adolescence on health status one must realize that almost all risk factors have a (large) genetic component; so the possible changes in health outcomes as a result of an increase in physical activity are generally small. Furthermore it must be taken into account that, for instance, the development of CVD risk factors during childhood and adolescence can be also the result of normal growth and development. Especially during adolescence, the rate of maturation can be a very important factor. A good example to illustrate the importance of this factor is the so-called 'adolescent dip' in total serum cholesterol levels, which can strongly bias the results of studies investigating the relationship between physical activity and total serum cholesterol in adolescents.

A third important issue is the problem of assessing the amount of physical activity. There are many different ways to measure physical activity; they vary from direct measurements (i.e. observation, diary, questionnaires, interview) to indirect measurements (i.e. physiological measurements, mechanical devices, 'doubly labelled water'). First of all the use of different methods to assess physical activity in different studies can lead to ambiguous results, and secondly the definition of physical activity is often different between studies. Sometimes physical activity is defined as total habitual physical activity, while in other studies physical activity is limited to sports activity. Also proxy measures such as the time an individual watches television are used. However, whatever method is used it is basically impossible to measure the amount of physical activity in children and adolescents correctly. The best one can do is to get a crude indication of habitual physical activity (probably achieved by a combination of different methods). The measurement error related to the assessment of physical activity is in general non-differential, i.e. not related to the health outcome. This non-differential misclassification will lead to bias towards the null, which causes relationships to be underestimated; a phenomenon that exists for both under-reporting and over-reporting.

Another important issue concerns the intensity of different activities. One is often interested in the total energy expenditure of a certain individual. With questionnaires or interviews (the methods mostly used in large population-based studies) it is very difficult to assess the intensity of different activities carried out by a particular subject. Data from questionnaires are often converted to an activity measure using standard tables in which a particular activity is related to a certain amount of energy expenditure. This certain amount of energy expenditure is often seen as an indicator of intensity. This method introduces a new source of bias: not only can the intensity of the same activity be extremely different for different individuals, but also different absolute levels of aerobic fitness between individuals can have important implications for the translation of certain activities into energy expenditure.

GENERAL REMARKS

Although theoretically physical activity can be beneficial for health, there is only marginal evidence that physical activity during childhood and adolescence is beneficial for health outcomes during childhood and adolescence and/or for health outcomes at adult age. Furthermore, there is no real evidence that a high physical activity level during childhood and adolescence will last for ever. If there are some indications that physical activity is beneficial for health, there is hardly any indication that these health benefits have some sort of threshold value. In other words, the proposed guidelines for physical activity are highly speculative. Probably the best illustration of this is the argument against the 'old' guideline for children and adolescents of 30 min of moderate physical activity on most days of the week. The argument was that: 'although most young people are currently meeting this old criterion, the incidence of overweight children and childhood obesity is increasing and many young people have been shown to possess at least one modifiable cardiovascular disease risk factor'. This argument ignores the fact that the aetiology of every chronic disease is highly multidimensional and not fully understood (i.e. the increased incidence of overweight children and childhood obesity and the existence of at least one modifiable cardiovascular disease risk factor is not per se caused by a decrease in physical activity), and also ignores the fact that there is only marginal evidence that physical activity is related to cardiovascular disease risk factors in children and adolescents (i.e. is caused by factors other than a decrease in physical activity).

What should be done to provide evidence-based guidelines for physical activity in children and adolescents? There is a need for experimental studies in which groups of children and adolescents with different frequencies, durations, modes and volumes of physical activity are compared with each other in relation to a certain health outcome. Although this is the ideal situation for a scientific basis to obtain evidence-based guidelines for physical activity in children and adolescents, these experimental studies are difficult to perform. Individuals will be physically active outside the experimental setting, so the different intensities of physical activity are biased by the amount of habitual physical activity. In adults, there are some nice studies in which this procedure is followed (e.g. Asikainen et al 2002). However, for children and adolescents this is much more complicated to achieve.

Based on the present scientific evidence, the proposed guidelines for the amount of physical activity in children and adolescents are as valid as stating that every increase in physical activity can have some beneficial effect for children and adolescents. The advantage of such a simple guideline is that this goal is much easier to achieve than the 30 or 60 min of moderate physical activity each day. This simple goal, when reached, probably leads to the same health benefits as those achieved by the guideline goals proposed by the expert committees. On the other hand, based on the possible relationships between physical activity and body fatness and aerobic fitness, one could also argue that not moderate but vigorous physical activity should be recommended. However, the question how frequently and for how long the child or adolescent has to be vigorously active to obtain health benefits remains unanswered with today's scientific evidence.

Another issue is that it is questionable whether guidelines for children and adolescents should be based on possible health benefits later in life. This is a long-term benefit, which will probably not have great influence on the behaviour of children and adolescents. This is perhaps best illustrated by the increase in smoking behaviour in youngsters all over the world at the beginning of this century, even though the long-term health burden of smoking behaviour is generally accepted and known by all children and adolescents. In light of this, perhaps physical activity guidelines should focus on other aspects than possible long-term health benefits (such as the joy or fun that physical activity can have or the social aspects of being physically active in groups, etc.).

SUMMARY

There is not much direct evidence that physical activity in childhood is related to adult health status. However, there is some indirect evidence. First of all, physical activity seems to be related to body fatness and body fat distribution and secondly physical activity seems to be related to aerobic fitness. For both these (indirect) health outcomes it is argued that the best evidence is found for high intensity physical activity. Furthermore, it seems to be important that physical activity levels during adolescence continue into adult age.

For the prevention of osteoporosis later in life, there is quite a lot of evidence that weight-bearing physical activity is important, while regarding mental health the results of studies with physical activity as a possible determinant are ambiguous.

KEY POINTS

1. There are three pathways in which physical activity during youth can influence health at adult age: (1) direct, (2) indirect, due to a relationship between physical activity during youth and health status during youth, and (3) indirect, due to a relationship between physical activity during youth and physical activity at adult age.

2. The latter (i.e. a relationship between physical activity during youth and physical activity at adult age) is also known as tracking.
3. Physical activity guidelines for children and adolescents are not based on scientific evidence.
4. Regarding CVD risk factors, the only evidence available is a relationship between physical activity and both aerobic fitness and body fatness/body composition. For both relationships, high intensity physical activity seems to be important.
5. Regarding the prevention of osteoporosis, weight-bearing activities are important, but there seems to be a saturation point above which an increase in weight-bearing physical activity is no longer effective.
6. There is much more evidence for a relationship between aerobic fitness during youth and health outcomes at adult age than for a relationship between physical activity during youth and health outcomes at adult age.

References

American Academy of Pediatrics 2003 Prevention of pediatric overweight and obesity. Policy statement. Pediatrics 112:424–430

American College of Sports Medicine 1988 Opinion statement on physical fitness in children and youth. Medicine and Science in Sports and Exercise 20:422–423

Asikainen T-M, Miilunpalo S, Oja P et al 2002 Randomised, controlled walking trials in postmenopausal women: the minimum dose to improve aerobic fitness. British Journal of Sports Medicine 36:189–194

Biddle S, Sallis J, Cavill N (eds) 1998 Young and active? Young people and health-enhancing physical activity: evidence and implications. London: Health Education Authority

Biddle S J, Gorely T, Marshall S J et al 2004 Physical activity and sedentary behaviours in youth: issues and controversies. Journal of the Royal Society of Health 124:29–33

Blair S N, Clark D G, Cureton K J et al. 1989 Exercise and fitness in childhood. Implications for a lifetime of health. In: Gisolfi C V, Lamb D R (eds) Perspective in exercise science and sports medicine. McGraw-Hill, New York, p 605–613

Cale L, Almond L 1992 Children's activity levels: a review of studies conducted on British children. Physical Education Review 15:111–118

Department of Health 2003 Health survey for England: The health of children and young people. The Stationary Office, London, UK

Ferreira I, Twisk J W, Van Mechelen W 2005 Development of fatness, fitness, and lifestyle from adolescence to the age of 36 years. Determinants of the metabolic syndrome in young adults: The Amsterdam Growth and Health Longitudinal Study. Archives of Internal Medicine 165:42–48

Office of Disease Prevention and Health Promotion (US Department of Health and Human Services) 2003 Healthy people 2010. Online. Available: www.healthypeople.gov

Paffenbarger R S, Hyde R T, Wing A L et al 1986 Physical activity, all cause mortality, and longevity of college alumni. New England Journal of Medicine 324:605–613

Pate R R, Prat M, Blair S N et al 1995 Physical activity and public health: a recommendation from the Centers for Disease Control and Prevention and the American College of Sports Medicine. Journal of the American Medical Association 273:402–407

Raitakari O T, Porkka K V K, Rasanen L et al 1994 Relations of life-style with lipids, blood pressure and insulin in adolescents and young adults. The Cardiovascular Risk in Young Finns Study. Atheroscleroris 111:237–246

Sallis J F 1993 Epidemiology of physical activity and fitness in children and adolescents. Critical Reviews in Food Science and Nutrition 33:403–408

Sallis J F, Patrick K 1994 Physical activity guidelines for adolescents: consensus statement. Pediatric Exercise Science 6:302–314

Twisk J W R, Boreham C, Cran G et al 1999 Clustering of biological risk factors for cardiovascular disease and the longitudinal relationship with lifestyle in an adolescent population: The Northern Ireland Young Hearts Project. Journal of Cardiovascular Risk 6:355–362

Twisk J W R, Kemper H C G, Van Mechelen W 1998 Body fatness: longitudinal development of body mass index and the sum of skinfolds with other risk factors for coronary heart disease. International Journal of Obesity 22:915–922

Webber L S, Osganian S K, Feldman H A et al. 1996 Cardiovascular risk factors among children after a two and a half year intervention – the CATCH study. Preventive Medicine 25: 432–441

Further reading

Armstrong N, Van Mechelen W (eds) 2000 Paediatric exercise science and medicine. Oxford University Press, Oxford

Eisenman J C 2004 Physical activity and cardiovascular disease risk factors in children and adolescents: an overview. Canadian Journal of Cardiology 20:295–301

Kemper H C G (ed) 2004 Amsterdam Growth and Health Longitudinal Study. A 23-year follow-up from teenager to adult about lifestyle and health. Karger, Basel, Switzerland

Licence K 2004 Promoting and protecting the health of children and young people. Child: Care and Development 30:623–635

Snel J, Twisk, J 2001 Assessment of lifestyle. In: Vingerhoets A (ed) Advances in behavioral medicine, assessment. Brunner-Routledge, Hove, p 245–275

Twisk J W R 2001 Physical activity guidelines for children and adolescents: a critical review. Sport Medicine 31:617–627

Van Mechelen W, Twisk J W R, Kemper H C G (eds) 2002 The relationship between physical activity and physical fitness in youth and cardiovascular health later in life. What longitudinal studies can tell. International Journal of Sports Medicine Supplement 23

Glossary

Acclimation The process of chronic adaptation due to artificially imposed stress, which mimics the natural environmental stress.

Acclimatization The process of chronic adaptation due to environmental stress.

Additive error Linear regression assumes additive error, i.e. the magnitude of the error term remains consistent throughout the range of values measured for the dependent and independent variables.

Aerobic fitness The ability to deliver oxygen to the exercising muscles and to utilize it to generate energy during exercise.

Afterload The ventricular pressure at the end of systole. Ejection stops because the ventricular pressure developed by the myocardial contraction is less than the arterial pressure; thus this determines the end-systolic volume.

Allometric equation Curvilinear relationship which takes the form: $Y = aX^b + \varepsilon$, where Y is a measure of physiological function, X is a measure of body size, a is a constant multiplier and b is an exponent.

Amenorrhoea The absence of menarche or menstruation.

Anorexia nervosa A psychological eating disorder which involves severe self-imposed weight loss.

Anaerobic fitness The ability to perform maximal intensity exercise.

Anaerobic threshold (TAN) Upper boundary of the moderate intensity domain and term used to denote the onset of a sustained increase in blood lactate concentration.

Analysis of covariance Statistical technique which combines linear regression and analysis of variance to compare the slopes and intercepts of regression lines describing relationships between two variables in different groups.

Arteriovenous oxygen difference The difference in oxygen content between arterial and venous blood.

b exponent   The numerical value of b in the allometric equation, when the allometric equation describes the slope of the log-linear regression.

Biacromial measure   The measurement of the width of the shoulder.

Bicristal measure   The measurement of the width of the hip.

Biopsy   The removal and examination of tissue.

Breath-by-breath   Variable, such as $\dot{V}O_2$, averaged over one entire respiratory cycle.

Breathing frequency (fR)   The number of complete respiratory cycles in one minute.

Body temperature and pressure, saturated (BTPS)   Gas volume standardized to barometric pressure at sea level, at body temperature and saturated with water vapour.

Bulimia nervosa   An eating disorder characterized by episodic binge eating followed by associated measures taken to prevent weight gain, such as self-induced vomiting.

Cart and Load Effort Rating (CALER) Scale   A pictorial version of the CERT depicting a person cycling along level ground towing a cart which is filled progressively with bricks. The number of bricks in the cart is commensurate with numbers on the scale. The five verbal descriptors are selected from the CERT.

Cardiac index   The expression of cardiac output in relation to body surface area $(\text{L} \cdot \text{min}^{-1} \cdot \text{m}^{-2})$.

Cardiac output ($\dot{Q}$)   The amount of blood pumped by each ventricle per minute $(\text{L} \cdot \text{min}^{-1})$.

Centile   Any of the numbered points dividing a set of scores into 100 points.

Children's Effort Rating Table (CERT)   A 1–10 perceived exertion scale which contains 10 numerically linked expressions of effort from 'very, very easy' to 'so hard I am going to stop'. The CERT was designed to contain 'developmentally appropriate' numerical and verbal expressions.

Chronological age   The age of a person counted from birth by standard units, such as months or years.

Chronotropic effect   Affecting rate or timing of heart rate normally due to autonomic nervous system stimulation or inhibition.

Cold environment   Air temperature lower than 10°C.

Cool environment   Air temperature between 16 and 20°C.

Compliance   Indicator of the buffering capacity of the arterial wall.

Critical power (CP)   Upper boundary of the heavy intensity exercise domain and the asymptote of the hyperbolic power–time relationship.

Cross sectional research   Studies that are carried out at one period of time.

Cycling peak power (CPP)   The highest power output over 5–8 s achieved in inertia-corrected force velocity tests, where the concomitant measurement of force and velocity during the acceleration phase of a single sprint is possible.

Dead space   The volume of gas taken into the lung that is not involved in gas exchange. The physiological dead space is composed of the anatomical dead space and the volume of the alveoli that are ventilated but not perfused.

Dehydration   A transient process of water loss from a state of euhydration (normal amounts of body water) to one of hypohydration (abnormal losses of body water).

Delay time (δ)   Time between the onset of exercise and the extrapolated onset of the exponential (when modelling the response to a step change function using an exponential function).

Dependent variable   Variable on the X axis (horizontal axis) of a bivariate plot.

Development   The acquisition of behavioural competence and/or differentiation and specialization of the embryo during prenatal life.

Differentiated rating of perceived exertion (RPE)   The RPE emanating from a specific area of the body, for example the legs or the lungs during cycling.

Distal   The segment of the body farthest away from the centre of the body; opposite of proximal.

Distensibility   Indicator of the elastic properties of the arterial wall.

Diurnal variation   The changes (fluctuations) that occur during an average day.

Dynamic muscle actions   Muscle generates force whilst the limb is moving at a given velocity causing lengthening and shortening of the muscle.

Ectomorphy   The classification of physique that assesses the degree of slenderness or thinness.

Effort continua   The subjective response to an exercise stimulus involving the interplay of three main effort continua – perceptual, physiological and performance.

Ejection fraction   The percentage of blood in the ventricles that is pumped out in one heartbeat.

Electronically evoked twitch   An electrical stimulus applied to a motor nerve near the muscle. Provides an indication of maximal intrinsic muscle force.

End-diastolic volume   The volume of blood contained within the heart at the end of diastole.

Endomorphy   The classification of physique that assesses the degree of roundness, or fatness.

End-systolic volume   The volume of blood remaining in the heart at the end of contraction.

Enzyme   A protein with specific catalytic activity. Almost all metabolic reactions are dependent on and controlled by enzymes.

Error/residual   The numerical value of the distance of an individual data point from a regression prediction line. Error is positive when the point falls above the line and negative when below.

Estimation paradigm   A passive process by which the individual provides a rating of perceived exertion in response to a request from the investigator to indicate how 'hard' the exercise feels at that moment in time. This information may then be used to compare responses between conditions after some form of intervention or to assist in the prescription of exercise intensity.

Estimation–production paradigm   In the estimation–production paradigm, expected or derived values of objective intensity measures derived from a previous estimation trial are compared to values produced during a subsequent exercise trial(s) in which the child actively self-regulates exercise intensity levels using predetermined RPEs.

Explanatory variable   Any independent variable entered into a multilevel regression model, e.g. stature, mass, age etc.

Fatigue index (FI)   An indicator of fatigue given by the difference between the highest and the lowest power achieved, expressed as a percentage of the highest power output.

Forced expiratory volume in 1 second (FEV$_1$)   The volume exhaled during the first second of a forced expiratory manoeuvre.

Forced vital capacity (FVC)   The volume of air exhaled during a forced maximal expiration following a forced maximal inspiration.

40% Δ   Forty per cent of the difference between ventilatory threshold and peak $\dot{V}O_2$.

Functional residual capacity (FRC)   The lung volume after a normal expiration.

Gain   Oxygen cost relative to the stimulus (exercise intensity).

Gluconeogenesis   The synthesis of glucose from non-carbohydrate precursors such as glycerol and amino acids.

Glycogenolysis   The breakdown of glycogen into glucose 1-phosphate by the action of phosphorylase.

Glycolysis   The anaerobic degradation of one molecule of glucose to two molecules of pyruvate.

Growth   Changes in size of an individual, as a whole or in parts.

Haematocrit   Volume of red cells usually expressed as a percentage of total blood volume.

Heat capacity   The quantity of heat needed to produce a unit rise of temperature in the body and measured in $J \cdot {}^{\circ}K^{-1}$.

Heteroscedasticity   Describes the spread in data around a regression line where the error term increases as the magnitude of the dependent variable increases.

Hot environment   Air temperature as high as 40–50°C.

High-density lipoproteins (HDL)   HDLs transport cholesterol from the tissues to the liver to be broken down and excreted. HDLs accelerate the clearance of cholesterol from the blood, reducing the likelihood of cholesterol becoming deposited in arterial walls to cause arteriosclerosis, and thereby reducing the risk of coronary heart disease.

Hydrolysis   A reaction in which large molecules are split by interaction with water into smaller molecules.

Hyperpnoea   Excessive ventilation due to an increase in breathing frequency and/or tidal volume.

Independent variable   Variable on the Y axis (vertical axis) of a bivariate plot.

Inotropic effect   Altered force of contraction in heart rate muscle normally due to autonomic nervous system stimulation or inhibition.

Intima media thickness   Thickness of the intima media of the artery, which can be seen as an indicator of preclinical atherosclerosis.

Lactate threshold (T_{LAC})   The point at which blood lactate accumulation increases non-linearly in response to progressive exercise.

Linear regression equation $Y = a + bX + \varepsilon$.

Lipolysis   The breakdown of triacylglycerols (triglycerides) into fatty acids and glycerol.

Lipoproteins   Organic compounds formed from lipids and proteins that transport fats and cholesterol in the blood.

Logarithm, natural   Obtained by multiplying a number by a factor known as Euler's constant (e = approximately 2.71828).

Log-likelihood (i.e. –2*log-likelihood)   Sometimes called the deviance statistic. Used to judge the goodness of fit of nested multilevel regression models.

Log-linear regression equation   The linear form of the allometric equation: $\log_e Y = \log_e a + b \cdot \log_e X + \log_e \varepsilon$.

Longitudinal research   Studies in which data are obtained on the same individual three or more times during a period of time.

Low-density lipoproteins (LDL)   LDLs transport cholesterol to all non-hepatic cells. Excess cholesterol tends to be deposited on the blood vessel wall and is associated with the development of arteriosclerosis.

Maturation   Process of being mature, or the progress towards the mature state.

Maximal intensity exercise   The performance of any type of exercise that requires an all-out effort and where the predominant, though not exclusive, energy supply for the accomplishment of the exercise is from anaerobic metabolism.

Maximal lactate steady state (MLSS)   The highest exercise intensity that can be maintained without incurring a progressive increase in blood lactate. It reflects the highest point at which the diffusion of lactate into the blood and removal from the blood are in equilibrium.

Maximal oxygen uptake ($\dot{V}O_2$max)   The highest rate at which an individual can consume oxygen during exercise.

Maximal voluntary ventilation (MVV)   Measurement of air exhaled over a period of time, usually 15 s, expressed in $L \cdot min^{-1}$ BTPS.

Mean power (MP)   The average power output achieved during maximal intensity exercise lasting between 1 and 60 s. MP is usually averaged over 30 s.

Mean response time (MRT)   Time from the onset of exercise to reach 63% of the final $\dot{V}O_2$ amplitude; equal to the sum of the delay time and time constant in an exponential model that incorporates a delay.

Mesomorphy   The classification of physique that assesses the degree of muscularity, and bone development.

Metabolic syndrome   Having three or more risk factors for CVD.

Minute ventilation ($\dot{V}E$)   The volume of air taken in or breathed out in 1 minute, usually expressed in $L \cdot min^{-1}$ BTPS.

Multilevel modelling   An extension of multiple regression analysis appropriate for analysing multilevel or hierarchically structured data such as longitudinal growth and exercise data.

Multiplicative error   Allometric models assume multiplicative error, i.e. the magnitude of the error term increases as the range of values measured for the dependent and independent variables increase (i.e. demonstrate heteroscedasticity).

Muscle action   The state of the muscle that is dependent upon the external force applied to that muscle.

Muscle moment arm   Perpendicular distance from the axis of rotation to the line of action of the intrinsic muscle force.

Normoxia   Normal levels of oxygen.

OMNI Scale   A 0–10 perceived exertion scale which depicts four characters at various stages of fatigue on a 20–25° incline. The scale is anchored with six equally distributed verbal descriptors along the scale, which utilize various states of feeling 'tired'.

Ontogenetic allometry   Allometric body size and exercise performance relationships examined at the individual level.

Optimized peak power (PPopt)   The highest power output obtained from force-velocity tests that involve a number of sprints lasting 5–10 s against a range of applied resistances.

Osmolality   The number of particles per kilogram of solvent.

Osteopenia   The state prior to the disease state of osteoporosis.

Osteoporosis   A condition characterized by enhanced skeletal fragility.

Oxygen deficit   The difference between the theoretical oxygen requirement and the volume of oxygen actually used during a period of exercise in which the level of oxygen uptake is insufficient to supply the energy required.

Peak oxygen uptake (peak $\dot{V}O_2$)   The highest oxygen uptake observed during an exercise test to exhaustion.

Peak post-exercise lactate   The highest lactate concentration achieved during or shortly after an exercise protocol.

Peak power (PP)   The highest power output achieved during maximal intensity exercise lasting between 1 and 60 s. PP is usually averaged over 1, 3 or 5 s.

Perceived exertion   The sensation of strain, aches and fatigue from the peripheral muscles and pulmonary system, among other sensory cues. This is mediated by the interplay of three main effort continua – perceptual, physiological and performance environment.

Perceptual continuum   The initial basis from which to explore the derivations of the ratings of perceived exertion. It is founded on the premise that perception plays a fundamental role in our behaviour and in how we adapt to a situation. It involves factors such as mood, understanding and motivation.

Performance/situational continuum   The interplay of the perceptual continua and the unique patterns of physiological responses on the RPE are influenced by the situational characteristics of the performance.

pH   A measure of the relative acidity or alkalinity of a solution. A pH of 7 indicates neutrality, values above 7 indicate alkalinity, and those below 7 indicate acidity.

Phase 1   Also termed the cardiodynamic phase. The initial increase in $\dot{V}O_2$ following the onset of exercise that is due to an increase in pulmonary blood flow and pulmonary ventilation.

Phase 2   The exponential increase in $\dot{V}O_2$ following the onset of exercise and phase 1. Represents oxygen uptake dynamics at the muscle, also termed the primary component.

Phase 3   The $\dot{V}O_2$ following the achievement of the asymptote of the exponential in phase 2.

Physiological continuum   Perceived exertion is related to heart rate, blood lactate, oxygen uptake, respiratory frequency, ventilatory volume and body temperature, among other factors. Some factors are characterized by linear growth of increases in intensity (e.g. heart rate) and some factors are characterized by a non-linear (positive accelerating) growth function.

Pictorial Children's Effort Rating Table (P-CERT)   The scale depicts a child running up a 45° stepped gradient at five stages of exertion, corresponding to CERT ratings of 2, 4, 6, 8 and 10. All the verbal descriptors from the original CERT are included in the scale.

Pneumotachograph   A device used to measure gas flow by measuring the pressure drop across a tube with known resistance to flow.

Poikilothermal   Having a varying body temperature.

Population attributable risk (PAR)   A risk estimate that combines the prevalence of the risk factor with the relative risk for the risk factor for a certain health outcome.

Power function ratio   The ratio Y/X^b where b is the slope of the log-linear relationship.

Preload   The end-diastolic volume at the beginning of systole.

Primary component   See Phase 2.

Production paradigm   An active process in which the individual is required to actively produce an intensity based upon his/her interpretation of effort sense and the cognition and understanding of the RPE prescribed.

Production-only or repeat-production paradigm   The assessment of perceived exertion using a repeat-production paradigm examines a child's ability to discern between different target RPEs while self-regulating exercise intensity on more than one occasion.

Proximal   The segment of the body closest to the centre of the body; opposite of distal.

Ratio standard   The variable constructed when a measure of physiological function is divided by body mass, e.g. mL $\cdot$ kg^{-1} $\cdot$ min^{-1}, W $\cdot$ kg^{-1}, etc.

Residual volume (RV)   The volume of gas remaining in the lung at the end of a maximal expiration.

Respiratory exchange ratio (R)   The ratio of the volume of carbon dioxide expired per minute to the volume of oxygen consumed during the same time in the lungs.

Saltation   Increase in the size of the body through unique time-constrained episodes that occur intermittently.

Scaling   The process of removing or controlling for the influence of body size upon physiological function.

Shortening fraction (SF)   The difference between the diameter of the ventricles at the end of systole (ESD) and the original diameter at the end of diastole (EDD), expressed as a percentage (SF = (EDD – ESD)/EDD).

Simple linear equation ($Y = bX + \varepsilon$)   The mathematical model assumed when the ratio standard is applied. This equation represents a straight line that passes from zero through the intersection of the mean values for the Y and X variables.

Slow component   Increase in oxygen uptake during phase 3 above the oxygen uptake predicted from the linear power–oxygen uptake relationship below the anaerobic threshold.

Somatotyping   The method of defining a person's body type or physique in terms of classifications of ectomorphic, endomorphic and mesomorphic components.

Specific latent heat of vaporization   The quantity of heat required to change a unit mass of a substance from liquid to vapour without a change in temperature and measured in J $\cdot$ g^{-1}.

Static muscle actions   Muscle generates force whilst remaining at a fixed length.

Statis   No measurable accretion in growth, or increase in size occurs; separates individual saltation events.

Stroke index   The expression of stroke volume in relation to body surface area (mL $\cdot$ m^{-2}).

Stroke volume   The amount of blood ejected from one ventricle per heartbeat (mL).

Syndrome X The clustering of dyslipidaemia, hypertension, hyperinsulinaemia and obesity.

$t_{1/2}$ Half-time of the response. The time taken to achieve 50% of the total change in the response.

Testosterone Circulating hormone that is responsible for the stimulation of the anabolic process of skeletal muscle growth.

The deadly quartet Another name for the clustering of dyslipidaemia, hypertension, hyperinsulinaemia and obesity.

Thermal strain The physiological and mental response to thermal stress.

Thermal stress An accumulation of environmental conditions that stress the thermoregulatory system.

Thermoneutral zone The temperature range where mammals do not have to use extra energy to conserve or dissipate heat.

Tidal volume (V_T) The volume of air that is inhaled or exhaled with each respiratory cycle.

Time constant (τ) Time taken to reach 63% of the final amplitude of an exponential function.

Torque A product of the muscle force and the muscle moment arm.

Total lung capacity (TLC) The volume of gas contained in the lung after a full inhalation.

Tracking Predictability of values measured at an early age for values of the same variable later in life.

Tricarboxylic acid cycle A series of chemical reactions occurring in the mitochondria in which carbon dioxide is produced and hydrogen and electrons are removed from carbon molecules. During the cycle energy is liberated and used to synthesize ATP from ADP and Pi.

Turbine flow meter A device used to measure gas flow by measuring the number of revolutions of a rotating turbine per unit of time.

Velocity The rate of change of position and direction over time, calculated by dividing distance by time.

Venous return The amount of blood that enters the heart from the venous circulation.

Ventilatory threshold (T_{VENT}) Point in an incremental exercise test at which ventilation increases disproportionately to oxygen uptake.

Very low-density lipoproteins (VLDL)   VLDLs transport triglycerides synthesized in the liver to the adipose tissue. VLDL residuals may become LDLs associated with the development of coronary heart disease.

Vital capacity (VC)   The volume change that occurs between maximal inspiration and maximal expiration.

Warm environment   Air temperature up to 8–10°C above skin temperature, ~30–40°C.

Wind chill   An index that quantifies the effect of cold upon the skin as well as overall heat loss. Wind chill is directly related to the velocity of the wind.

Index